Color Atlas of

Gynecological Surgery

Volume 5: Infertility Surgery

David H. Lees
FRCS(ED), FRCOG
Honorary Consultant Obstetrician and Gynecologist,
Jessop Hospital for Women, Sheffield

Albert Singer
Ph.D, D.Phil (OXON), FRCOG
Former Reader in Obstetrics and Gynecology,
University of Sheffield

Consultant Gynecologist to the Whittington
and Royal Northern Hospitals, London

with a contribution from

Robert M. L. Winston
MB, BS, MRCOG
Senior Lecturer and Consultant Gynecologist,
Institute of Obstetrics and Gynecology, Hammersmith Hospital,
The Royal Postgraduate Medical School, London

Year Book Medical Publishers, Inc.
35 East Wacker Drive, Chicago

To our wives
Anne & Talya

Printed by Royal Smeets Offset b.v., Weert, Netherlands

Distributed in Continental North, South and
Central America, Hawaii, Puerto Rico, and the
Philippines by
Year Book Medical Publishers, Inc
By arrangement with Wolfe Medical Publications Ltd
Library of Congress Catalog Card Number: 77 90543
International Standard Book Number: 0 8151 5355 4

Contents

Acknowledgements

This six-volume Colour Atlas of Gynaecological Surgery was produced at the Jessop Hospital for Women, Sheffield as part of a postgraduate project to teach operative surgery by edited colour slides. We are indebted to all who took part in the exercise, but there are some whom we would particularly like to mention.

Mr Alan Tunstill, Head of Department of Medical Illustration, The Royal Hallamshire Hospital, Sheffield Area Health Authority (Teaching), organised the whole of the photography. Mr Stephen Hirst, of the same Department, took nearly all of the photographs; the colour diagrams are all the work of Mr Patrick Elliott, Medical Artist of the Department.

Many colleagues provided material for this volume. In Sheffield, Professor Ian D. Cooke generously gave full access to clinical material in his unit; he and Dr Elizabeth Lenton gave information, hormone assay profiles and advice for Chapter 1. Dr Frank Comhaire of Gent, Belgium supplied the authors with the thermograms (page 18) and details of his protocol for the investigation of the infertile male which allowed the construction of the flow chart on page 20. Professors Ian Craft (London) and Michael Baggish (Connecticut, USA) provided the hysteroscopic photographs that appear on page 36, while Winthrop Pharmaceuticals provided the diagram of endometriotic 'sites' on page 73. Mr Robert Sawers, Dr Fernando Zegers and Dr Sandra Niak of Sheffield helped in obtaining some of the photographs that appear in Chapters 11 and 12 while Dr Lorna Kidd and Dr John Mills of Dundee, Scotland generously supplied the ultrasonographs on page 172.

Professor John Newton, formerly of Kings College Hospital, London kindly provided the authors with details of the documentation manual as featured in Part 8 of Appendix E. Professor Pepperell and associates from Melbourne, Australia gave permission for the reproduction from their recent publication 'The Infertile Couple' of Tables 5 and 6 in Chapter 1. Professor J-G Forsberg of the Anatomisk Institutt, Bergen, Norway gave us help and advice on embryological matters and the use of the diagrams to illustrate points in fetal development.

The anaesthetists at all levels were very co-operative. Dr A G D Nicholas, Dr D R Powell and Professor J A Thornton were the consultants involved. Of the numerous senior registrars we remember particularly Doctors Bailey, Birks, Burt, Clark, Dye, Mullins, Saunders and Stacey.

Miss J Hughes-Nurse, Mr I V Scott, Miss P Buck, Miss V Brown and Dr H David were the senior registrars and lecturers in obstetrics and gynaecology during the time and greatly assisted by keeping us informed of suitable cases and in the organising of operations. Doctors Katherine Jones, E Lachman, Janet Patrick, K Edmonds, A Bar-Am and C Rankin were involved in the management of the cases and assisted at operations.

Miss M Crowley, nursing officer in charge of the Jessop Hospital operating theatres ensured that we had every facility, and Sisters J Taylor, M Henderson, E Duffield, M Waller and A Broadly each acted as theatre sister or 'scrub' nurse at the individual operations. Mr Leslie Gilbert and Mr Gordon Dale the operating room assistants, were valuable members of the team. We particularly wish to thank the whole theatre staff for their courtesy and efficiency.

A large amount of secretarial work was involved. We are grateful to Mrs Gillian Hopley of the University Department who dealt with most of it. Mrs Valerie Prior and Mrs Talya Singer were responsible for typing the manuscript.

In view of the increasing complexity and diversity of the whole project we have had to enlist the further assistance of our wives. Colour matching, proof-reading, spot typing and slide organisation have all demanded much extra time both at home and when travelling overseas.

The photographs in this book were taken on Kodachrome 25 colour reversal film. The camera was a 35 mm Nikkormat FTN fitted with a 105 mm f2.5 Nikkor auto lens. A PK-3 extension ring was used for close-ups and a 55 mm f3.5 Micro-Nikkor auto lens for general views. Illumination was provided by a Sunpak auto zoom 4000 electronic flash unit, set on full power. An exposure setting of 1/60th of a second at f16 was used.

Introduction

There is probably no substitute for the type of personal tuition provided by teacher and pupil working together in the operating theatre as surgeon and assistant, with knowledge and experience being passed on directly. There is, however, the disadvantage that such a relationship is not available to everyone and is, at best, transient. In addition the learner is frequently not at a stage in his career when he can take full advantage of what is available. The majority, therefore, have to look elsewhere for such instruction.

Textbooks of operative surgery provide the principal source of information, but these are only as good as their illustrations. The occasional colour plate does not instruct and there is something unreal about the well-executed drawings prepared by a medical artist to the specification of the author. The one worthwhile teaching aid is the simple line diagram or sketch, which demands considerable skill and ingenuity and allows the student to see and follow what is required. But to carry that information in one's mind and apply it in practice is another matter. In surgery, with all its accompanying distractions, the real life structures are frighteningly different from those which the simple diagrams have led one to expect, and these same structures obstinately refuse to adopt the position and behaviour expected of them.

Cine films are excellent but the cost of their production in time and money is high, besides which they are clumsy to use. This series of atlases offers what we consider to be the next best thing: a series of step-by-step colour photographs accompanied by an appropriate written commentary. This form of presentation follows almost exactly the colour slide plus commentary method most often used to teach surgery. Using slides, of course, it is necessary to have projection apparatus and access to a library or bank of suitable material. The method adopted in this series – of using high quality colour reproduction processes – retains the advantages of the slide and commentary method while avoiding its drawbacks.

The present series of atlases sets out to provide detailed instruction in the techniques of standard gynaecological operations. Its methodology is straightforward. The technique of each operation is clearly shown, step-by-step, using life-size photographs in natural colour, and with liberal use of indicators and accompanying diagrams. Where a step is repetitive or there is a natural sequence of steps, grouping has sometimes been used, but the natural size of the structures is maintained.

The accompanying commentary is concise and is printed on the same page as the photograph or photographs to which it refers. Every effort has been made to include only necessary material, but in situations where experience and special training have provided additional information and knowledge, that has been included.

The illustrations are selected and the accompanying commentaries so arranged as to carry the reader forward in a logical progression of thought and action in which he becomes involved. Occupied with one step he is at the same time anticipating the next, and in due course confirms his foresight as logical and correct. The photographs are those of a real patient having a real operation and the picture seen is exactly what the reader will see in the operation theatre when he does it himself. Interest is concentrated on the one step of the operation being taken at that time.

In any form of medical teaching there is the inevitable problem of pitching instruction at the level required by the audience and the presumption that the reader has insight into the specialist knowledge of the author is just as irritating as being patronised. We do not think there is a problem in this context because an atlas is by definition a guide and therefore for general use. It is just as likely to be consulted by a junior house surgeon about to assist at his first hysterectomy as by a senior colleague seeking an alternative method of dealing with a particular problem. That, at least, is the spirit in which it has been written.

Certain assumptions have had to be made to avoid verbosity, tediousness and sheer bulk of paper. It is hoped that the reader will be kind enough to attribute any omissions and shortcomings to the acceptance of such a policy. No one should be embarking on any of the procedures described without training in surgical principles, nor should he attempt them without knowledge of abdominal and pelvic anatomy and physiology.

Several areas have purposely been avoided in preparing the Atlas. There is no attempt to advise on the indications for operative treatment and only in the most general terms are the uses of a particular operation discussed. Individual surgeons develop their own ideas on pre- and post-operative care and have their personal predilections regarding forms of anaesthesia, fluid replacement and the use of antibiotics.

Even on the purely technical aspects the temptation to advise on the choice of instruments and surgical materials is largely resisted and it is assumed that the reader is capable of placing secure knots and ligatures. Each volume of the Atlas contains a photograph of the instruments used by the authors and some of these are shown individually. Most readers will have their own favourites but the information may be useful to younger colleagues. We do not consider the choice of suture material to be of over-riding importance. The senior author has used PGA suture material since its inception and although generally preferring it to catgut does not consider it perfect. It has disadvantages and can be very sore on the surgeon's hands but it does have advantages in that it is particularly suitable for vaginal work and for closing the abdomen.

There are, of course, several methods of performing the various operations but those described here have consistently given the authors the best results. It need hardly be reiterated that the observance of basic surgical principles is probably more important than anything else.

The Atlas is produced in six volumes, each of which relates approximately to a regional subspecialty. This is done primarily to keep the size of the volumes convenient for use but also to allow publication to proceed progressively.

From what has been written it might appear that the authors think of gynaecologists as necessarily male. The suggestion is rejected: the old-fashioned usage of the inclusive masculine gender is merely retained for simplicity and neatness. Anyone questioning the sincerity of this explanation would have to be reminded that every gynaecologist must, in the very nature of things, be a feminist.

Introduction to Volume 5

In compiling this volume it has been necessary to remember that the Atlas is primarily concerned with surgical operations and techniques. Otherwise it would be easy to become involved in the many aspects of a huge subject on which there are both wide differences of opinion and a vast literature. The subject and content of each chapter in this volume is influenced by the various considerations and requirements set out below. The major causes of infertility are either as a result of tubal obstruction, disorders of ovulation or an abnormal semen specimen. This being so the active treatment of ovulatory disorders is almost without exception non-surgical and it frequently involves the administration of drugs to induce ovulation. Surgery, although the major treatment method in tubal obstruction, usually plays a secondary role in the overall management of the problem as a whole and this must be emphasised. To do so and at the same time put the matter in perspective Chapter 1 has been given over to a review of current thought regarding the investigation and treatment of infertility resulting from ovulatory or male factors. Total management of the infertile couple is considered since it is essential for the surgeon to know the scope of the problem in relation to all methods of management.

Treatment is necessarily preceded by careful clinical investigation of both partners and includes a comprehensive series of hormone assays with a number of minor surgical investigative procedures on the female partner. These surgical techniques, described in Chapter 2, are in all essentials standard gynaecological teaching and practice in the United Kingdom.

Congenital defects in the female genital tract can sometimes have an important bearing on infertility. Chapter 3 consequently includes a short revision of developmental anatomy in the female and also indicates the aberrations most likely to affect fertility.

Before considering the various surgical options it is important to remember that the infertility patient is very often under considerable emotional and psychological stress and this must be taken account of. General advice on this aspect of management is therefore offered in Chapter 4.

The completed clinical investigation may reveal congenital or acquired anatomical abnormalities of two kinds. A minority are severe or sufficiently clear cut to interfere with conception; the vast majority are much less severe and it is well nigh impossible to say whether they are causal factors in infertility. Many of the latter are present in patients who are not infertile and their importance must therefore be questioned. The minority group is treated surgically by whatever method is indicated; the majority group should have non-surgical treatment in the first place. In this volume of the Atlas the emphasis is on the various techniques used in surgical treatment. These are presented on a regional basis and vagina, cervix, uterus, ovary and fallopian tube are considered in Chapters 5 to 9.

Operations involving the vagina, cervix, uterus and ovary are macroscopic procedures and with the exception of cerclage, trachelorrhaphy and uteroplasty have already been described in other volumes of the Atlas. Key photographs are selected from operations already illustrated to provide quick reference or revision of the procedure. The legend is abridged and the reader given the volume and page reference of the full description should that be required. New photographs are employed where required or for clarification. Cerclage, trachelorrhaphy and two types of uteroplasty are illustrated in detail.

Tubal surgery presents difficulties not encountered in routine gynaecological practice and these arise from the fact that the tubes are small, mobile, thin-walled, vascular and easily traumatised by ordinary surgical instruments and handling. To minimise this trauma advantage has been taken of the magnified illumination provided by the operating microscope. Whether or not this type of surgery (microsurgery) should be performed by specialists is arguable; the realities are that practising gynaecologists continually see patients needing such surgery and neither in the UK nor most other countries are there facilities for transfer to special centres. Surgeons frequently have to operate upon such cases without the benefit of special equipment and the authors believe that they can do so quite adequately provided they observe and follow principles and practice such as those described in Chapter 9. Operating microscopes and specialist training are desirable but not essential and very worthwhile results can be obtained from the orthodox macroscopic operations described and illustrated. The colposcope as an operating microscope is sometimes used for the important purpose of checking that sutures are properly placed and suture lines intact. Purpose-built operating microscopes, however, are becoming less prohibitive in price and should be available to most surgeons in the not too distant future.

New advances in the treatment of infertility have resulted in a huge literature which it is frequently essential to consult. Rather than overload the text by adding long reference lists at the end of each chapter, these have been included with the appendices.

Microsurgical techniques clearly have an important application in infertility surgery and no one can doubt that in certain situations they must lead to improved results. The operation of tubo-cornual anastomosis for example is more logical and scientific than tubal implantation especially if the blockage is near the tubal end of the interstitial portion. It is also a great advantage to obtain precise approximation of the cut ends when anastomosing the fallopian tube and only the magnification of the microscope gives this facility. Procedures such as fimbriolysis, extensive salpingolysis and the various forms of salpingostomy all benefit from the increased precision of working under magnification. The authors do not intend to join in controversy as to who should actually do tubal microsurgery. Some take the view that it is an expensive and specialised field, so different from routine gynaecological surgery that it should be in the hands of specially trained experts. Others maintain that given the necessary equipment these operations are only extensions of recognised gynaecological techniques which the average surgeon can quickly absorb and adequately perform. The routine use of microsurgical procedures in sister disciplines is cited as a logical example to follow.

For those interested and concerned with full microsurgical techniques Mr Robert Winston has contributed Chapter 10 of this volume. He sets out the principles and practice in this specialised field and illustrates and describes the various tubal operations.

The undoubted future importance of in vitro fertilisation and embryo transfer makes the inclusion of a short chapter on the surgical technique quite essential. This is provided in Chapter 11.

Artificial insemination scarcely involves actual surgical procedures but this important aspect of infertility management demands full consideration. The basic clinical techniques are described in Chapter 12 to serve as a guide to those unfamiliar with such management and as a reference in circumstances where the guidance of laboratory colleagues may not be available.

Appendices have been used as an economical method of presenting certain detailed information on some subjects covered in the general text. These include a suggested schema for recording details of history, investigation and treatment of the infertile couple. Advice is also given on the collection and examination of the semen specimen. A synopsis of recommendations for institutional planning to set up an AID service is also included.

1: The problem of the infertile couple – A guide to diagnosis and management

The treatment of the infertile couple is a difficult problem which commonly ends in disappointment and sometimes with success. Numerous doctors and services are involved in solving this problem; from the family doctor to whom the couple first present to the specialist gynaecologist, endocrinologist or urologist to whom the couple may be referred for investigation and eventual treatment. If the infertility continues for any length of time the psychological stresses on the marriage may lead to a need for psychiatric attention. Besides the clinical specialists a large number of other and non-clinical specialists such as radiologists, histopathologists and microbiologists, are involved in helping to determine the cause of the couple's infertility.

The role of the gynaecological surgeon in this team effort is important, not only in respect of alleviating the mechanical aspects of the infertility, but in appreciating the many associated facets of the problem. He is in the unique position of being able to obtain an overview of the situation; a position not readily available to other members of the team. He must therefore be familiar with not only normal tubal physiology and pathology but with its emphasis on gamete and embryo transport, ovum pick-up and nutritional status of the ovum. He will already have a knowledge of disorders of ovulation, abnormalities in semen sample and the uncommon cervical and immunological factors in infertility. It is important not to concentrate on the surgical aspects of the problem to the exclusion of the other factors of the infertility. In this chapter an attempt will be made to present the many basic mechanisms which together make up the physiology and pathology of the infertile couple.

Definition

Infertility is defined as the 'incapacity of a man, woman or couple to participate in reproduction, i.e. the production of a live child' (Belsey 1980). The inability to conceive or impregnate, and the ability to carry a conceptus to a live birth, reflect different processes and aetiologies, with distinct implications for their solution or prevention. Without contraception it is estimated that three-quarters of couples should achieve a conception within one year.

Prevalence of infertility

The normal biological variations of human populations with respect to chromosomal, congenital and endocrinological disorders affecting both men and women can be represented as a base rate or core of infertility. To these rates might be added the occurrence of acquired conditions such as pelvic inflammatory disease, postpartum sepsis or the long term consequences of mumps orchitis. These latter conditions which vary between communities, both on a geographic and socio-economic basis, sometimes occur in epidemic proportions so that infertility becomes a major health problem as has recently been shown to occur in various regions of Africa.

The prevalence rate of involuntary infertility is traditionally estimated at about 10 per cent although recent census data, from a number of developed and developing countries, show a range which extends from 1–1.5 per cent (never pregnant) for married women of age 35–39 in Korea and Thailand to levels of up to 24 per cent for similar women in areas of Columbia and Africa (Belsey 1980). In Africa rates vary enormously within different countries and tribal regions, reflecting the prevalence of particular 'acquired' factors. It also seems that secondary infertility (i.e. a previously fertile woman unable to conceive after a period of two years, excluding period of lactation) in many countries, especially in Africa, may be more frequent than primary infertility and probably again represents the operation of specific factors such as postpartum sepsis.

Causes of infertility

Despite differences that may be attributable to geographic or socio-economic factors as outlined above, there are three major definable causes of infertility. These are:

1 Tubal obstruction
2 Disorders of ovulation
3 Oligo or azoospermia

In approximately 15–20 per cent of infertile couples there may be an abnormality in both partners.

The incidence of these factors in various countries is shown in Table 1 but the validity of such comparisons between countries is doubtful as many clinical reports represent self-selected couples or couples referred to centres of expertise. Variations also occur as a result of different diagnostic techniques. For example, Chatfield et al (1970) in a Kenyan study showed that 49 per cent of cases of secondary infertility were due to tubal occlusion as diagnosed by tubal insufflation; the

TABLE 1

CAUSES OF INFERTILITY (%)

Country	Tubal Obstruction	Ovulatory Disorders	Mixed Gynaecological Problems	Total Female	Total Male
England	19	25	34	78	22
Australia	11	43	26	80	20
Israel	16	33	23	72	28
West Africa*	62	21	13	96	45
Kenya†	56	2	2	60	—
Brazil	35	11	27	73	27
Bulgaria*	77	12	11	100	41

*Categories >100% since multiple factors present in some couples.
†Information for males unavailable.

same group when submitted to laparoscopy showed a rate of 73 per cent.

Variation in aetiological causes is greatest in women and may reflect on diagnostic accuracy and interpretation of results. A significant number of 'mixed gynaecological problems' exist in many studies and these represent the occurrence of certain conditions whose diagnosis depends on the completeness of the investigation. Such conditions include endometriosis, fibroids, cervical and immunological factors and so-called ovulatory infertility.

Each of the three major factors will now be discussed in detail after which a plan for the comprehensive evaluation of the infertile couple will be given.

1. Tubal obstruction

The majority of identifiable tubal disorders result from genital tract infection which is usually of subclinical type. Tubal distortion at micro or macroscopic level usually follows an inflammatory process (**Figures 1** and **2**) with varying degrees of fibrosis resulting. This may take the form of peritubal or ovarian adhesions or outright obstruction to any part of the tube. In its gross form complete fibrosis may completely envelop both tubes and ovaries.

These distortions result in interference with ovum pick-up and transport and scanning electron microscopy as recently reviewed by Vasquez et al (1980) shows a loss of cilia in the endosalpinx with associated fine adhesions developing between the tubal lumen and fimbria. These adhesions may well be the cause of disturbed tubal function in women with mild or even subclinical evidence of pelvic inflammation. The value of prompt diagnosis and treatment of these early conditions is essential if tubal function is to be preserved.

The authors feel that only by a full understanding of the aetiology and diagnosis of pelvic infection can effective treatment be instituted, thus leading to a reduction in the incidence of tubal obstruction.

Aetiology: the role of pelvic infection

Any form of acute pelvic infection inevitably involves the fallopian tubes. The source of the infection in nearly all cases is from a focus within the genital tract; either from exogenous organisms transmitted by venereal or iatrogenic means (i.e. following either a termination of pregnancy, dilatation and curettage, a hysterosalpingogram, or associated with an intra-uterine device), or endogenous organisms, usually of the anaerobic type. Although it is difficult to culture organisms from the tube in the presence of acute infection, there have been some recent studies where this has been possible. Westrom (1980) found on culture of the tube and associated serological studies in acute salpingitis the following organisms:

Chlamydia trachomatis	60%
Neisseria gonorrhoea	10–15%
Mycoplasma	10–15%
Anaerobic	5%
Not able to culture	15–20%

Occasionally and especially in underdeveloped countries genital tract tuberculosis, secondary to pulmonary TB may occur and cause blockage and eventual gross distortion of the oviduct as can be seen clearly in the hysterectomy specimen in **Figure 5**.

Natural history

The influence of tubal infection on the incidence of female infertility and on ectopic pregnancy is not well documented. The study of Westrom (1975, 1980) on this subject is unique in that he has been able to follow reproductive events after salpingitis in 900 women (age 13–34 years) who were treated for laparoscopically verified acute non-tuberculous salpingitis between 1960 and 1974. Of the total cases, 77.1 per cent of women had one infection, 17.1 per cent two and 5.8 per cent three infections. After excluding 192 women who were voluntarily infertile (i.e. used contraception), he found that 19.1 per cent of these remaining 708 women were infertile because of tubal occlusion.

The *infertility rate* increases significantly with the number of infections (Table 2) and the severity of the laparoscopically diagnosed inflammatory change (Table 3). He also found that of all the first pregnancies after salpingitis, 6.6 per cent were ectopic. This is equal to one ectopic per 15 intrauterine pregnancies compared with the usual rate of one per 300 in women with no salpingitis history. The rate of ectopic pregnancy did not seem to depend on the age of the women or the severity of the infection. It is of interest that since 1960, 46.2 per cent of all ectopic pregnancies in Westrom's clinic had a past history of salpingitis.

TABLE 2

INFERTILITY DUE TO TUBAL BLOCKAGE AFTER 1–3 EPISODES OF SALPINGITIS

Number of episodes	% Infertility (age groups) 15–24	25–34	Total
One	9.4	19.2	11.4
Two	20.9	31.0	23.1
Three	51.6	60.0	54.3

from Westrom (1980)

TABLE 3

INFERTILITY DUE TO TUBAL BLOCKAGE DEPENDENT ON SEVERITY OF SALPINGITIS

Severity of salpingitis	% Infertility (age groups) 15–24	25–34	Total
Mild	5.8	7.8	6.1
Moderate	10.8	22.0	13.4
Severe	27.3	40.0	30.0

from Westrom (1980)

Diagnosis of pelvic infection

(1) Clinical: difficulties in accurate diagnosis

Since acute salpingitis is one of the most common acute gynaecological disorders, and a disease mainly confined to the young and nulliparous woman, the need for early and correct diagnosis is evident. It is now accepted that laparoscopy, used routinely, fulfils all the criteria of a highly accurate, safe, simple and time-saving diagnostic aid in confirming the presence of salpingitis. From a number of studies over the last decade it would seem that the gynaecologist should be very cautious in making or excluding a diagnosis of acute salpingitis without visual verification.

Jacobson and Westrom (1969) in their large laparoscopic study of 905 women presenting either with classical symptoms and signs of acute salpingitis (814) or in whom laparoscopy unexpectedly found acute salpingitis, concluded that 'diagnosis by conventional clinical criteria implies an unsatisfactory low accuracy rate due to their unspecific characteristics and the wide range of symptom occurrence'. Reference to Table 4 shows that without the liberal use of laparoscopy a considerable number of true salpingitis cases would have been clinically misinterpreted or subjected to expectant treatment and the fact that an acute salpingitis may be consistent with scarcity of symptoms would not have been evident. The most common errors in one direction or another were found to be acute appendicitis, intrapelvic haemorrhage or pelvic endometriosis. Mistakes were also made when tumours were misinterpreted as inflammatory masses and vice versa.

The minimal criteria for the provisional clinical

TABLE 4

COMPARISON BETWEEN CLINICAL AND LAPAROSCOPIC DIAGNOSIS OF ACUTE SALPINGITIS

Clinical diagnosis (pre-exploration)	No.	Laparoscopic diagnosis: Acute salpingitis	Other disorders*	Normal
Acute salpingitis	814	532 (65%)	98 (12%)	184 (23%)
Other than acute salpingitis†	91	91		
Total	905	623	98	184

*This included acute appendicitis (24), pelvic endometriosis (16), corpus luteum haemorrhage (12), ectopic pregnancy (11).
†This included ovarian tumour (20), acute appendicitis (18), ectopic pregnancy (16), chronic salpingitis (10).

from Jacobson (1980)

diagnosis of acute salpingitis or acute pelvic inflammatory disease must be the presence of:

- acute low seated abdominal pain *with two or more of the following symptoms or signs*
- abnormal (or increased) vaginal discharge
- fever (>38°C) or chills
- irregular bleeding
- urinary or rectal symptoms
- marked tenderness of the pelvic organs on bimanual examination
- palpable adnexal mass
- erythrocyte sedimentation rate exceeding 15 mm/hour.

Bacteriological confirmation of the infection must be sought; this can be done preoperatively by taking swabs from the urethra, cervix and rectum and searching for N. gonorrhoea, pyogenic and anaerobic organisms. The culture of chlamydial and mycoplasma organisms is difficult and requires specialised techniques. Swabs must be placed in appropriate transport media and kept refrigerated at 4°C until analysed, preferably within 12 hours. At the same time a wet saline swab taken from the endocervix should reveal predominantly leucocytes on examination. It would be rare to find an infection in the upper genital tract without evidence of such (i.e. leucocytes in the swab) in the lower tract.

(2) Laparoscopic

Laparoscopy should be performed within 24 hours of admission and before treatment has started. Salpingitis seen at laparoscopy can be graded as follows:

- Mild: tubes reddened, swollen and covered by discharge (1 in **Figure 1**), 'violin string' adhesions or fibrin deposits, but freely movable and with open abdominal ostia.
- Moderate: as for mild but more marked changes, tubes not freely movable, patency of abdominal ostia uncertain. These changes are obvious in the tube (1) in **Figure 2**. Dense adhesions have already formed at (2).
- Severe: pelvic peritonitis and/or abscess formation; ostia closed (**Figures 3** and **4**). In this case leakage of a pyosalpinx necessitated laparotomy with drainage of the pyogenic material (**Figure 4**).

For those particularly concerned with the diagnosis and management of pelvic inflammatory disease the proceedings of the international symposium on that subject held at the Center for Disease Control, Atlanta, Georgia, is recommended. (*American Journal of Obstetrics and Gynecology* 1980, **138**, 7, pp. 845–1112.) The importance of early diagnosis in relation to subsequent infertility is stressed and the particular role of laparoscopy is again emphasised.

1

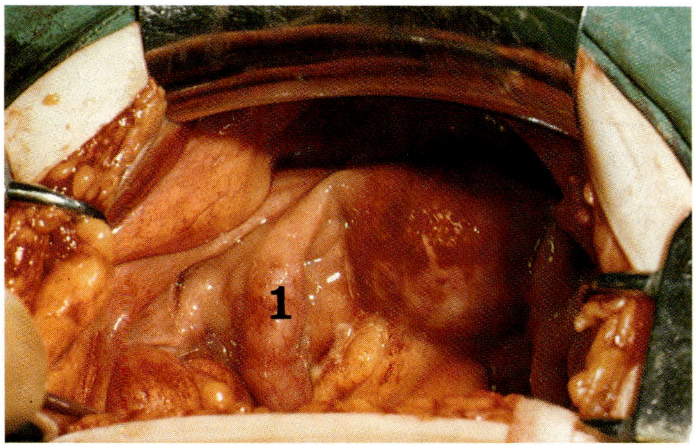

2

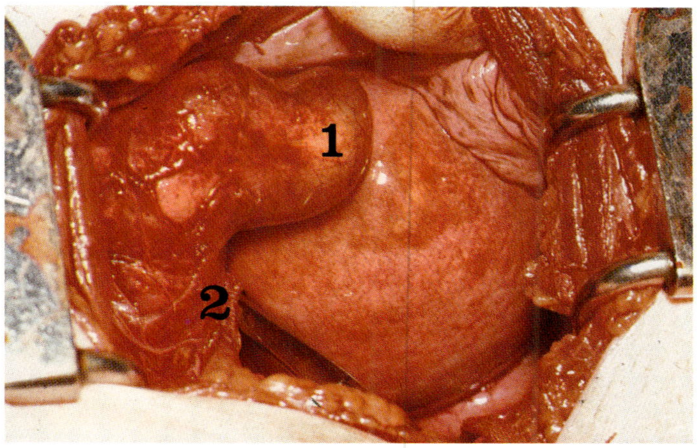

1 and 2 Mild (left) and moderate (right) pelvic sepsis
These views, and those in the following figures (**2–5**), were taken at laparotomy; identical views would be seen via the laparoscope. Bacteriological specimens can be obtained by aspiration through the palpiteur sheath.

3 Severe pelvic sepsis
The tube is seen (1) with purulent exudate (2) in the pouch of Douglas.

4 Rupture of a pyosalpinx with seepage of purulent exudate into the pelvis
Aspiration and drainage is being undertaken; a bacteriological specimen (1) is being obtained.

3
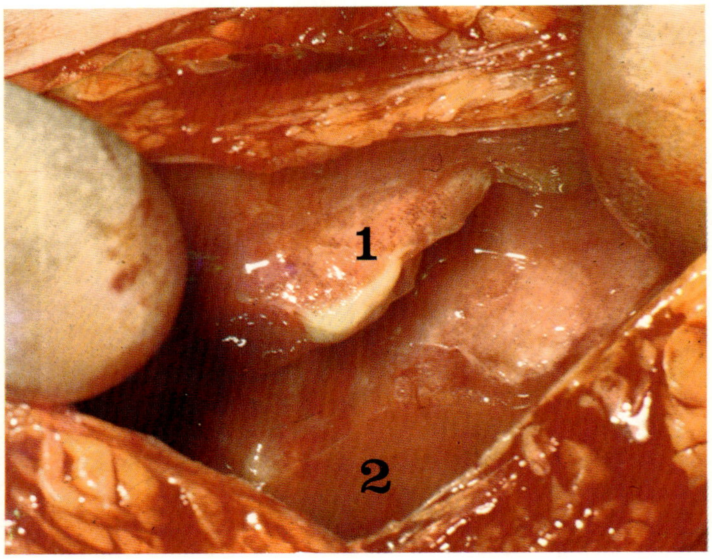

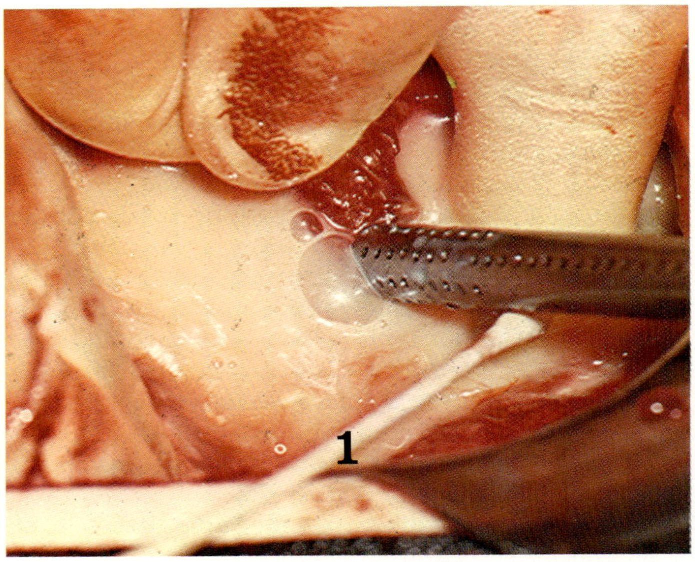

4

Treatment of pelvic infection

As can be seen from the long-term follow-up of Westrom's cases, the best hope of preventing tubal obstruction is by the early treatment of the mild inflammatory process; only 6.1 per cent of the group became infertile compared to 30 per cent of those with a severe infection. Laparoscopy is an invaluable aid in the diagnosis of these early mild cases. Antibiotics must be commenced as soon as the diagnosis is made with the patient hospitalised and at rest. The preparation used will depend on the predominant organism. For gonorrhoeal infections procaine penicillin intramuscularly is the universal choice, with kanamycin, tetracycline or erythromycin reserved for the resistant case. In non-gonorrhoeal cases much will depend on the severity of the condition, with ampicillin and doxycycline given for mild cases and a combination of gentamycin (intravenously), ampicillin and metronidazole for severe cases. Surgical drainage is necessary in cases where intraperitoneal rupture of a pyosalpinx has occurred (**Figures 3** and **4**).

5
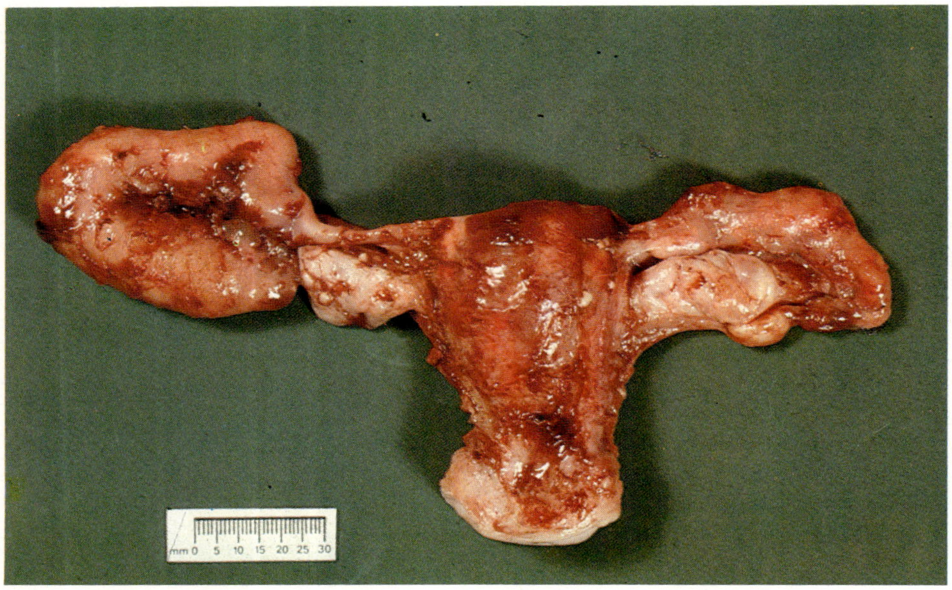

5 Chronic pelvic tuberculosis
Bilateral tuberculous caseosalpinges showing gross destruction of the tubal structure. This condition, particularly common in underdeveloped countries, accounts for a significant proportion of tubal obstructive disease in these areas.

2. Disorders of ovulation

In the investigation and treatment of the disorders of ovulation, an understanding of hormonal control of ovulation is essential. It is proposed to examine the regulatory mechanisms involved and then review those tests of ovarian function which are of benefit to the clinician.

Regulation of ovulation

Normal ovulation depends primarily on the satisfactory function of the pituitary-ovarian axis; there is a secondary influence on this axis by various endocrine organs and neural connections. An average 28 day menstrual cycle is initiated by an early follicular phase rise of follicle stimulating hormone (FSH) with a peak of FSH and luteinising hormone (LH) occurring at the mid-cycle in association with ovulation. Both these hormones (**Figures 6** and **7**) as measured in blood are present throughout the cycle; the early rise of FSH in the cycle commences as a result of the fall in progesterone and oestrogen secretion in the preceding cycle. An adequate FSH secretion at this time is essential for follicular maturation and, with a small amount of LH, is necessary for oestrogen secretion from the rapidly growing follicle which is about to ovulate. In **Figure 8** this rise in oestrogen in the latter part of the first half of the cycle is seen and this increase in oestradiol is responsible for an obvious surge of LH (**Figure 7**) associated with a smaller rise in FSH (**Figure 6**). The LH surge peaks on 1 or sometimes 2 days and is responsible for ovulation and subsequent luteinisation of the ruptured follicle, which has released the ovum at ovulation.

The corpus luteum continues to secrete both oestradiol (**Figure 8**) and progesterone (**Figure 9**) in large amounts and their high concentration suppresses the further secretion of FSH and LH. In the absence of pregnancy the corpus luteum will involute and the subsequent reduction of steroid secretion (i.e. oestradiol, progesterone) is followed by a rise in FSH. The secretion of FSH and LH from the pituitary is in the form of short episodic bursts which are maximal at mid-cycle (one/two hourly) and this characteristic can lead to possible errors when attempting precisely to date ovulation by the mid-cycle peak of LH.

A possible role in the ovulatory cycle of the hormone prolactin (**Figure 10**) secreted by the pituitary is still unclear. It does however induce disorders of ovulation when it is produced in excess. This will be discussed later.

Tests of ovarian function

(1) Hormonal

Serial measurement of urinary or plasma FSH/LH
These are measured by radioimmunoassay and the normal levels are shown in **Figures 6** and **7**. In the clinical situation their levels are of practical benefit. For example when ovarian inactivity is present as indicated by low oestrogenic secretion, the presence of a high FSH indicates that primary ovarian failure is present whereas a normal or low FSH indicates that the failure is at the hypothalamus or pituitary; perhaps suppressed by hyperprolactinaemia.

The rise of plasma LH at mid-cycle implies ovulation but its episodic release as mentioned above may cause an error of ± one day in timing the peak by daily blood estimations. Multiple blood samples or measuring urinary LH would reduce this error. About 20 hours separates the LH peak from actual ovulation.

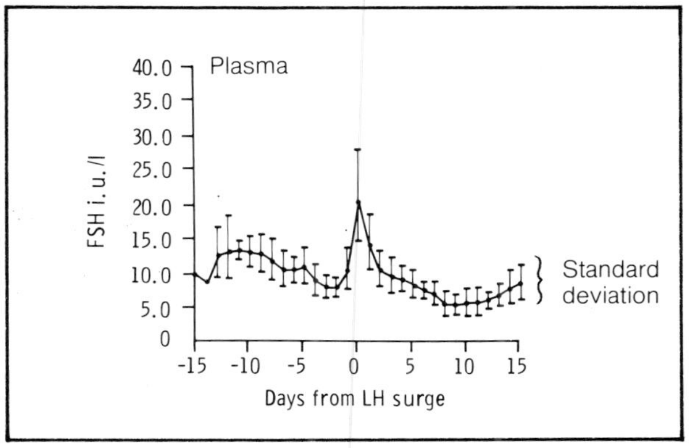

6

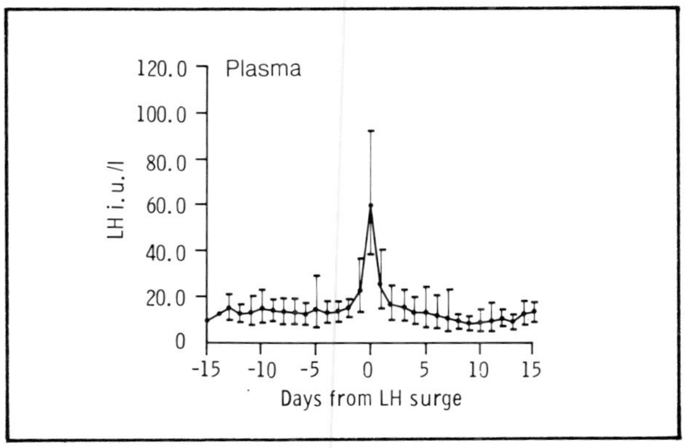

7

Oestrogen assay
Whether measured in plasma or urine, oestrogen assays are of some value when assessing ovarian function and timing ovulation. The preovulatory peak of oestrogen (**Figure 8**) occurs about 37 hours before ovulation and the urinary peak may be 1 or 2 days before (45 per cent) or on the same day as the LH peak (55 per cent). One can use daily oestrogen assays to identify the rise to the oestrogen peak followed by frequent LH assays for the first sign of a rise as an indicator of ovulation. This system would be seen to be of value when employing artificial insemination, a technique in which accurate ovulation timing is important. Total oestrogen levels (urinary) below 10 μg/24 hours are indicative of minimal ovarian activity while levels above 15 μg/24 hours are evidence of early ovarian follicular activity.

Plasma progesterone or urinary pregnanediol
Ovulation produces a rise in progesterone production with the increase beginning one or two days after ovulation (**Figure 9**). Its peak is reached some 5 days following ovulation and the rise represents a 20 to 40-fold increase above the follicular phase levels of plasma progesterone. This rise in progesterone and pregnanediol is the most reliable indicator of ovulation because rises in LH and oestrogen concentration may occur in anovulatory cycles. Although it is assumed that this rise is indicative of ovulation, it is still theoretically possible for the ovum to be entrapped in the follicle with subsequent anovulation, and a seemingly ovulatory pattern of progesterone secretion. Plasma values of above 10 ng/ml or urinary pregnanediol levels of >2 mg/24 hours are evidence of ovulation and remain at this level for approximately 7 days. A measure of these substances in plasma or urine 7 days prior to menstruation should give reasonable evidence of ovulation.

Progesterone assays may be of value in women with 'ovulatory infertility'. This state exists in women found to be ovulating and menstruating regularly but in whom no specific factor responsible for their infertility can be found. Previously many of these women were regarded as normal but a recent long-term follow-up of a number of these couples in Sheffield over a minimum of 5 years has shown that their spontaneous conception rate is very markedly lower than that of the general population. Comparison of hormonal parameters in normal women and those with ovulatory infertility shows that differences in the two groups are small except for the lowered progesterone concentration over the first half of the luteal phase of the cycle. In the infertile cycles mean progesterone concentrations rose slowly following the LH surge to reach a plateau at about 7 ng/ml and were significantly lower than the control cycles for days +1 to +7 after the LH surge. This evidence suggests that their infertility could be the result of a subtle endocrine abnormality in the luteal phase.

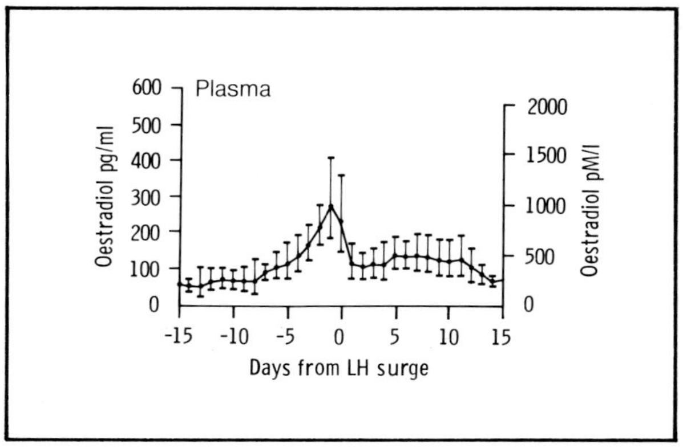

8

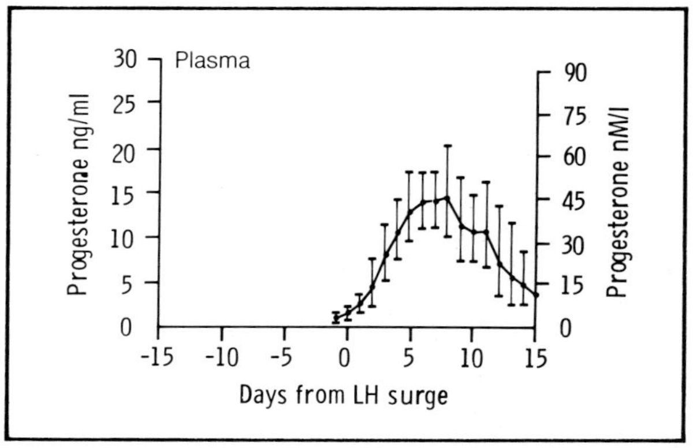

9

(2) Clinical
The only proof of ovulation is conception but a number of clinical observations indicate the possible presence or absence of ovulation and ovarian activity.

Cervical mucus
Cervical mucus is produced as a result of oestrogen; it is maximal at the time of the preovulatory surge of oestrogens and changes abruptly with the first output of progesterone. The preovulatory mucus is clear and acellular with a high water content and low viscosity and can be readily stretched to form threads (spinnbarkeit) and when dried on a slide will produce a ferning effect. The cervical os is open at this time. The mucus will allow the free entry of sperm both in vivo and in vitro. After ovulation the cervical os will close, the mucus will become scant, viscid and impenetrable to sperm, with reduced spinnbarkeit and ferning potential.

Basal body temperature charts (BBT)
The secretion of progesterone is accompanied by an approximate rise of 0.5°C in body temperature between the follicular and luteal phase of the cycle. This rise occurs after ovulation and is universally employed as a crude indicator of ovulation. The temperature may be taken orally, vaginally or rectally and is recorded by the patient on rising in the morning. Erroneous results are obtained in women employed in evening/night occupations.

A recent study in Sheffield (Lenton et al 1977) shows that a substantial error may occur when using this chart as an indicator of ovulation. In this study a group of trained observers correctly interpreted either an ovulatory or anovulatory chart in 80 per cent of cases; the day of ovulation was reckoned in only 34 per cent. The thermal nadir was found retrospectively to coincide with the LH surge in only 43 per cent of charts from normal and from 25 per cent of those from infertile women. In **Figures 10** to **12** three typical patterns of BBT charts are seen with **Figure 10** showing a normal ovulatory pattern, **Figure 11** a pattern not uncommonly seen which may or may not be associated with endocrine abnormality and **Figure 12** a typical anovulatory pattern. The LH surge is marked by a perpendicular arrow in the first two cases.

Despite its drawbacks the use of the BBT chart in an infertility clinic is probably justified as a means of providing a concise visual record of menstrual times, times of hormone assay, results of biopsy and treatment dosages. It should not be used to draw detailed conclusions about the progress of hormonal events.

10

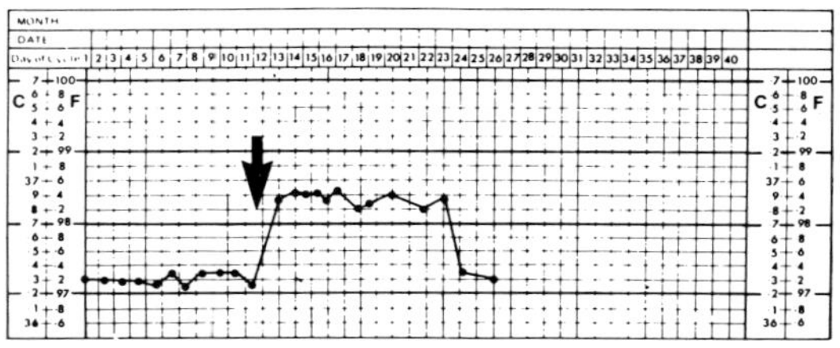

11

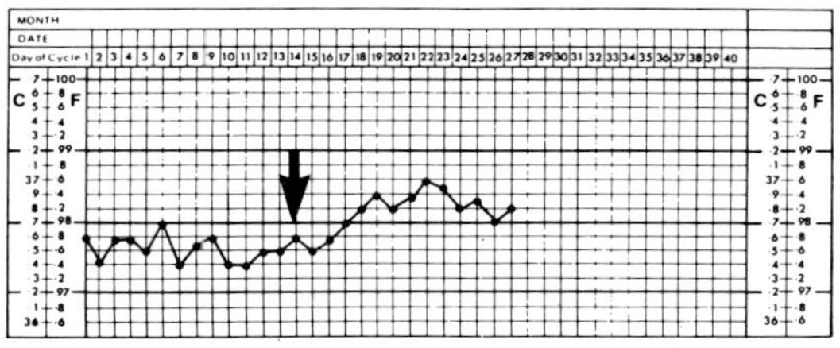

12

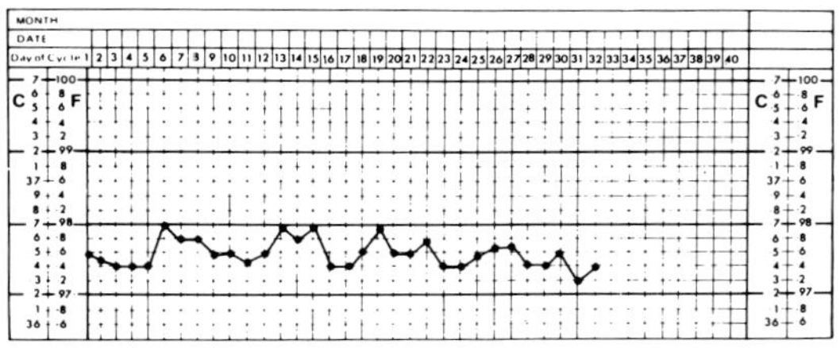

Endometrial biopsy

This is discussed later (pages 26 to 27). The presence of secretory endometrium indicates the presence of progesterone and evidence of ovulation.

Disorders of ovulation: clinical conditions

Classification *(after Brown et al 1980)*

These are best divided into the clinical conditions of:

(a) Primary amenorrhoea – no spontaneous bleeding up to age 18 years.

(b) Secondary amenorrhoea – no spontaneous bleeding for a period of 6 months or more.
– amenorrhoea 6–12 months.
– amenorrhoea >12 months.

(c) Oligomenorrhoea – cycles occurring between 5 weeks and 6 months and may be ovulatory or anovulatory.

(d) Anovulatory cycles – cycles of usually 3–6 weeks duration.

(e) Ovulatory infertility – ovulation occurs and in the absence of any other explanation for the infertility, this is presumed to be due to some abnormality of the follicle or corpus luteum.

Before failure of ovulation can be assumed local uterine causes such as uterine absence or intrauterine synechiae (adhesions) must be excluded. All investigations are directed towards elucidating the cause of the disorder so that the appropriate therapy can be given.

Primary amenorrhoea

The majority of these patients have either a disorder of the hypothalmic pituitary axis, gonadal agenesis or a major chromosomal abnormality. Investigation of the first condition is identical to that for those with secondary amenorrhoea. The other conditions are usually clinically obvious and recognised before infertility becomes a problem.

Secondary amenorrhoea (oligomenorrhoea)

The possible causes are shown in Table 5 (overleaf) and usually involve disturbances in hypothalamic-pituitary function or ovarian failure. The former is the commoner cause of anovulation in women presenting with these symptoms. Changes in weight* caused by or associated with either gross obesity, anorexia nervosa, drug ingestion (oral contraceptive steroids, tranquillisers) and psychological disturbances all act on the hypothalamic region. The absence of ovarian function is indicated by low basal urinary oestrogens and tests for anovulation are not necessary.

Anovulatory cycles

Disorders of oestrogen production lead to recurrent anovulatory cycles. In one type there are fluctuating variations in oestrogen levels, often in the normal preovulatory range, but without luteinisation occurring. Bleeding however occurs as a result of oestrogen withdrawal. In another type a constant elevated

*Optimum weight has been defined by Garrow (1979) using the formula of $\frac{\text{weight}}{\text{height}^2}\left(\frac{\text{Kg}}{\text{metre}^2}\right)$, with the result lying between 19 and 24.

TABLE 5

CAUSES OF SECONDARY AMENORRHOEA

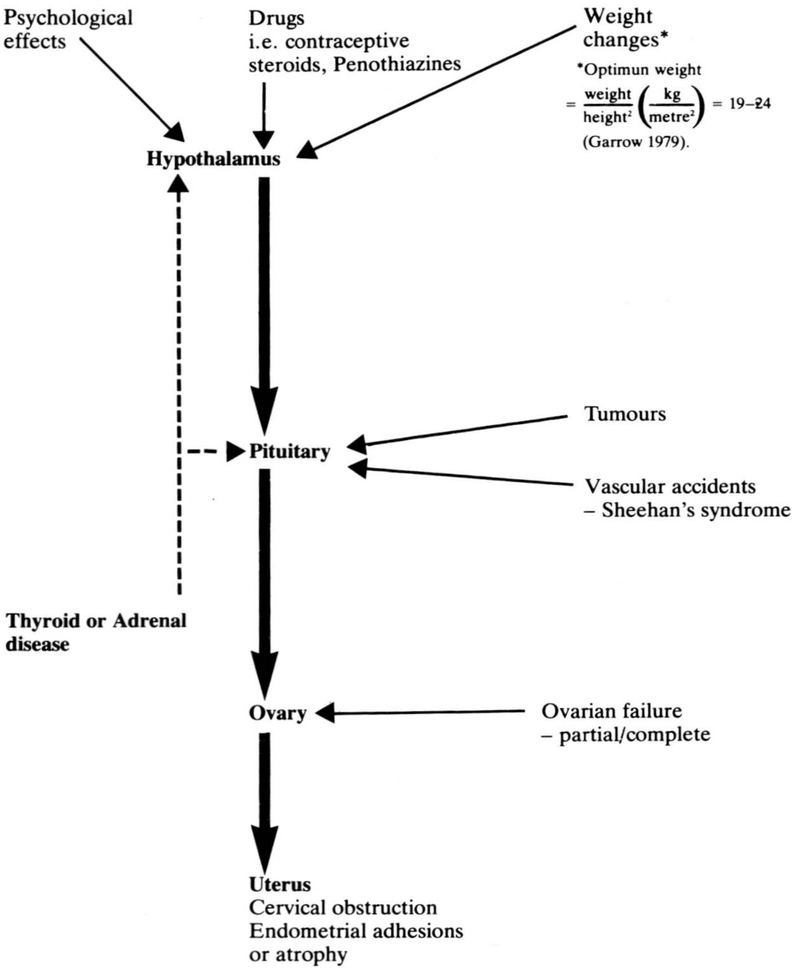

oestrogen level exists (approximately 20–40 μg/24 hours) and bleeding occurs as a breakthrough phenomenon.

Disorders of follicular or corpus luteum function
Many of these women ovulate and menstruate regularly but remain infertile. It is only by detailed hormonal evaluation (i.e. FSH, LH, prolactin, oestrogen and especially progesterone) that this condition can be fully evaluated. Exclusion of a male or tubal cause of infertility is important.

Hormonal investigation

Investigation of patients with primary and secondary amenorrhoea associated with hypothalamic-pituitary disorders is similar. The tests for the anovulatory patient are:

(i) Plasma FSH and LH.
(ii) Plasma prolactin.
(iii) Thyroid function which includes – serum thyroxine T_4 and tri-iodothyronine resin uptake T_3; minor abnormalities of thyroid function affect ovulation and hypothyroidism may be a cause of hyperprolactinaemia.

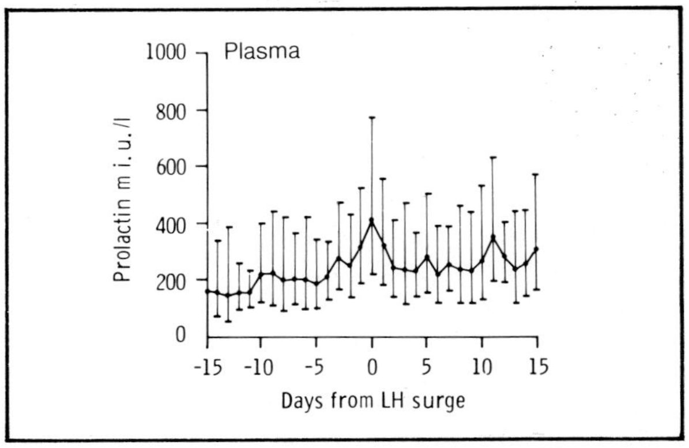

13

Plasma prolactin is estimated by radioimmunoassay and the normal levels are given in **Figure 13**. Elevation of the level above 800 m.i.u./l (M.R.C. 75/504) alerts the clinician to the very uncommon presence of a pituitary tumour, but this is more likely to be associated with concentrations of the order of 2500 m.i.u./l. Radiographic visualisation of a normal 'floor' to the sella tursica of the pituitary fossa will exclude a large tumour but more sophisticated screening in the form of computerised axial tomography (CAT scan) may be necessary to exclude suprasellar extension of the tumour. However, more commonly, oligomenorrhoea and/or amenorrhoea in nearly 10–20 per cent respectively of cases is associated with hyperprolactinaemia. In these the element of stress and the operation of drugs, two potent causes of prolactin elevation, must be excluded. This necessitates the collection of three basal resting blood samples and the simultaneous suspension of drugs like reserpine, benzamides, phenothiazines, methyldopa and oestrogens.

Treatment

Obviously a detailed investigation of the couple as given on page 20 will have been performed before treatment of ovulatory disorders is contemplated. Causes of ovulatory failure i.e. premature menopause, or gross endocrine abnormalities (i.e. of the thyroid or adrenal glands) which contribute to anovulation will have been likewise corrected by appropriate (replacement) therapy. Treatment for the remainder will be directed towards the induction of ovulation with drugs. As readers are aware a high rate of spontaneous ovulation occurs in many oligomenorrhoeic and amenorrhoeic women while under investigation. There is probably a significant placebo effect of drug management.

The drugs currently used for ovulation induction are:

Clomiphene citrate

Bromocriptine

Gonadotrophins (obtained either from human pituitary or from postmenopausal urine).

A detailed description of the various treatment regimes employing these drugs is outside the scope of this text and the reader is referred to the references for further information.

3. Oligo and azoospermia

The investigation of the male partner involves initially the collection of one but preferably two semen samples. If this is normal then no further tests are necessary, but if it is abnormal then further investigations are needed. The female partner in such a situation must still be fully investigated in case there exists an eventual need for artificial insemination.

The management of the male with an abnormal semen test is difficult as in no more than 50 per cent can a definite cause be found. Therefore it is very important that an adequate clinical examination be undertaken to detect those few conditions that are amenable to treatment.

Definitions of oligo and azoospermia

Azoospermia is understood to mean a complete absence of spermatozoa in the semen sample; oligozoospermia a reduction in the sperm numbers to below that assessed as normal (cf. Appendix A).

The aetiology of oligo and azoospermia is multifactorial and a comprehensive list (as described by Hudson et al 1980) is given in Appendix A.

Investigation of the male partner

The semen specimen

The criteria for normality are based on data from men whose partners were very recently fertile. With this in mind it is stressed that more than one factor in the semen sample (i.e. total count, motility, morphology) must be considered before a decision on the potential fertility of the man can be made. A detailed account of the collection and assessment of the semen specimen is given in Appendix A.

Clinical examination and investigation

Prior to a full physical examination, a detailed history should be taken. A suggested questionnaire incorporating important points in such a history, can be found in Appendix E.

14

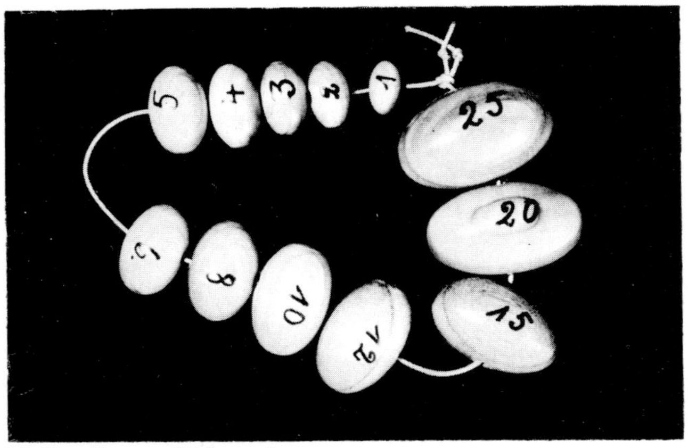

14 Prader orchidometer

Physical

The physical examination is initially general and then more specific; the former concentrating on features of hypogonadism with complete or partial absence of pubertal development and/or poorly developed secondary sexual characteristics.

The specific genital examination includes:

- penile abnormalities; hypospadias or phimosis.
- testicular size; this should be measured objectively using a Prader orchidometer (**Figure 14**) which is composed of a series of ellipsoids corresponding to various testicular volumes (from 1–25 ml). The adult testis exceeds 15 ml in volume.
- vasal and epididymal abnormalities. There may be congenital absence of the vas (and seminal vesicles). Irregularities in the epididymides suggest past infection, or obstruction and/or impairment of sperm maturation.
- varicocele identification. The patient must stand for this examination and the cough impulse be obtained. The latter can be accentuated by a valsalva manoeuvre.
- rectal examination and palpation of the prostate in suspected cases of chronic genital tract infection.

Hormonal

In the presence of an abnormal semen specimen certain hormone estimations are valuable. These include, FSH, LH, testosterone and prolactin.

- FSH; in azoospermia the finding of a high level is presumptive evidence of severe testicular damage to the Sertoli cells, whereas a normal level indicates a less severe degree of damage or duct obstruction.
- LH and testosterone; these tests are of limited value with subnormal levels indicating a pituitary or hypothalamic cause of the abnormal semen sample.
- prolactin; in the rare case of a prolactin secreting pituitary tumour, this hormone will be elevated. Some authors report hyperprolactinaemia in cases of oligospermia.

Testicular biopsy

It is now possible to correlate hormone levels (as described above) with the histological severity of the spermatogenic abnormality. This makes the need for biopsy unwarranted in most cases. It is suggested that it be reserved for patients in whom obstruction is suspected where an abnormal semen sample is present with normal hormone levels and testicular size.

Cytogenetic studies

Cytogenetic abnormalities in infertile men occur in 2 per cent of studied groups. It is mainly employed for diagnosing an additional X chromosome in Klinefelter's syndrome, multiple X chromosomes or mosaicisms. Simple buccal smears and Barr body analysis will often be adequate but formal karyotype analysis is preferable.

Postcoital test

The usefulness of this commonly performed test is now in some doubt. Done usually 24–36 hours prior to ovulation, it assesses the quality of sperm motility and of cervical mucus. Ideal timing is essential to obtain optimum mucus and it is suggested that serial daily observation of mucus be made so as to choose the best quality mucus for the ‘test’. The result is highly dependent on a normal sperm count; the absence of sperm in the postcoital test where the semen specimen was normal would suggest a possible psychosexual problem.

Abnormal tests are difficult to interpret and could be due to poor timing with poor quality mucus, or an ‘inferior’ semen. There is a small possibility of immunological immobilisation of the normal ejaculated sperm by the otherwise optimal mucus. If this is so then further examination of the ‘ovulatory’ mucus is indicated with in vitro cross-over tests with donor sperm or donor mucus. These are rarely done in any ordered manner that would allow the often given diagnosis of ‘cervical hostility’, an exceedingly rare condition in our experience, to be made.

There seems to be very little correlation between the results of postcoital tests and the ultimate fertility outcome (Kovacs 1978). Thus a poor test does not exclude examination of the semen sample or of testing for ovulation nor does a satisfactory result imply that both partners are necessarily normal.

Special tests to detect varicocele

Varicoceles are not infrequently found in those males presenting with their female partner to an infertility clinic and are reckoned to occur in between 8–16 per cent of adolescents. The detection and surgical management of this condition leads to a significant improvement in fertility with Comhaire (1980) estimating that within one year after surgical cure the sperm quality improved by 60 per cent in his cases and between 30–50 per cent fathered a child.

Varicoceles are due to reflux of renal venous blood into the spermatic vein and pampiniform plexus, with the refluxed blood containing a high concentration of the vasoactive catecholamines. The latter may result in chronic vasoconstriction of the testicular arterioles with consequent tubular dysfunction and interference with hormone production. Prognosis after surgery is probably dependent on the degree of pre-existing tubular change.

Diagnosis is simple and relies on observation and palpation of the distended pampiniform plexus when the patient is standing and undertakes a valsalva manoeuvre.

However the detection of small or even subclinical varicoceles is important as their cure can improve

15

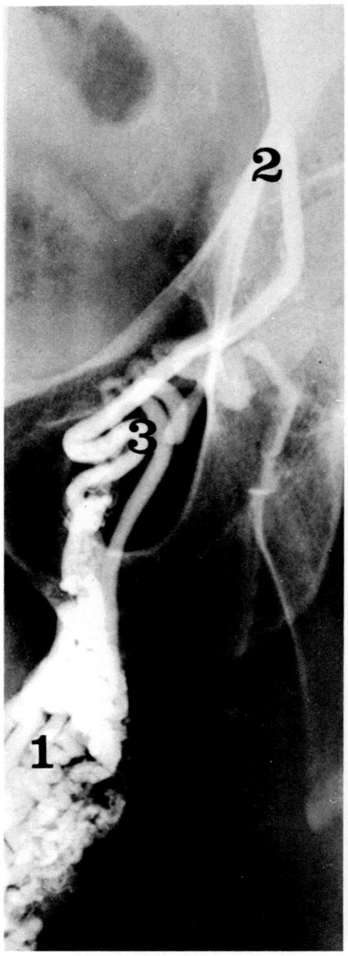

16

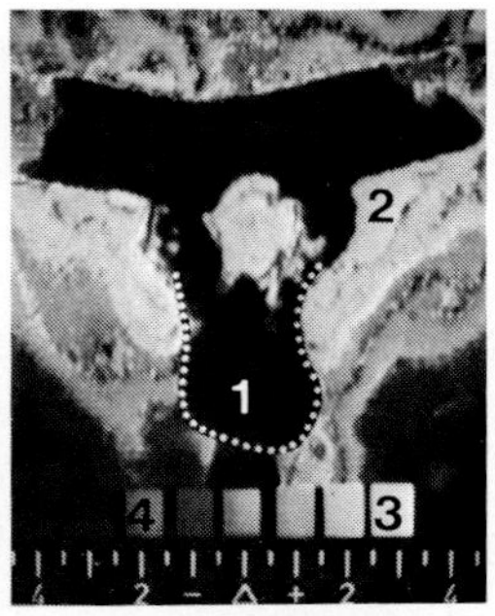

17

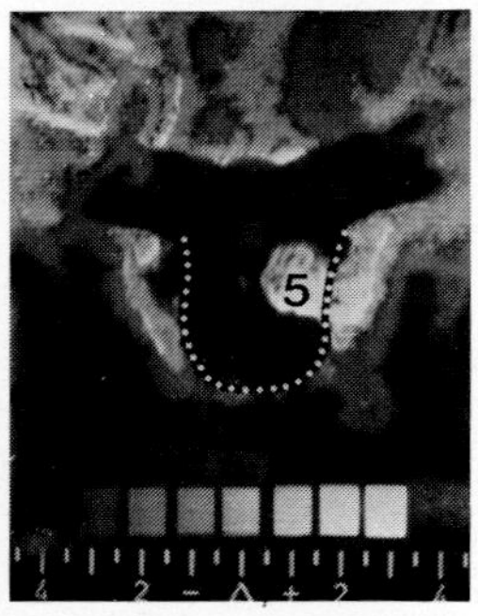

18

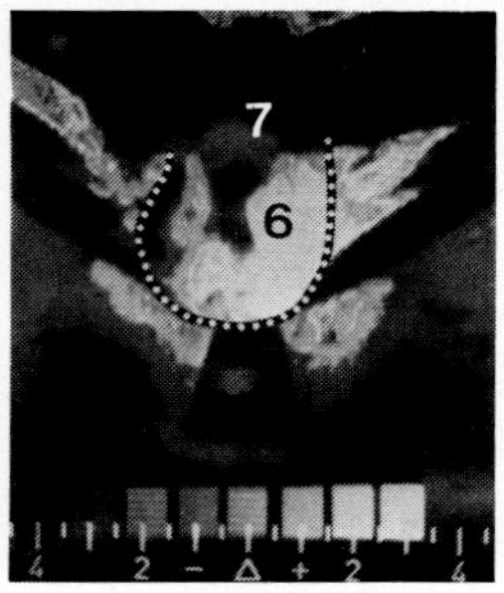

15 Retrograde venography of the internal spermatic vein
An obvious varicocele is seen (1) with an associated incompetent spermatic vein (2). Variations in the venous anatomy are common and may include a duplicated paravertebral entrance into the renal vein or multiple closely arranged sinusoid channels in the inguinal canal region (3). Left to right shunts occur in 20 per cent of venograms, making visualisation of the right side imperative.

16 to 18 Thermograms of scrotal area used in detection of subclinical varicocele
Figure 16 shows a normal scrotal area with the scrotal skin (1) 3.5°C cooler than the skin of the groin (2). Temperature differences are normally recorded in various colours (although these figures have been reproduced in black and white only). Each 0.5°C isotherm, situated at the bottom of the figure, is represented by a different colour ranging from white (warm, 3) to purple/black (cold, 4). In **Figure 17** a clinically undetected varicocele is shown. The zone of increased temperature is present at (5) in the upper left quadrant of the scrotal area overlying the pampiniform plexus. **Figure 18** is of a moderately sized varicocele with the skin of the left hemiscrotum excessively warm (6). The scrotum is isolated from the thigh by means of gauze (7) in order to clearly demonstrate the hyperthermia of the scrotal skin.

subsequent fertility. A number of special tests are now available to aid in their diagnosis. These are:

Doppler blood flow measurement.

Retrograde venography of the internal spermatic vein (**Figure 15**).

Scrotal (tele) thermography (**Figures 16** to **18**).

The *doppler blood flow measurement* is used to detect the inversion of blood flow in the internal spermatic vein in patients with varicocele. This simple test relies on the detection of an audible murmur when the probe of either an ordinary doppler device (i.e. as used to detect fetal heart sounds) or better when a smaller more sensitive pencil probe shaped doppler device is placed over the region of the spermatic artery in men with varicoceles. The man should be recumbent and the doppler device is placed as cranially as possible over the spermatic funicle at the base of the scrotum. The patient should then undertake the valsalva manoeuvre and in the absence of a varicocele, no murmur is heard.

This method, because of its cheapness and non-invasive nature is highly recommended in the screening of the subfertile male.

Retrograde venography of the internal spermatic vein will visualise the small and the abnormal venous channels which comprise the varicocele. This latter is of great assistance to the urological surgeon when undertaking ligation. The technique is by percutaneous puncture of the right femoral vein under local anaesthesia and television control and necessitates the passage of a Cobra catheter into the left renal vein via the vena cava. Valsalva manoeuvre in the half erect position in the normal male will result in no reflux visualisation of the spermatic vein. A typical example of a varicocele is seen in **Figure 15**.

Scrotal (tele) thermography. This specialised technique developed by Kormano (1970) is valuable in detecting the subclinical varicocele; Comhaire (1980) believing that 1 in 5 are subclinical. Before the test is undertaken the man stands upright and the genital area is uncovered for 15 minutes. In normal men the scrotal skin temperature is 3–5°C less than the upper thigh (**Figure 16**). If blood of body temperature is refluxed into the pampiniform plexus, the scrotal skin overlying this area will be warmer than normal so that on the thermogram this can be recognised as a 'hot spot' (**Figures 17** and **18**). Hyperthermia may extend over the whole affected hemiscrotum with a temperature difference often exceeding 2.5°C. Comhaire (1980) states that falsely normal or abnormal thermograms are uncommon; the latter possibly occurring in 1 in 20 cases.

Clinical disorders of male infertility

A comprehensive list of aetiological causes is given in the introduction to this section. The mode of clinical presentation of these disorders depends on the severity of the sperm deficit and testicular volume. Hudson et al (1980) have recently suggested a clinical classification based on these two parameters (Table 6).

Management

Although it is beyond the scope of this text to deal with details of management, a general guide will be given based on the clinical conditions as listed in Table 6. The factors leading to the infertility of the male partner can be classified into treatable and non-treatable and this determines management. A general plan is given in Appendix A.

Before any treatment is begun it is important to emphasise the value of counselling and the psychological assessment of the couple. The presence of undue tension, anxiety and general stress factors as well as possible psychosexual difficulties should be diagnosed and corrected where possible.

TABLE 6

A CLASSIFICATION OF SEMEN DISORDERS*

Sperm Count	Testicular Volume		
	Normal (15–30ml)	Slight to Marked Reduction (10–15ml)	Marked Reduction (<10ml)
Azoospermia	OBSTRUCTION	Germinal cell arrest Cytoxic drugs Irradiation	KLINEFELTER'S SYNDROME SERTOLI CELL ONLY Gonadotrophin deficiency
Severe Oligospermia $<5\times10^6$/ml	IDIOPATHIC HYPOSPERMATOGENESIS	Varicocele CRYPTORCHIDISM	Orchitis
Moderate Oligospermia $5–20\times10^6$/ml	Recent illness VARICOCELE IDIOPATHIC HYPOSPERMATOGENESIS	Infection Chronic illness	
Normal Motility defect	Infection Varicocele Immunologic Accessory gland dysfunction Absent dynein arms (Kartagener's syndrome)		

from Hudson (1980)

*Some disorders appear twice in this Table and those which occur more commonly in a particular category are shown in capitals.

Suggested schema of investigation and treatment of the infertile couple

Female

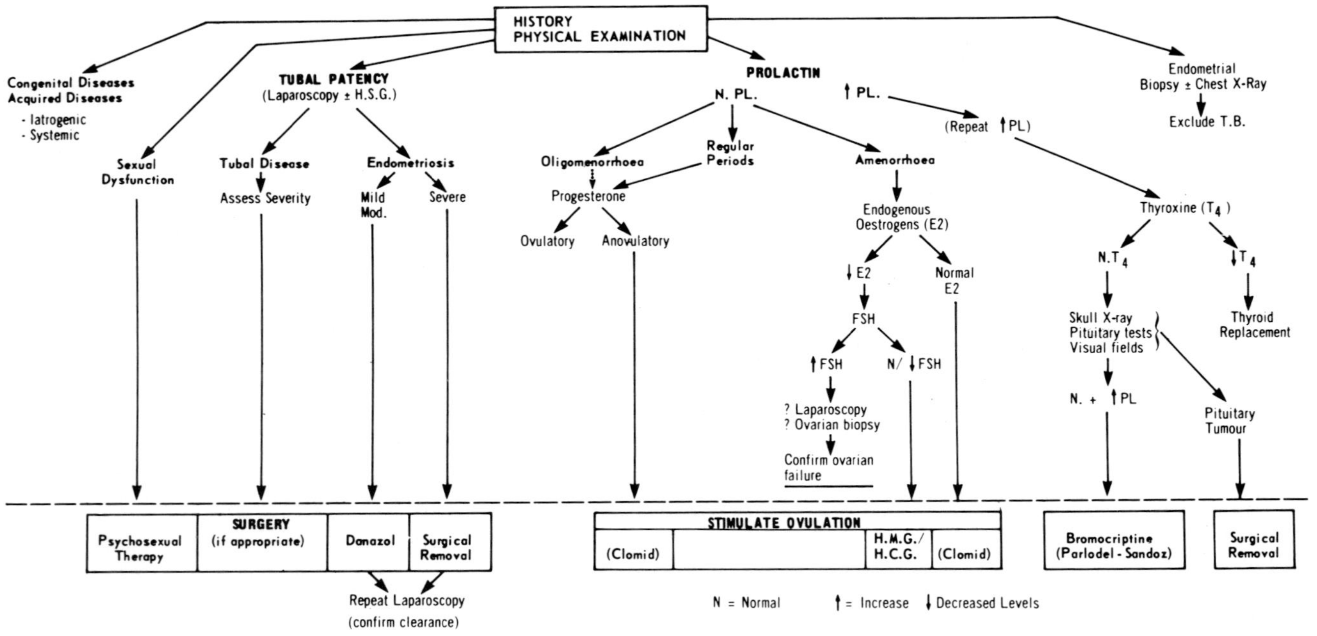

Male

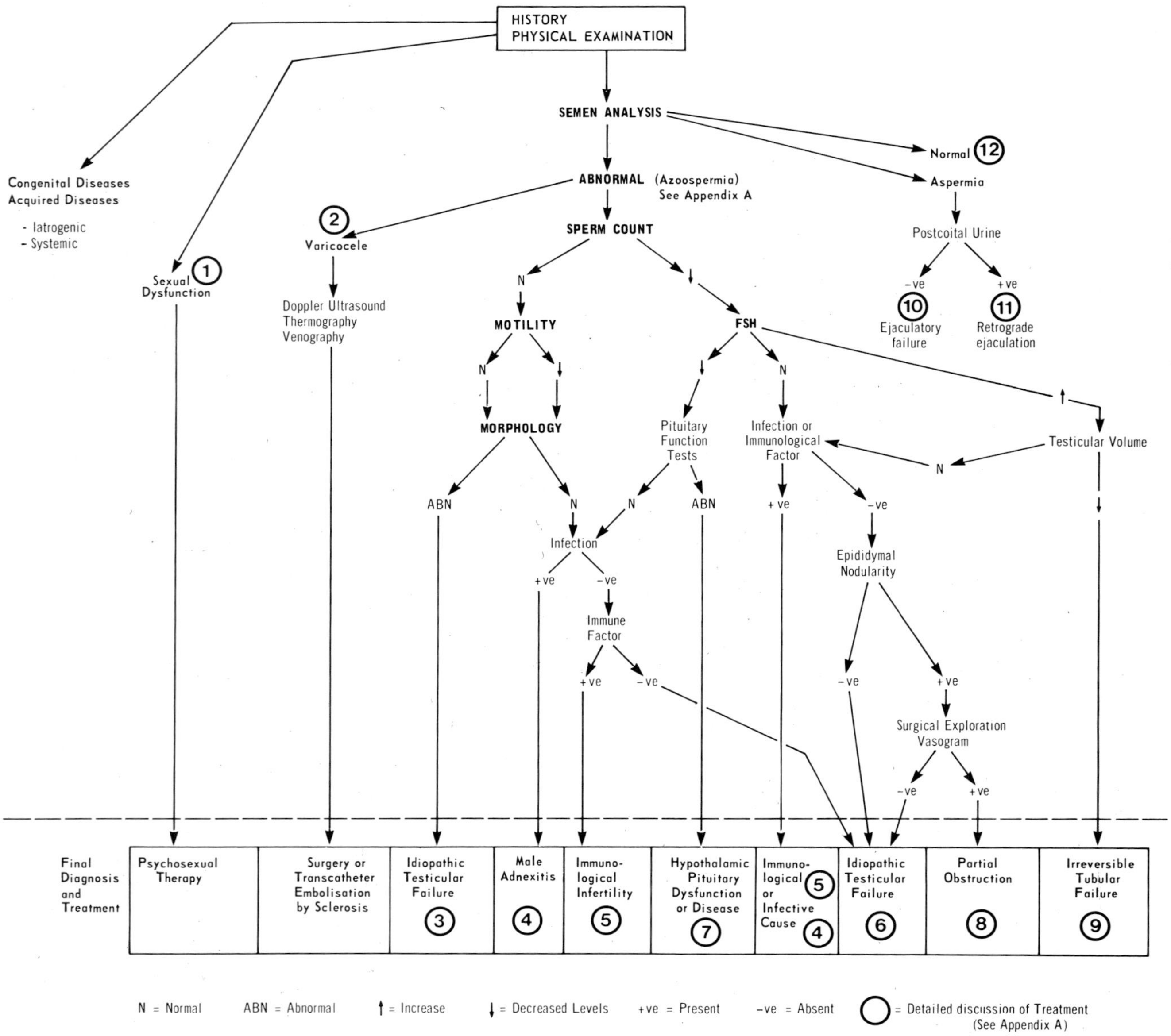

2: Techniques for the investigation and diagnosis of utero-tubal disease

Partial or complete blockage of the fallopian tubes or the presence of an intra-uterine abnormality can be demonstrated by a number of tests. These include:

Rubin's test
Hysterosalpingography (HSG)
Laparoscopy
Hysteroscopy
Endometrial biopsy

Laparoscopy is the optimal technique with which to ascertain the presence of tubal and peritubal disease. It can also assess tubal patency, and study muscular and fimbrial motility but the status of the intratubal ciliary surface, which is so important as a guide to prognosis in tubal surgery (see page 149) cannot be determined by laparoscopy. Its employment in all cases of infertility is an ideal which is not practicable in many centres. Apart from the question of availability many women fear anaesthetics and the expense of the procedure, usually done as a hospital inpatient, is not inconsiderable. This being so hysterosalpingography and the Rubin's test are still employed in many centres as a screening test for tubal patency.

Rubin's test

This technique has limited value because of its inherent high false positive rate and its inability to give any information on the site and extent of tubal blockage. The insufflation of carbon dioxide into the uterus at 60–90 ml/minute for two minutes with the pressure measured and recorded on a kymograph forms the basis of this test. Normally gas enters the peritoneal cavity via the fallopian tubes at less than 100 mm of mercury pressure; readings between 100–200 mm being abnormal. The method has possible complications which include: gas embolism, introduction or reactivation of pelvic sepsis, vasovagal stimulation, uterine and/or tubal perforation and pain.

Hysterosalpingography (HSG)

This is a technique in which a radio-opaque material is introduced into the uterus while simultaneously screening and viewing by fluoroscopy the passage of dye from the cervix to the peritoneal cavity. A water soluble medium meglumine iodipamide (Endografin) has replaced the more viscous media such as lipiodol.

The picture obtained by HSG can provide evidence of uterine, tubal and peritubal disease and is used by many gynaecologists as a primary screening procedure in women with primary infertility. There are certain contraindications to HSG which include:

- acute/subacute pelvic sepsis
- past pelvic sepsis with an adnexal mass
- sensitivity to radio-opaque medium as determined by previous experience

Patency is demonstrated by the free spillage of radio-opaque medium into the peritoneal cavity. The medium (1 in **Figure 1**) can be introduced via the cervix through a rigid Spackman cannula (2 in **Figure 1**) anchored to the cervix by a long volsellum forceps (3 in **Figure 1**) or by the use of a vacuum attached cap (4 in **Figure 1**).

Dye accumulates proximal to the block if the tube is partially or totally occluded and may also pass into the peritoneal cavity after some delay if a partial block is present. In the presence of a hydrosalpinx spherical drops of medium appear in the tube; calcification indicates the past presence of tuberculosis. Examples of tubal and peritubal disease demonstrated by HSG are shown in **Figures 7–12**.

False positive results may be due to tubal perforation by the medium and false negatives result from tubal spasm, reflux of dye, leakage around cannula and excessive pain causing the procedure to be abandoned. The subject has recently been reviewed by Philipp and Carruthers (1981).

1

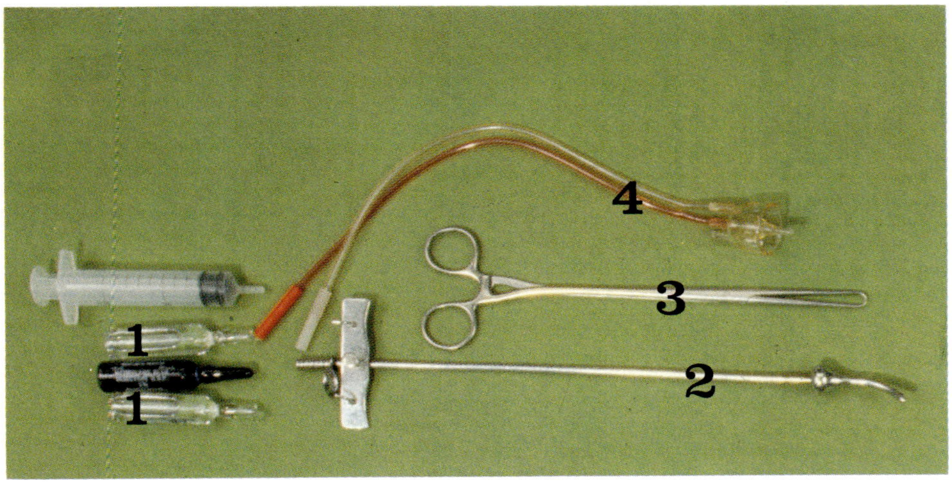

1 Instruments used in hysterosalpingography
1 Water soluble contrast medium
2 Spackman cannula
3 Volsellum for attachment of cannula to cervix
4 Cervix adaptor. The radio-opaque dye is injected along the red tube while vacuum is applied by suction through the clear tube.

Comparison of HSG and laparoscopy

A number of studies (Maathuis et al 1972, Swolin and Rosencrantz 1972, Duignan et al 1972, Taylor 1977) have investigated the accuracy of HSG by subsequently performing a laparoscopy. In the comprehensive investigation by Duignan et al, 273 women were submitted to both investigations. In 70 per cent of cases similar information was obtained; in 22 of 79 in whom HSG suggested bilateral tubal occlusion, patent tubes were subsequently shown at laparoscopy. Conversely, tubal patency was demonstrated by HSG in 10 patients in whom it could not be shown at laparoscopy. In these 10 the tubes appeared normal at laparoscopy and it was concluded that the inability to demonstrate tubal patency with dye was due to leakage into the vagina and subsequent loss of filling pressure in the tubes. Six patients in whom HSG appearances indicated peritubal adhesions had none when examined laparoscopically.

The major discrepancy between the HSG and laparoscopy findings concerned women in whom the HSG had shown patent tubes with no apparent pelvic abnormality, whereas laparoscopy revealed endometriosis (20 patients), peritubal or periovarian adhesions (18), small subserous fibroids (4), unilateral hydrosalpinx (1) and small ovarian cyst (1).

The technique

The examination is carried out in a fully equipped radiography department with fluoroscopy screening facilities. Contraindications to the procedure are obviously determined prior to attendance. The steps in the procedure are shown (**Figures 2 to 6**).

2

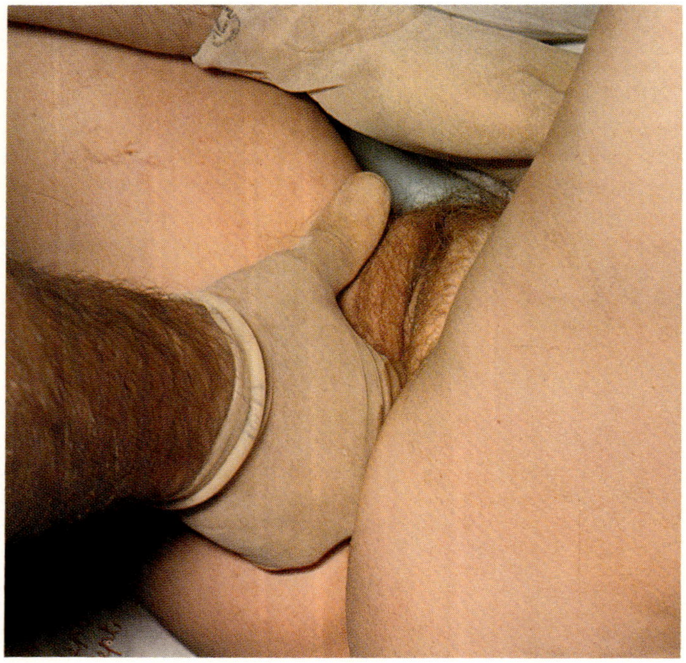

2 Preliminary pelvic examination
This is undertaken not only to determine the position of the uterus, but also to discover evidence of any recent sepsis that would be indicated by pain and/or tenderness at the examination.

3

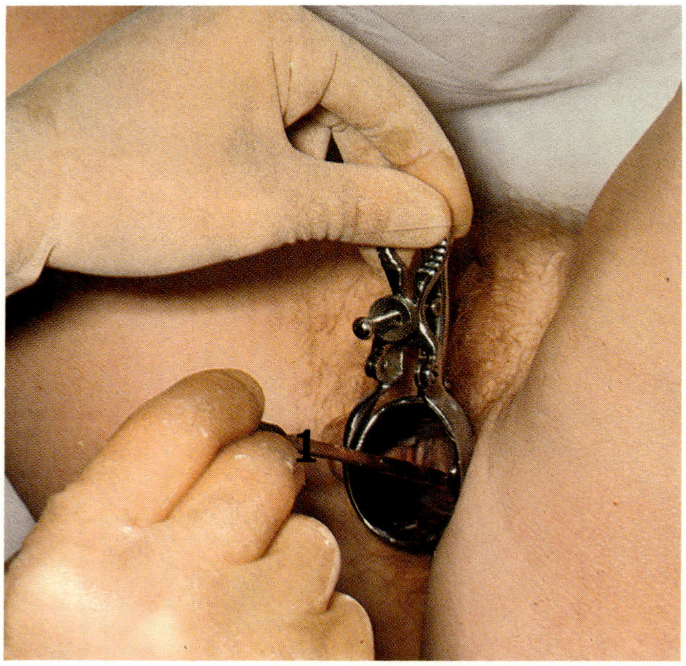

3 Passage of uterine sound
A self retaining Cusco vaginal speculum has been inserted and a uterine sound (1) determines the direction of the cervical canal and the uterine length. Excessive pain at passage of this sound could indicate the presence of a small endocervical canal and the need to use the vacuum attached cervical cap through which to inject dye rather than the endocervical fitting Spackman cannula (as seen in **Figures 24–25**).

4

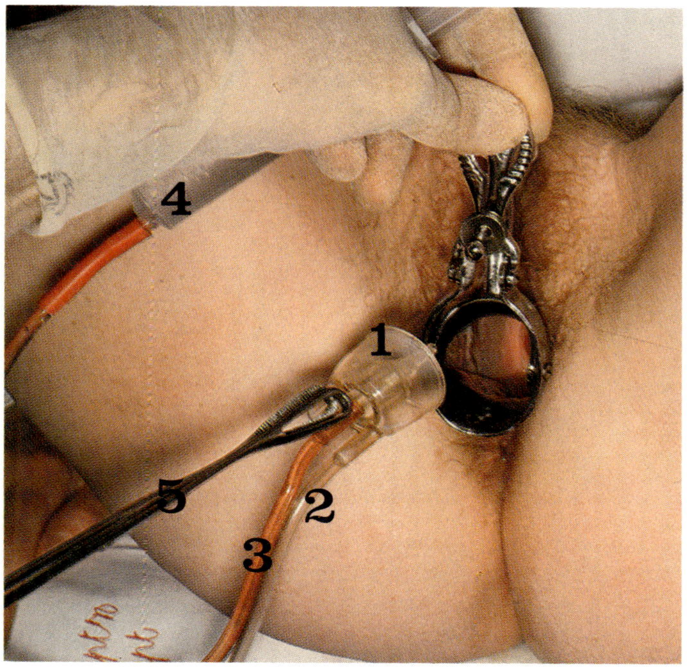

5

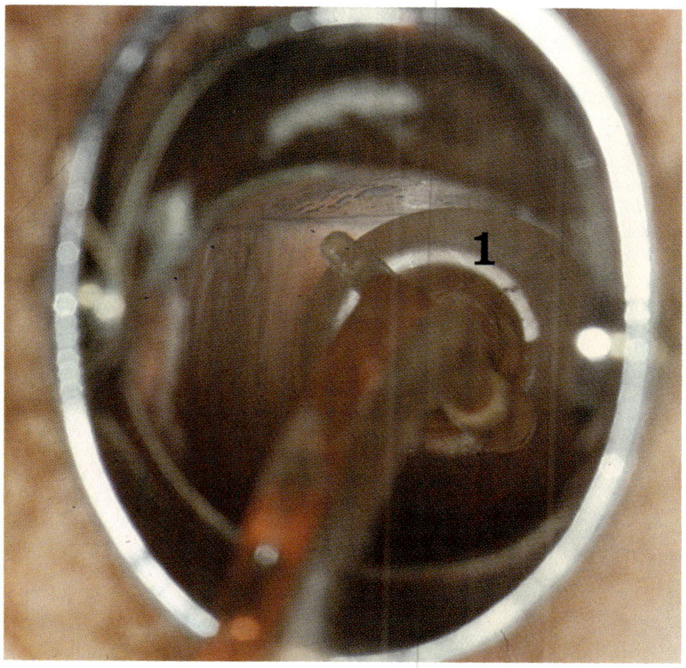

4 and 5 Application of vacuum attached cervix adaptor
The flexible airtight system for introduction of media was devised by Fikentscher and Semm and involves the application by suction of a transparent plastic cervical adaptor (1 in **Figure 4**) on to the cervix. Vacuum can be generated via a hand-held pump by an assistant or a small suction machine. The clear tubing (2) in **Figure 4** is attached to the vacuum device and the dye inserted via a separate tube (3) from a 20 ml syringe (4) held by the operator. In **Figure 5** the rim of the adaptor (1) is seen being manoeuvred on to the external cervical os; if the adaptor does not draw up at once then it indicates that its rim does not fit the cervix. In this case the introducing forceps (5 in **Figure 4**) can be lifted, lowered or partially rotated until it does. Before application of the adaptor to the cervix it is important to fill the delivery tube (3) with medium so as to remove air space and avoid air shadows in the uterine cavity.

6

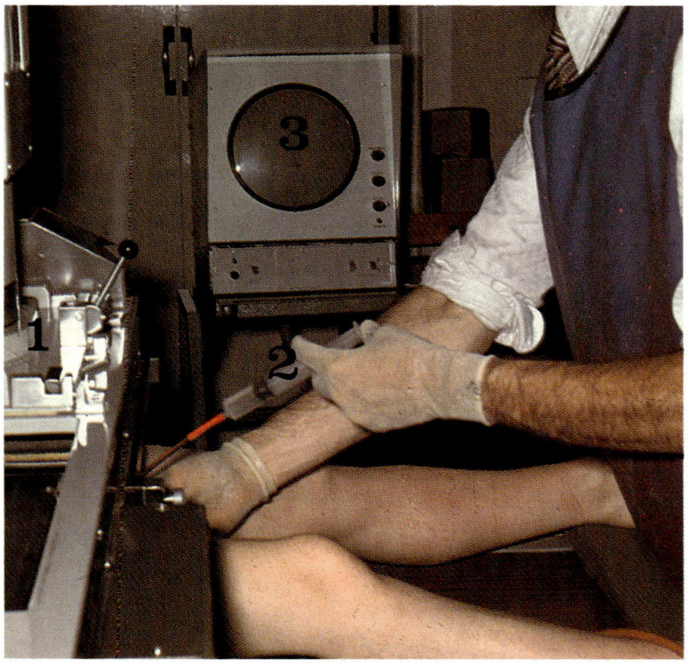

6 Insertion of medium and fluoroscopic screening
As soon as an airtight seal is obtained and the adaptor fixed to the cervix, the speculum and introducing forceps can be removed and the patient adjusted underneath the screening table (1). The medium can then be introduced from the syringe (2) at a slow rate. The simultaneous screening can be seen on an adjacent television screen (3). The introduction of medium in cases in which an intrauterine abnormality is suspected is extremely slow as too rapid filling of the cavity may obliterate the characteristic signs of a submucous fibroid, polyp, or adhesion. Film exposures are requested by the operator at frequent intervals during the procedure. A delay film is taken 30 minutes after the introduction of the radio-opaque medium; the patient being allowed to move from her recumbent and uncomfortable position on the screening table.

7

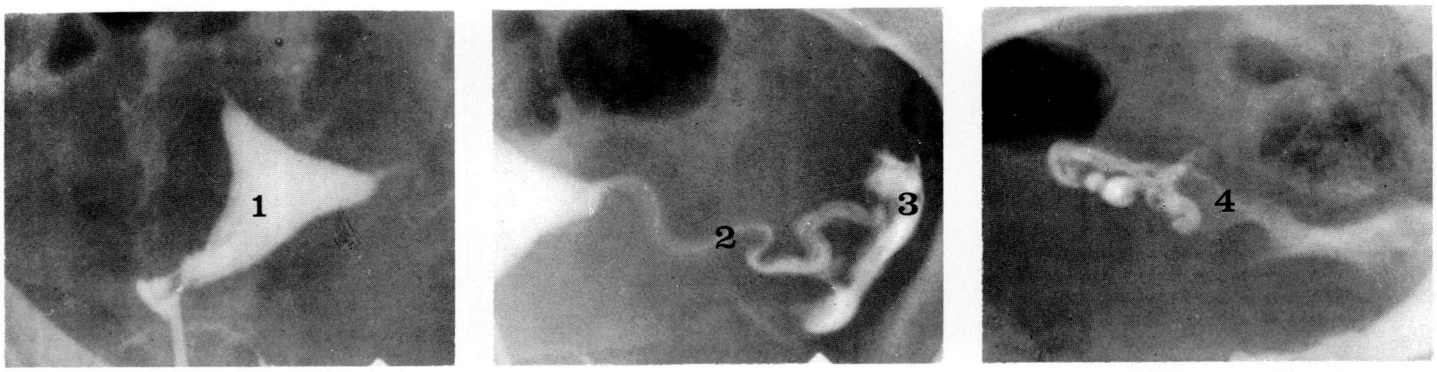

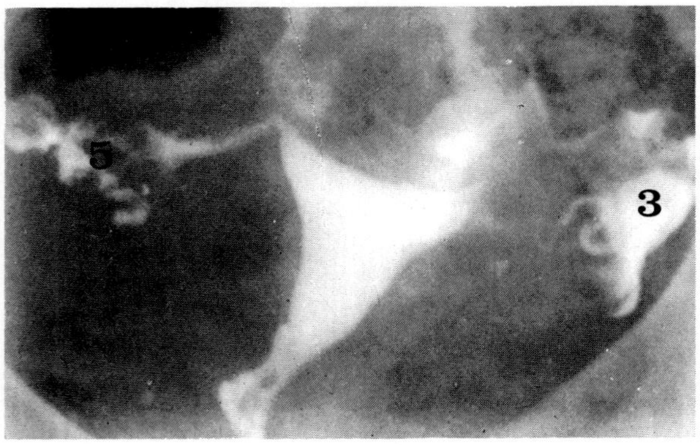

7 Stages in the screening of a normal uterus and tubes
These four exposures show the stages of sequential filling of the uterus and tubes. In the first, the uterine cavity (1) has filled and its smooth outline is noted. Once filling has occurred the medium immediately passes along the left tube (2) with spillage just commencing from the left ostium (3). The same process occurs simultaneously in the right tube (4) and in the last exposure spillage has occurred from left (3) and right (5) tubal openings. Only 8 ml of medium was needed to procure evidence of these normal tubes. Radioscopic screening was performed after every 2 ml had been injected; repeated screening like this assures that intravascular extravasation has not occurred. The total number of ml injected can be taken as a measure of the physiological capacity of the uterus.

8

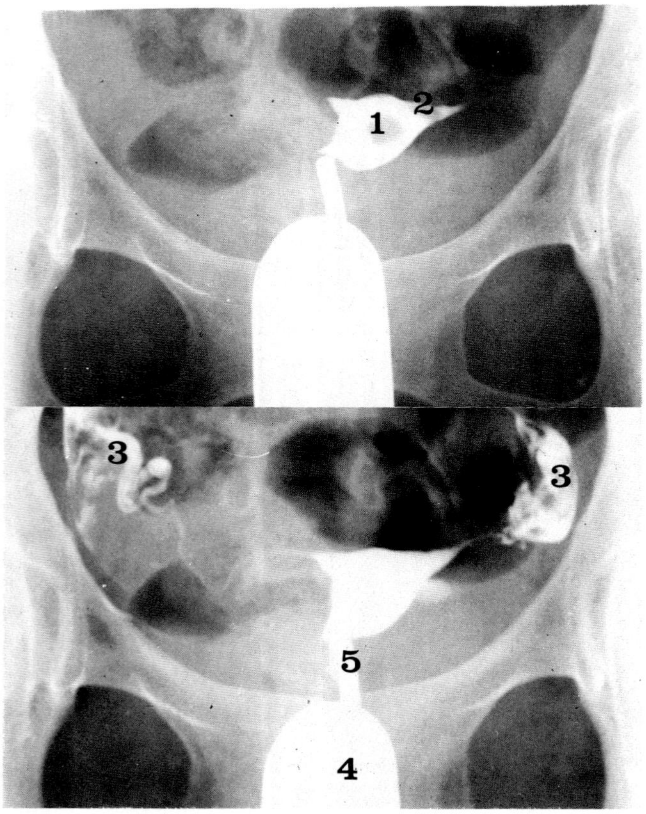

8 Screening to show the presence of a submucous polyp
A small filling defect, compatible with, and subsequently proven to be a submucous polyp is seen at (1) after the instillation of only 3 ml of medium. Another slightly darker area (2) occluding the left cornual region is an air bubble. In the lower exposure the uterine cavity is now full and the filling defect difficult to visualise; tubal patency indicated by spillage has occurred at (3) and (3). The vaginal speculum is at (4) with the tip of the metal cannula (5) in the endocervical canal.

9

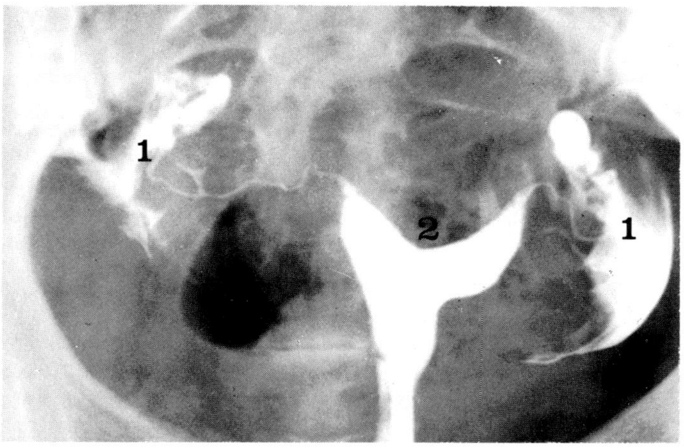

9 Normal tubal patency in an arcuate uterus
Bilateral tubal spillage is obvious (1) and (1) from an arcuate shaped uterus (2).

10

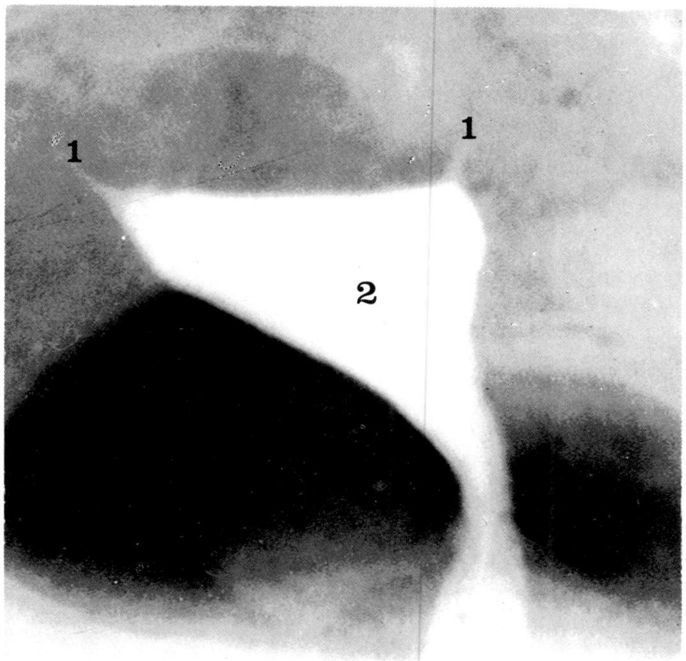

10 Tubal obstruction
Obstruction to the passage of dye has occurred at the utero-tubal junctions (1) and (1). The cavity of the uterus (2) appears normal. A considerable portion of the interstitial tube is patent on both sides; this finding would suggest anastomosis rather than implantation as the treatment of choice. This subject has recently been reviewed by Siegler (1980).

11

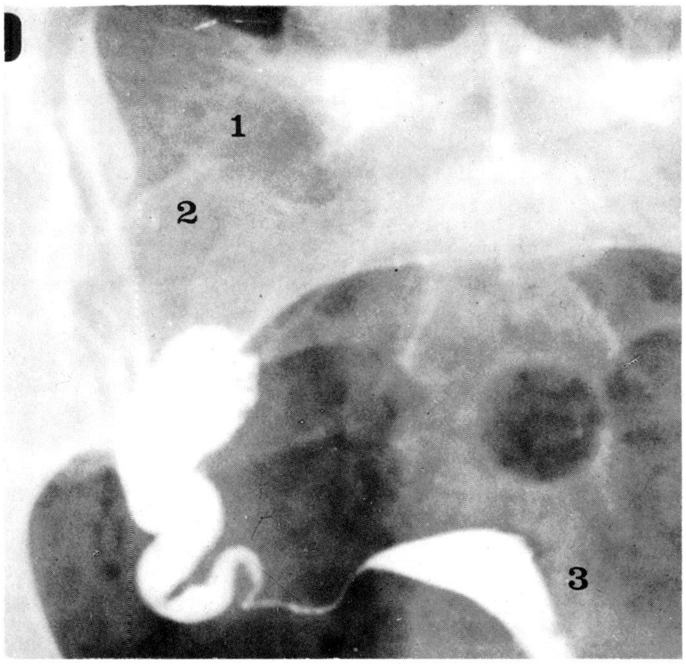

11 Tubal obstruction
Obstruction at the right tubal ostium (1) has prevented the passage of medium. A small hydrosalpinx (2) is clearly outlined. The tube is attached to the brim of the pelvis and the uterus itself seems to be deviated to the right as if retained in this position by possible chronic pelvic inflammatory disease. The operator should gently retract downwards on the introducing cannula (3) so as to determine if the uterine deviation is fixed or mobile.

12

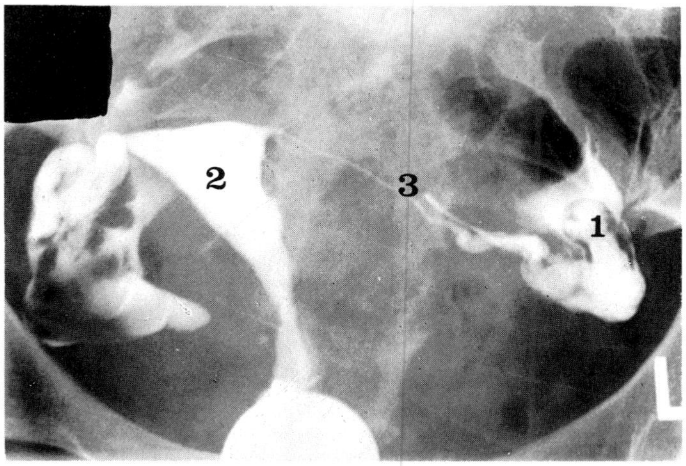

12 Tubal patency associated with peritubal adhesive disease
Spillage of dye has occurred, with loculation occurring in the area surrounding both tubal ostia. On the right side there is minimal extravasation. The uterus (2) is retracted to the right in the region of the pelvic brim. On the left, the tube is elongated (3) and although spillage has occurred, the medium seems to be loculated around the tubal opening (1). Severe peritubal adhesive disease was subsequently found at laparoscopy.

Endometrial Biopsy

It is customary in some centres to perform endometrial biopsy in the latter part of the cycle so as to obtain presumptive evidence of ovulation by the finding of secretory endometrium. There are definite histological features which allow accurate dating of the endometrium within the menstrual cycle. Dating is estimated on a 28 day cycle with ovulation occurring at day 14. Thus variable cycle lengths must be taken into account and it must be remembered that the normal luteal phase lasts for 14 days irrespective of the duration of the proliferative phase. Identification of these changes allows ready dating of biopsy material to within approximately 2 days. Dating may provide confirmatory interpretation of a basal temperature chart as being anovulatory or delayed ovulation. It is also helpful in a common form of ovulatory infertility which presents with a defective luteal phase. Endometrial biopsy is a convenient screening mechanism to select those patients in whom more extensive endocrine investigations are required, particularly if the basal temperature record is not grossly abnormal.

The histological appearance of the endometrium only indicates the hormonal response of the cycle in which it is obtained. Many women have variable ovulatory activity even with a regular cycle and a single biopsy which is normal or abnormal for the time at which biopsy was taken does not categorise a woman's ovulatory status. It would seem more rational to follow basic endocrine changes with a long term temperature chart and select those cycles in which biopsy would be most helpful. This may apply on two or more occasions depending on the fluctuation of the temperature record. Used in this way it may be a valuable tool in assessing the progressive response to an ovulation induction programme as a supplement to steroid activity.

Endometrial biopsy for the diagnosis of mycobacterium tuberculosis is used in many centres. The biopsy material should be divided so that one part can be specifically stained for the organism and the other reserved for guinea pig innoculation and culture.

Technique

A single strip of endometrium may be readily obtained from the uterine fundus by using either a Sharman curette or the finer aspiration tube curette (vabra or milex) attached to a simple suction pump. The procedure is undertaken without anaesthesia although in the nervous patient an intravenous injection (10 mg) of diazepam is helpful.

The aspiration is performed with the patient in lithotomy position by a non-touch technique; the steps of the procedure are shown in **Figures 13 to 15**.

13

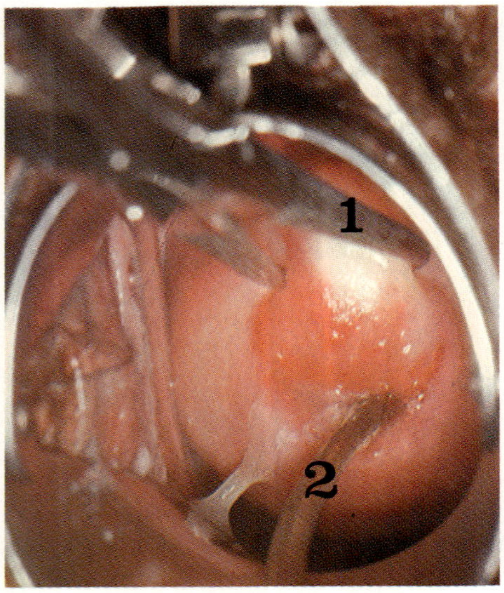

14

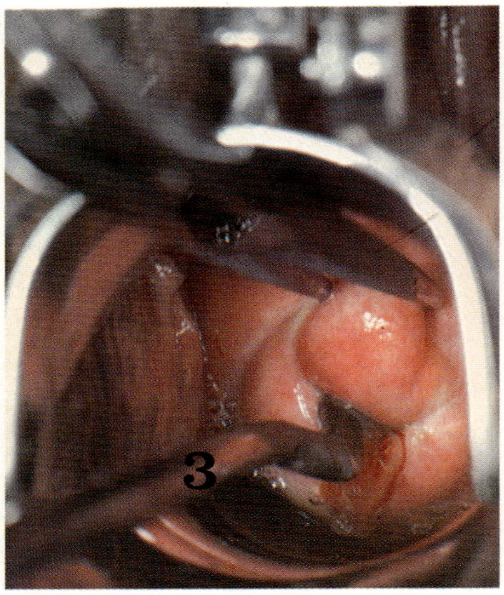

15

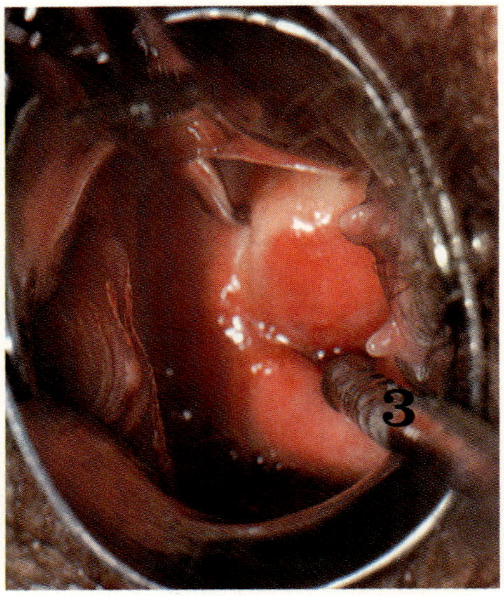

13 to 15 Safe passage of endometrial curette
A self retaining vaginal Cusco speculum has been inserted in **Figure 13** and the cervix and upper vagina cleaned with chlorhexidine solution. The anterior cervical lip is picked up with a single tooth volsellum, seen at (1), after which a uterine sound is passed to measure the length and direction of the uterine cavity (2 in **Figure 13**). The aspiration cannula is inserted into the uterine cavity (3 in **Figure 14**). The cannula is passed lightly up and down in the cavity and rotated slowly through 360 degrees (3 in **Figure 15**) so as to keep the cut out surface facing the uterine wall so that the whole surface of the endometrium is sampled. This latter manoeuvre is of importance if a search is being made for endometrial polypi. It is important to keep gentle downward traction on the volsellum to reduce uterine angulation (i.e. ante- or retro-version) thus avoiding perforation.

16
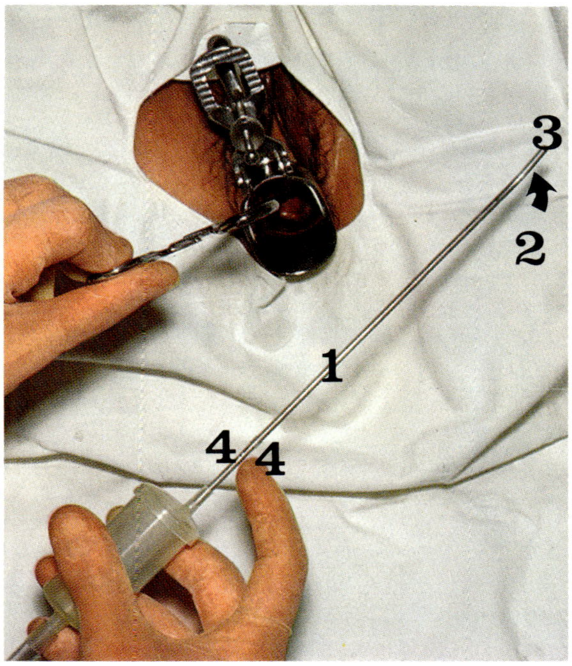

17
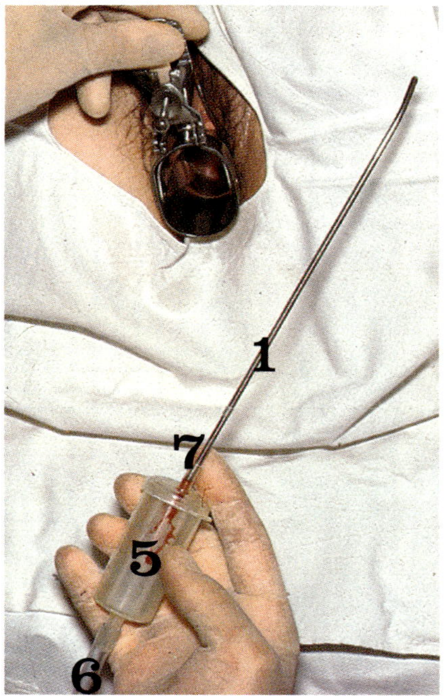

18
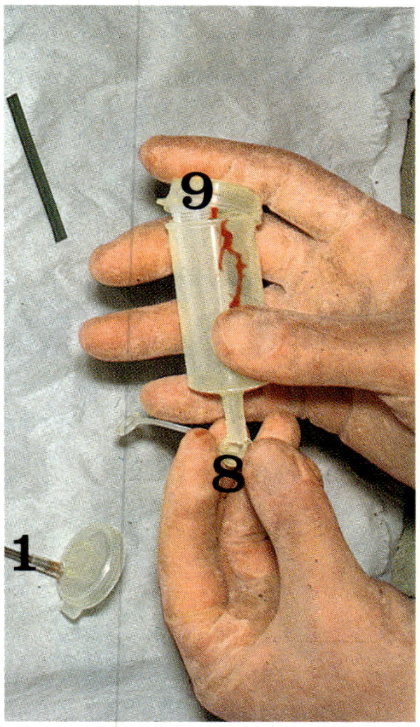

16 to 18 The endometrial aspiration curette
The apparatus consists of a stainless steel aspiration cannula (1 in **Figures 16 to 18**), 3 mm in diameter and slightly angled at the distal end. There is a cut out opening (2) 1.5 mm × 16 mm, a few mm from the rounded distal end (3). At the proximal end are two pressure equalising holes (4) (4). The aspirate is collected into a plastic chamber (5) fitted with a filter of sufficiently fine mesh to prevent the endometrium being sucked away. The apparatus is prepacked and sterilised and is connected by plastic tubing (6) to an electric suction pump which is capable of producing a negative pressure of 600 mm Hg within 3 seconds and is foot operated.

Once the cannula is inserted into the uterine cavity, the pressure equalising holes are covered with a forefinger (7 in **Figure 17**) and the pump switched on. At the end of the procedure the tubing is detached from the collecting chamber as in **Figure 18** and the bottom aperture closed with the attached cap (8 in **Figure 18**). The cannula (1) is removed and the chamber filled with formalin solution; the chamber being closed with a separately provided cap (9). The specimen is labelled and sent for histology.

19
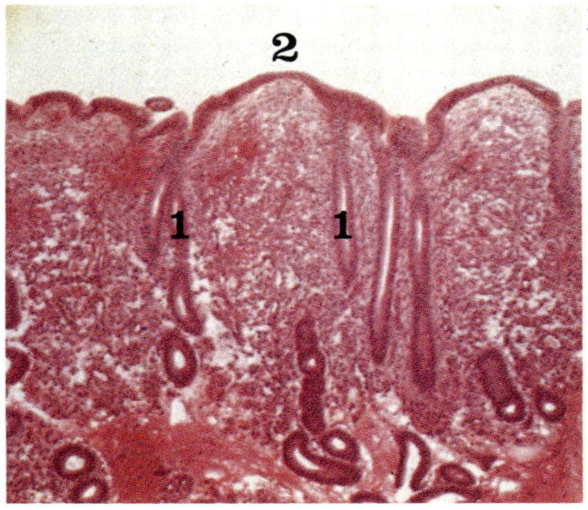

20
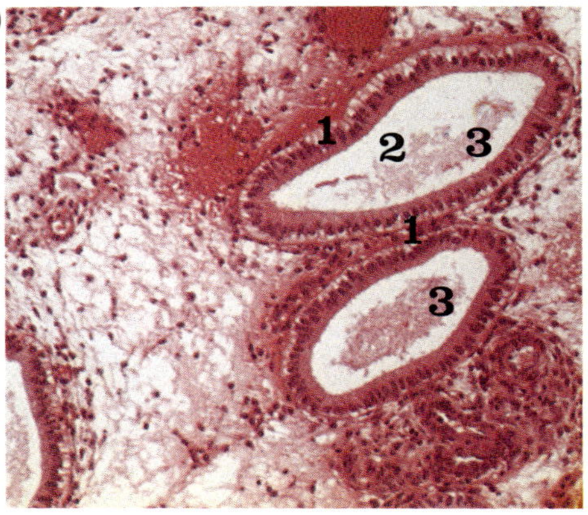

21
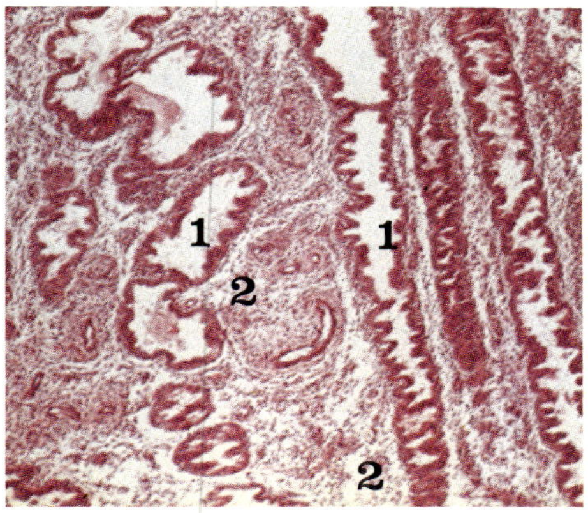

19 to 21 Endometrial histology
Figure 19 shows an endometrial biopsy taken at day 7 in the menstrual cycle and shows a typical proliferative endometrial pattern with straight glands (1) extending into the endometrial cavity (2). In **Figure 20**, taken two days after ovulation (day 16–17) subnuclear vacuolation (1) has already appeared in the tortuous glands (2). Some secretion (3) is present in the gland lumen. In **Figure 21** taken at day 25 there is marked tortuosity of glands (1) associated with oedematous stroma (2).

Laparoscopy

Laparoscopy may be used in the following ways in the investigation of infertility.

1. Observation of external features of the fallopian tubes and ovaries and their relationship to each other.

2. Tubal wall external appearance and muscular and fimbrial activity can be observed.

3. Recognition and assessment of extrauterine general pelvic pathology,
   (i) acute and chronic pelvic inflammatory disease
   (ii) pelvic endometriosis.

4. Estimation of tubal patency. This is established by the injection of dye through the uterine cervix and observing its escape through the fimbrial ends of the tube. It is a more accurate technique for determining patency than tubal insufflation (Rubin's test) with its 50 per cent inaccuracy rate (Frangenheim 1972), or hysterosalpingography with its 25–70 per cent inaccuracy rate (Swolin and Rosencrantz 1972, Leeton and Talbot 1973, and Keirse et al 1973). However, the latter technique still has much value in that it is the only means of determining the exact site of blockage in the fallopian tube.

5. Preoperative examination and assessment of all patients undergoing abdominal operations for infertility. The authors agree with others (Kistner and Patton 1975, Israel and March 1976, and Mattingley 1977) that laparoscopy should be used in all cases undergoing abdominal operations for infertility.

6. Postoperative examination of treated cases allows objective assessment of the results of tubal surgery and enables the surgeon to evaluate and thereby improve or refine his technique. It also has a therapeutic role in allowing lysis of postoperative adhesions.

Many clinicians are convinced that laparoscopy should be the primary method in assessment of the genital tract in the subfertile woman. Two large studies by Duignan et al (1972) and Templeton and Kerr (1977) support this claim. In both studies laparoscopy was undertaken on presumed infertile women with no clinically detectable abnormality. In both studies (summarised in Appendix B, page 181) nearly one-third of those with primary, and between two-fifths to one-half of those with secondary infertility, had a problem likely to affect tubo-ovarian function (oocyte pick-up). The high incidence of pelvic adhesions (as seen at laparoscopy) further strengthens the claim for the employment of laparoscopy as a primary routine procedure.

22

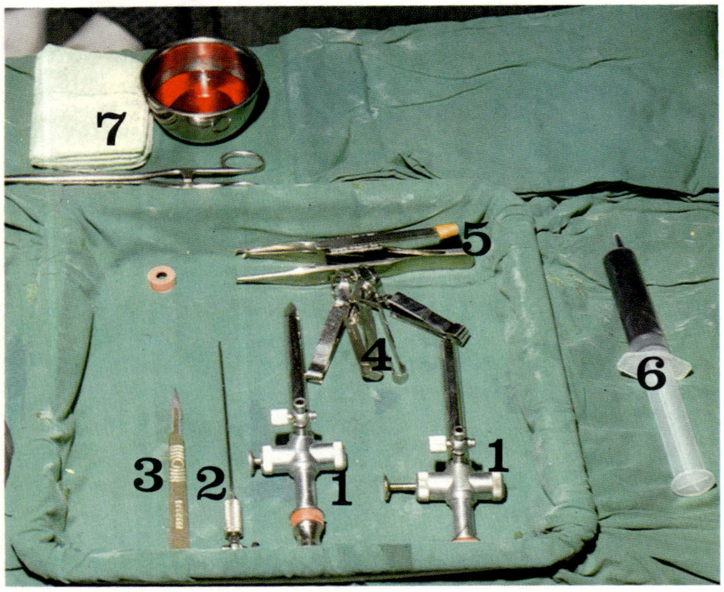

23

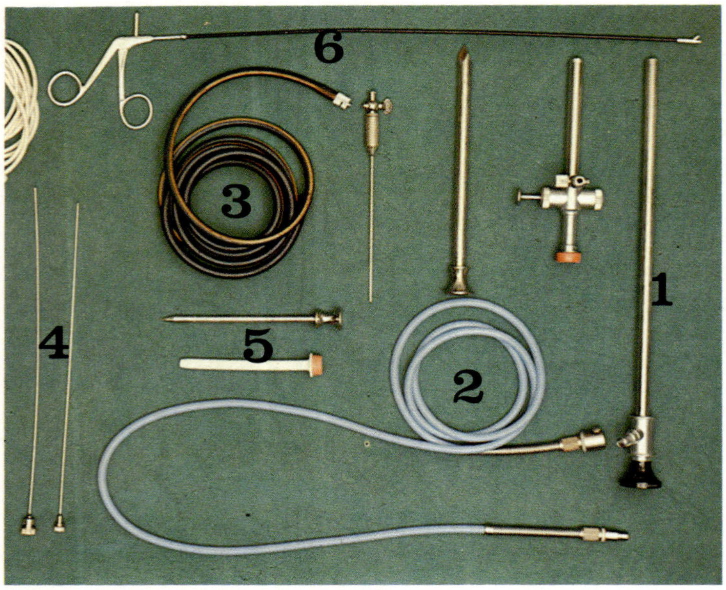

22 and 23 Laparoscopic equipment
The items in **Figure 22** are mainly concerned with the introduction of the instrument into the abdominal cavity and include:
1 Trochar and cannula
2 Verres needle
3 Sharp pointed scalpel
4 Towel clips
5 Michel clip forceps
6 Methylene blue dye
7 Skin preparation equipment.

Those in **Figure 23** are used in visual examination and intraperitoneal manipulation.
1 Examining telescope
2 Fibreoptic cable
3 CO_2 gas tube
4 Stilette needles as probes, or for aspiration
5 Trochar and cannula for second portal, if required
6 Ovarian biopsy forceps.

Anaesthesia. Laparoscopy is normally done under general anaesthesia and this is discussed by Alexander and Coe (1969), Peterson (1971) and Wadhwa et al (1979). In the outpatient department it obviously requires the use of local anaesthesia. There are several methods and nitrous oxide is frequently used as an insufflation gas while the subumbilical area and the abdominal wall are infiltrated with local anaesthetic. A paracervical and cervical block is also induced and a local anaesthetic agent is subsequently applied to the tubes. The technique is reviewed by Brown et al (1976) and Penfield (1977).

24
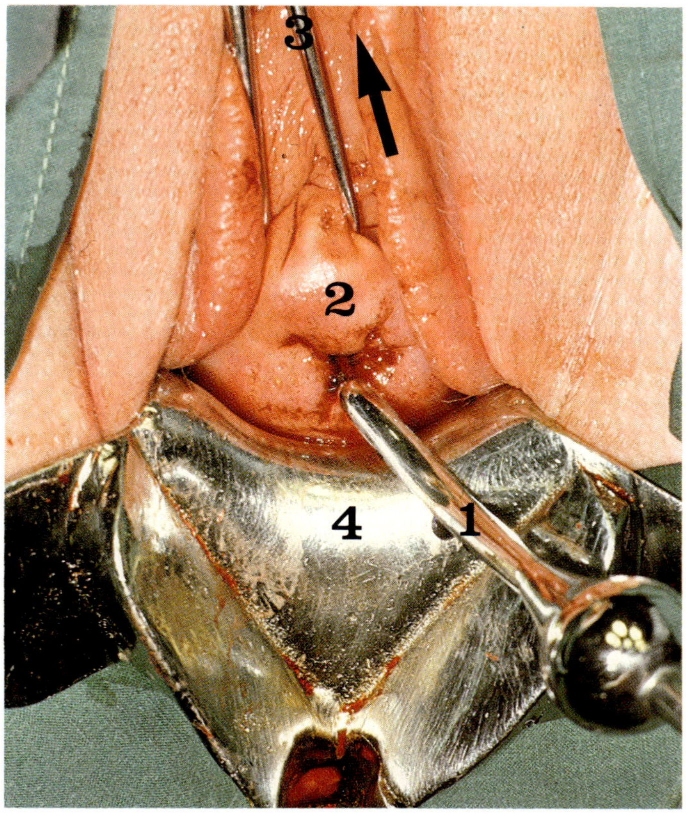

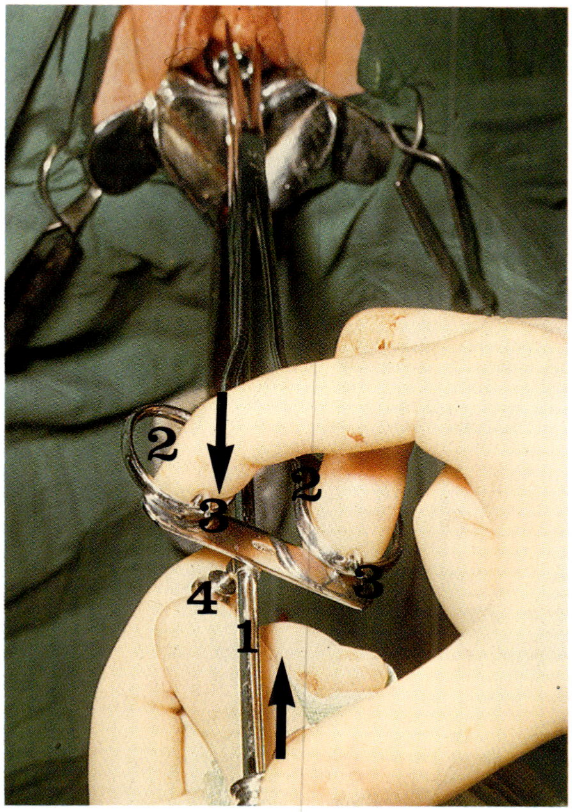

25

Stage I: Preparations for laparoscopy with patient in lithotomy position

24 Introduction of Spackman cannula
The cone-shaped end of the cannula (1) is about to be introduced into the cervical canal, the cervix (2) being held forwards and upwards in the direction of the arrow by the tissue forceps (3). The Auvard speculum retracting the posterior vaginal wall is numbered (4).

26
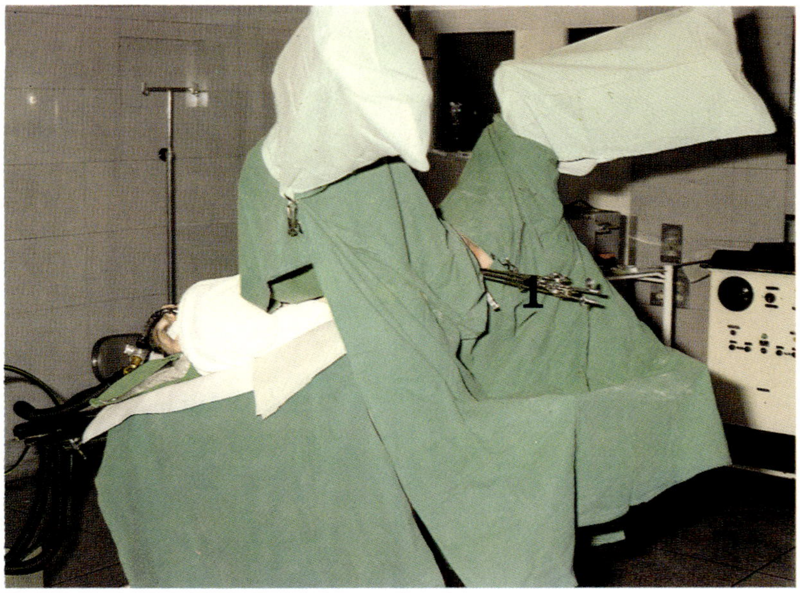

25 Locking the Spackman cannula in position
The surgeon keeps the Spackman cannula (1) firmly implanted in the cervical canal by thumb pressure (as arrowed) while drawing the ring handles of the cervical tissue forceps (2) firmly in the opposite direction (arrowed) with index and middle fingers. The handles of the forceps engage on the hooks of the mobile transverse rod of the cannula (3). With the forceps tensioned on to the hooks the end of the cannula is firmly held in the cervical canal. The surgeon maintains the position while the assistant tightens the screw (4) to fix the transverse bar to the cannula thus locking the cannula in position.

26 Patient prepared for laparoscopy
The patient is in lithotomy and moderate Trendelenberg position. The bladder has been emptied and the intrauterine cannula (1) is in position. The patient has been intubated and is being maintained on artificial respiration.

The assisted hyperventilation also tends to eliminate absorbed carbon dioxide.

27

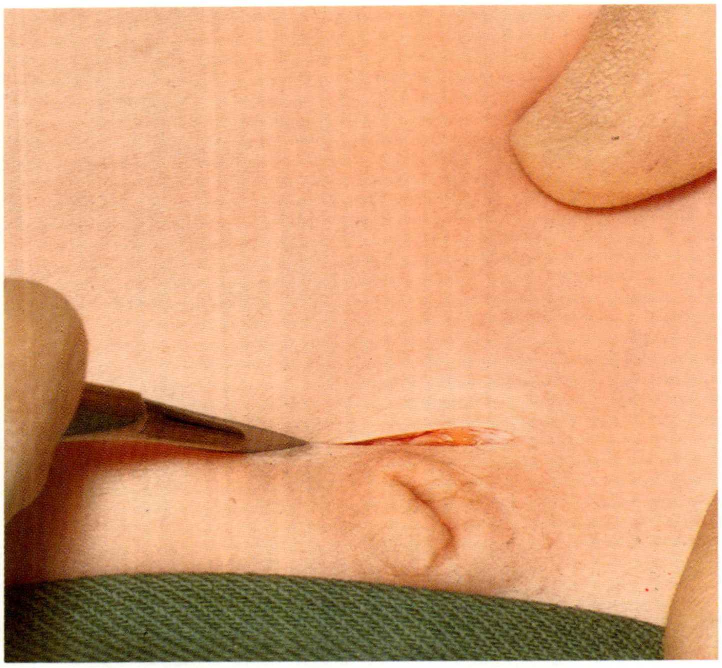

28

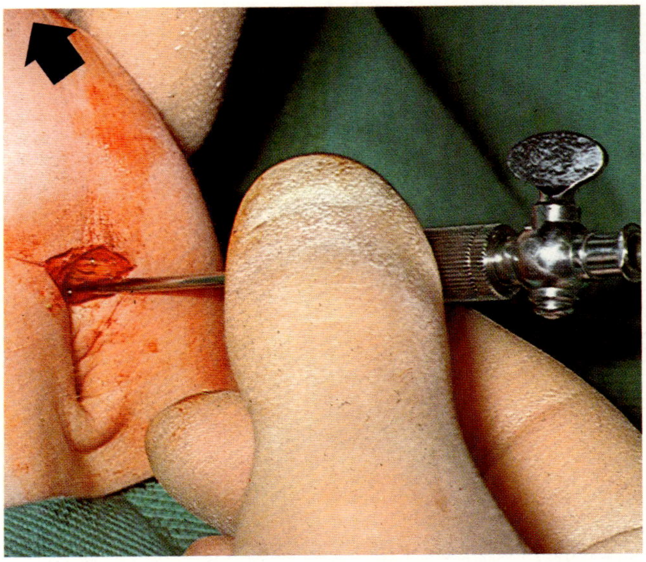

Stage II: Establishing a pneumo-peritoneum

27 Skin incision
The incision for the insertion of the laparoscope is made just on the lower edge of the umbilicus to the depth of the rectus sheath and is about 2 cm long.

28 Insertion of Verres needle
The Verres needle has a spring loaded and perforated blunt trochar within a sharp cannula to avoid visceral damage. The loose tissues of the lower abdominal wall are held upwards (as arrowed) in the left hand and the needle introduced in a direction which is clear of the sacral promontory and aimed towards the coccyx. This is felt to traverse first the rectus sheath and then the peritoneum during insertion.

29

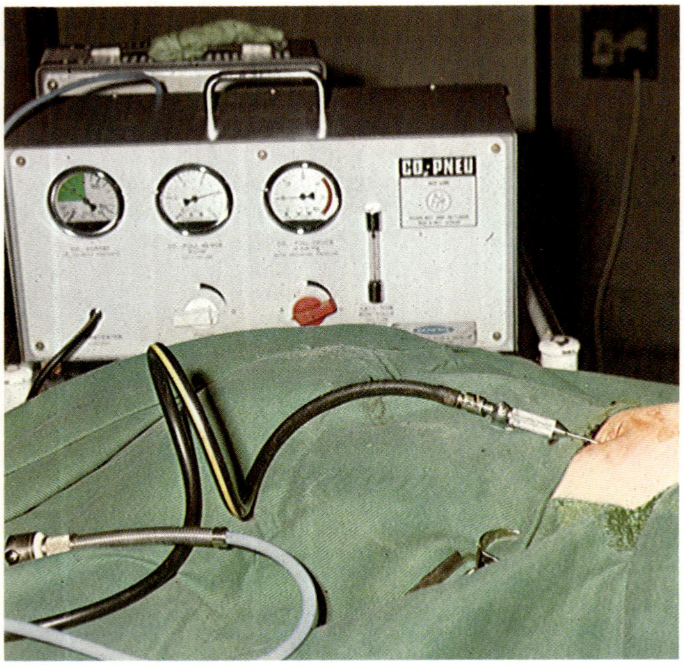

30

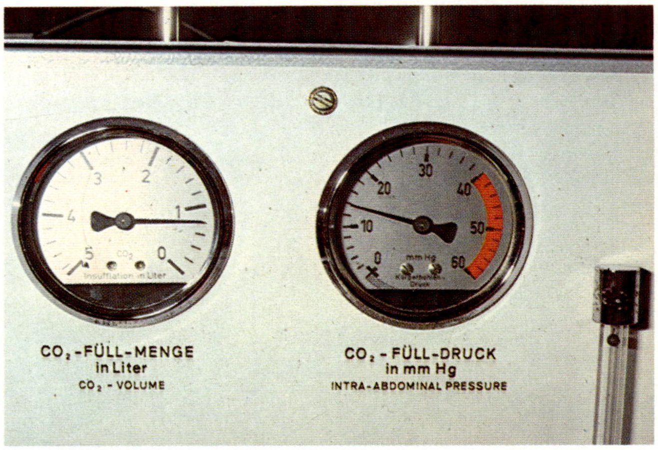

29 Recording intra-abdominal pressure
The gas flow is coupled to the Verres needle and the intra-abdominal pressure is carefully observed on the pressure dial of the laparoscope monitor. This pressure should not exceed 15–20 mm Hg and if it does this indicates that the end of the needle is not free in the peritoneal cavity. It is gently manipulated lest it be lying against a coil of bowel or the omentum; if the pressure still remains above 20 mm Hg the needle should be reinserted.

30 Observation of gas flow and volume
The right hand dial of the laparoscope monitor shows the intra-abdominal pressure and the left hand dial the volume of gas introduced into the peritoneal cavity. The CO_2 is run in at a speed of 1 litre per minute; the amount used is very much a question of the surgeon's individual preference. The authors prefer a total of 3 litres of gas.

31

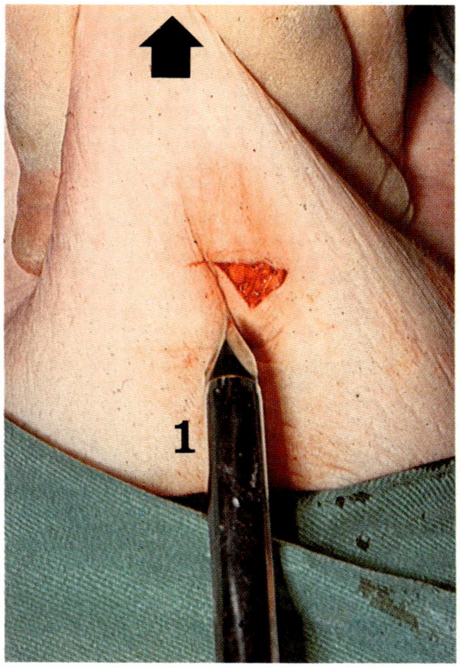

32

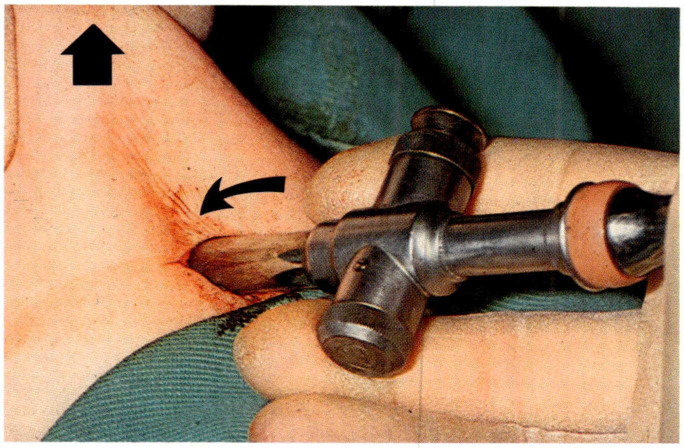

Stage III: Insertion of laparoscope

31 to 34

The Trendelenburg position is increased steeply at this stage and with the loose tissues of the lower abdominal wall held firmly upwards in the left hand as shown in **Figure 31**, the surgeon prepares to insert the trochar and cannula (1). It is advisable to make a small incision in the rectus sheath with the scalpel; this makes entry easier and more controlled and avoids the sharp trochar injuring the viscera as it forcibly comes through the abdominal wall. In **Figure 32** the upward lift of the left hand is maintained while the trochar is inserted by a pushing and partially rotating

33

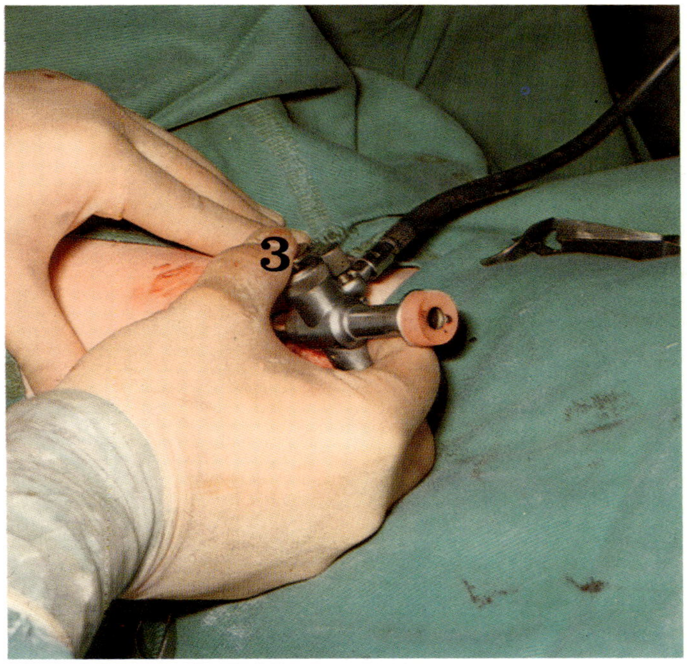

34

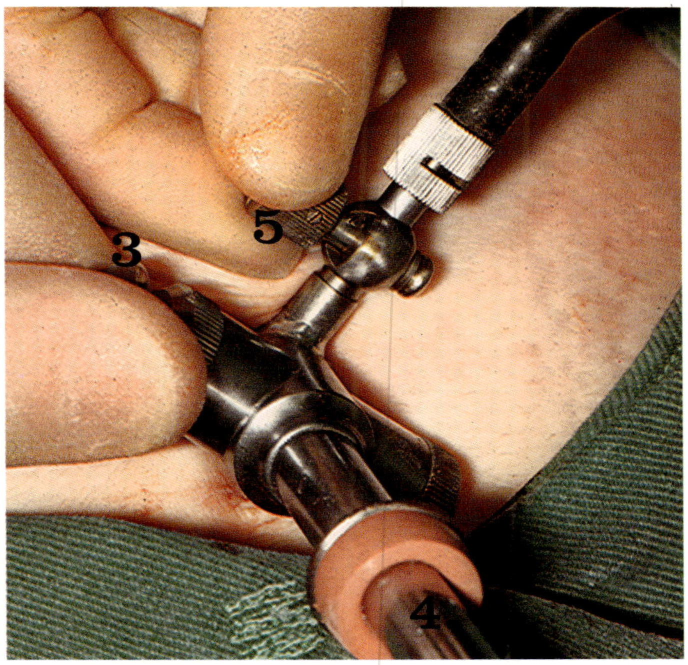

movement (arrowed). No great pressure is required and passage through the layers is easily recognised. The direction of insertion is towards the coccyx and the trochar and cannula traverse the abdominal wall obliquely. In **Figure 33** the trochar has been removed and the CO_2 tube connected. The cannula valve (3) is depressed and a rush of gas indicates that the end of the cannula is in the peritoneal cavity. The telescope can be introduced into the cannula when the valve is depressed and in **Figure 34** it is seen in place (4). The CO_2 control knob (5) is being opened to keep up the intra-abdominal pressure by a slow flow of 250 ml/min of gas.

35
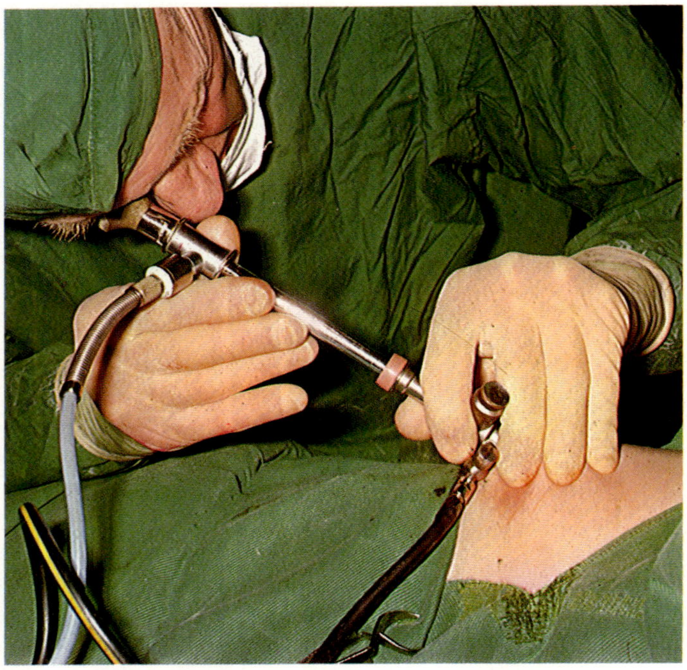

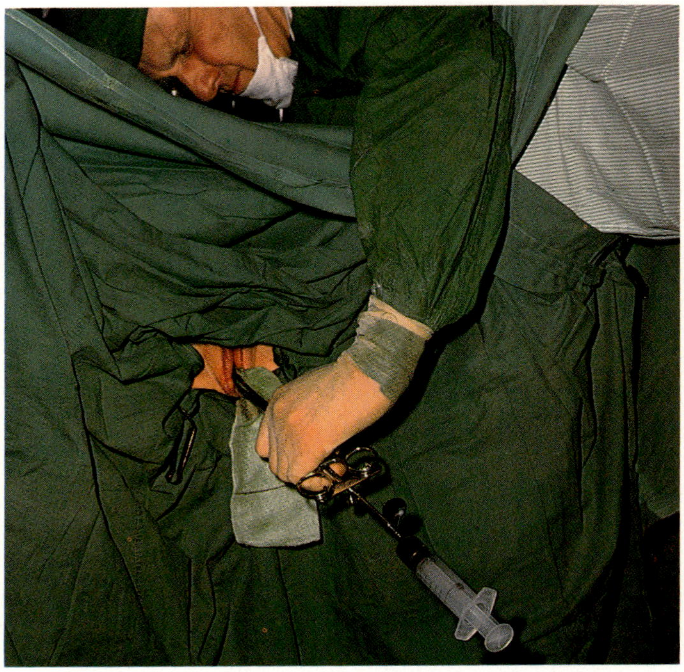
36

Stage IV: Laparoscopic examination

35 to 38
Examination is made as illustrated in **Figure 35**; two telescopes giving direct and right angled views are available. The tip of the telescope is dipped in warm water and a drop of glycerine applied to it before insertion. This generally avoids intraperitoneal clouding but if that still occurs it can usually be dispersed by holding the end of the telescope against a coil of bowel for a few seconds. In **Figure 36** the locked-in Spackman cannula with the uterus firmly impaled on its end is manipulated by the surgeon to obtain clear views of the pelvis as a whole. If the tubes and ovaries are

37
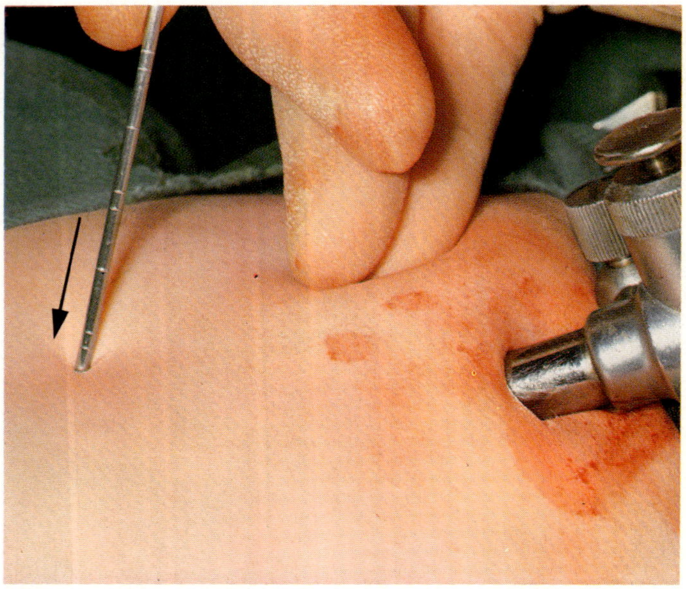

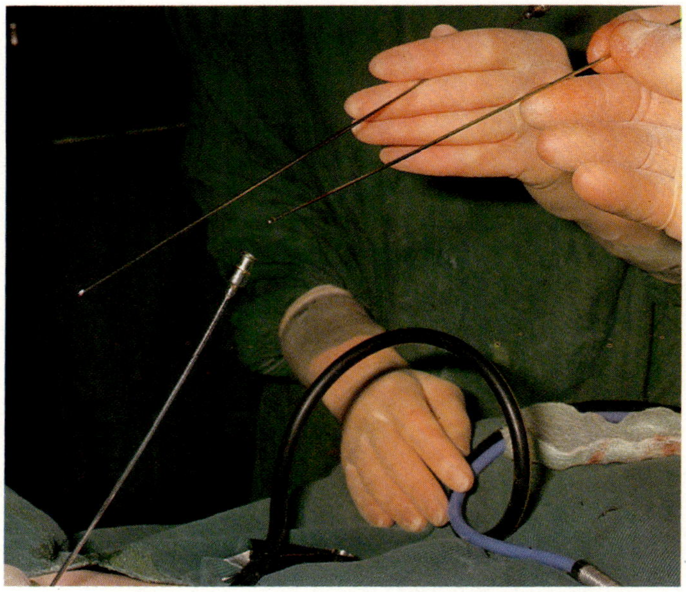
38

adherent to the posterior uterine wall or prolapsed in the pouch of Douglas it may not be possible to examine them without the help of a manipulating probe or palpateur. This can most conveniently be provided by inserting a Tuohy needle through a tiny scalpel prick in the skin at the lateral border of the rectus muscle on the line between the umbilicus and the anterior superior iliac spine. The needle is seen being introduced in the direction of the arrow in **Figure 37**, making sure by observation through the laparoscope that it does not encounter inferior epigastric or other vessels. Once in the peritoneal cavity the needle may be used to take a solid round-ended stilette which projects beyond the needle end and acts as a safe palpateur. A hollow blunt-ended cannula of the same diameter is also available and may be used for aspiration. The equipment is seen in **Figure 38**. The second puncture site is used for insertion of the smaller trochar and cannula when biopsy or diathermy forceps are required.

Laparoscopic appearances

39

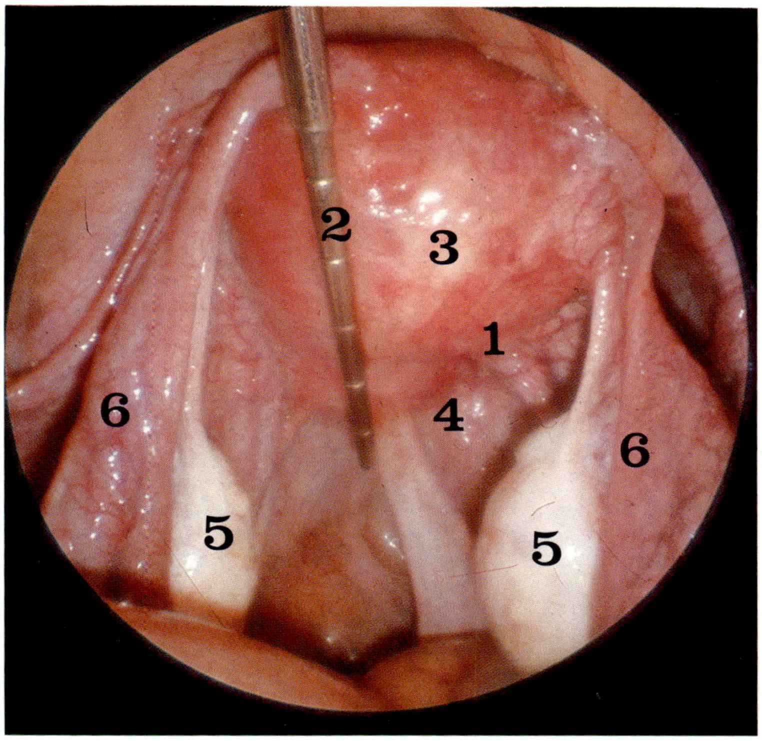

39 Chronic pelvic endometriosis
A frequent early site of endometriosis (1) is at the attachments of the uterosacral ligaments. The palpateur (2) is required to antevert the uterus (3) which is already being drawn backwards towards the pouch of Douglas (4) by fibrosis. The ovaries are numbered (5) and the fallopian tubes (6). This area always merits careful laparoscopic scrutiny.

40 Demonstration of tubal patency by injecting dye into uterus
Dye is seen flooding the photograph in the left lower quadrant as it escapes from the normal looking fimbrial end of the left fallopian tube (1). The left ovary is numbered (2). Dye appeared simultaneously on the right of the photograph indicating that the right tube is also patent. The surgeon has to be fairly expeditious in transferring his examination from one tubal ostium to the other; once a few ml of the dense and very pervasive dye spills into the pelvis visualisation is lost.

41 Difficulty in interpretation
This photograph illustrates a difficulty in diagnosis as referred to in **Figure 40**. In this case rapid spillage of dye from the direction of the left tube (arrowed) is filling the pouch of Douglas (1) before a corresponding efflux of dye from the right ostium (2). Such a situation could compromise interpretation of patency on the opposite side.

40

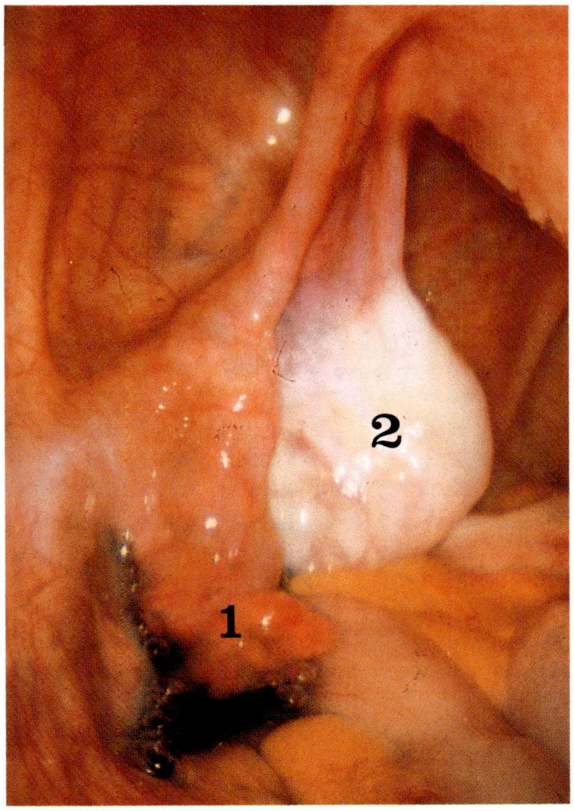

41

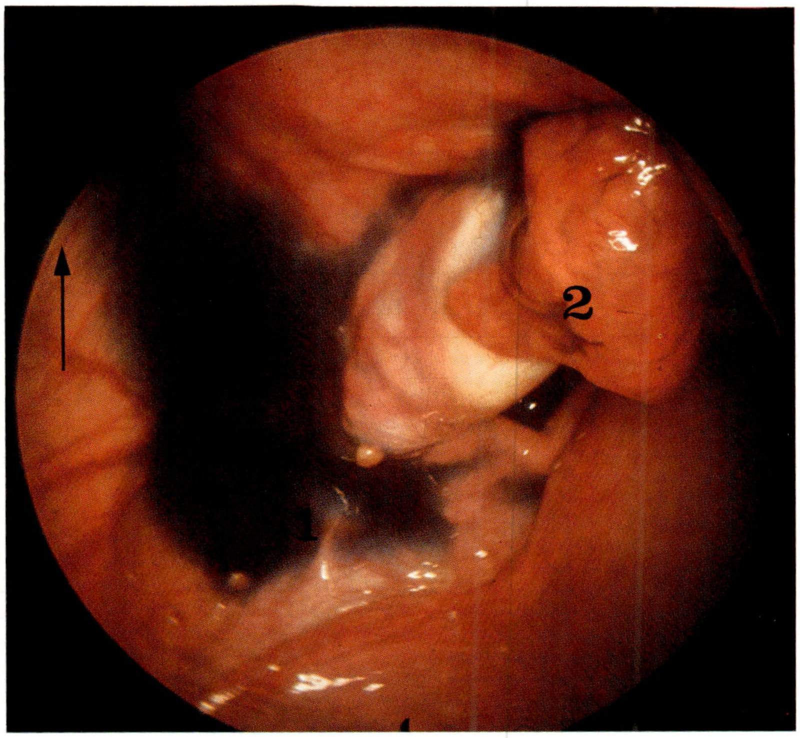

42

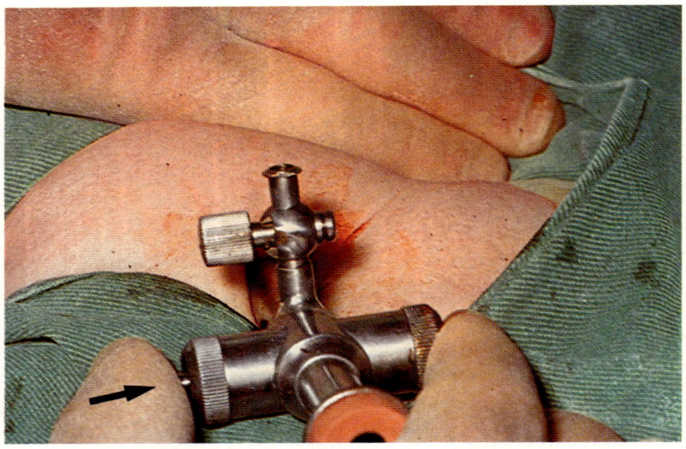

43

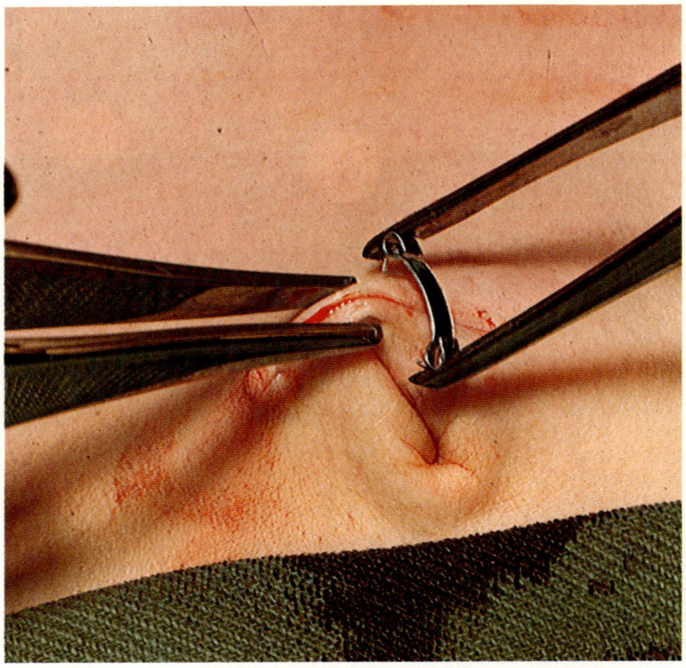

Stage V: Withdrawal of laparoscope

42 and 43 Expulsion of gas from peritoneal cavity and skin closure
When examination has been completed and the telescope removed the table is levelled. The valve on the cannula is depressed by the right thumb (as arrowed) while the left hand presses on the lower abdomen to expel as much gas as possible. The cannula is withdrawn and a fine figure of eight suture closes the rectus sheath where it was incised. Skin closure is by two narrow clips or a subcuticular stitch.

Hysteroscopy

Hysteroscopy, the technique of intrauterine visualisation, is being increasingly used by gynaecologists for the diagnosis and treatment of several intrauterine conditions related to infertility. Its acceptance followed the resolution of problems which related to satisfactory intrauterine illumination, the avoidance of uterine bleeding and adequate uterine distension by a satisfactory medium. Edström and Ternström popularised the technique in 1970 and in their study employed dextran 30 per cent w/v as the uterine distending medium. Since then others have used substances such as dextran 70, 32 per cent w/v, (Hyskon), 5 per cent dextrose in water and gas distension with CO_2. The dextran 32 per cent w/v solution is the most frequently used, it being a crystal clear thick solution of 70,000 molecular weight with a high refractory index. It does not readily mix with blood and because of its viscosity only a small quantity is needed for examination. Proper cleansing of the instrument is important immediately after use so as to avoid hardening and caramelisation of the substance around the device.
The instrument itself is a modified cystoscope with its distal sheath rounded to conform to the cervical anatomy (**Figures 44** to **45**). Most hysteroscopes have a 7 mm outer diameter and encase a 5–7 mm telescope. There are some devices with separate channels which allow for instrumentation, irrigation and uterine distension. Light is provided via a fibre-optic cord from an external light source with a 150, 300 or 1000 volt lamp.

A new endoscopic instrument has been developed which differs from the regular hysteroscope in that it does not require liquid or gas to distend the uterine cavity. Designed by the Institut d'Optique de Paris, the contact hysteroscope (**Figure 47**) is manufactured by the MTO Company of Paris. The light source is provided by surrounding room or directed light. With a diameter of either 6 or 8 mm and a magnification range of 1.6× to 2× it can easily be directed through the cervix and allows adequate viewing of the endocervical canal and all uterine surfaces.

With a focal distance of only 4 mm to point of contact the contact hysteroscope gives a close detailed image of tissue surfaces rather than the panoramic view of conventional hysteroscopes. The viewer must interpret tissue changes by colour, contour and consistency. Its advantage lies in its simplicity of use with no extraneous electrical cables and no distending medium required. This latter point obviously reduces the risk of disseminating a potential ascending infection.
Hysteroscopy employing a distending medium is painful and therefore a paracervical block using about 8–10 ml of a 2 per cent solution is required. If an extensive therapeutic procedure is to be undertaken, such as removal of polypi, biopsies or division of intrauterine septa then general anaesthesia may be preferred. Contact hysteroscopy using the 6 mm model is usually accomplished without anaesthesia (Barbot 1980) but the 8 mm device requires a paracervical block for painless passage.

Technique

Figures 44 to **46** show the insertion and positioning of the distending medium hysteroscope.

44

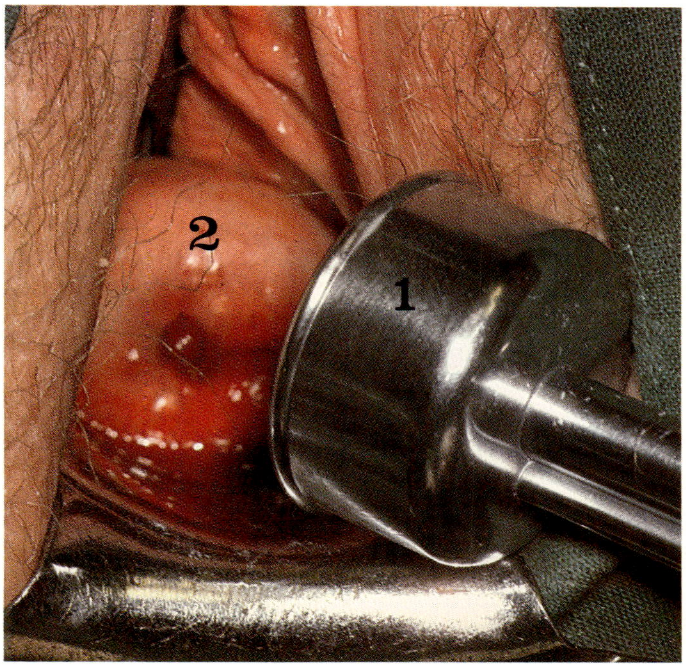

45

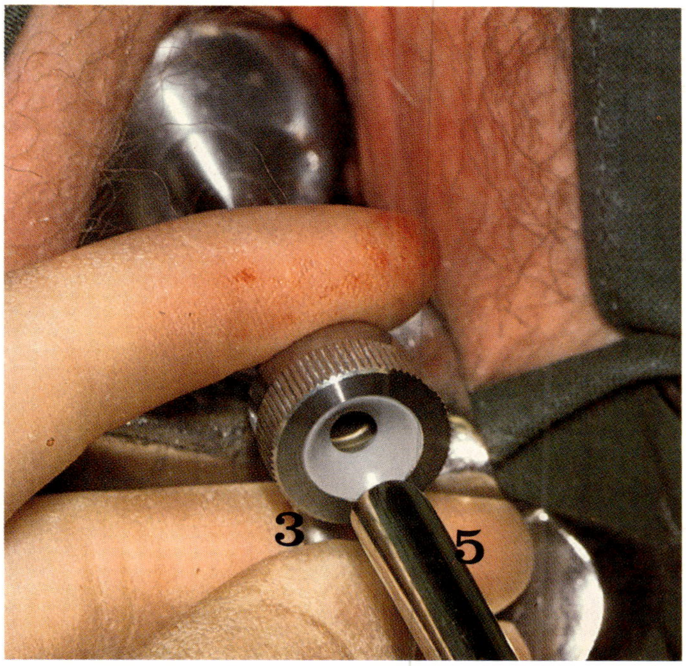

44, 45 and 46 Insertion of hysteroscope
In **Figure 44** the metal suction cap (1) is about to be placed on to the ectocervix (2); the cervical canal having already been dilated to a Hegar 7 size. Once in position suction is maintained via a small metal cannula (3 in **Figures 45** and **46**) to which rubber tubing (4 in **Figure 46**) is attached and connected to a suction apparatus. In **Figure 45** the telescope (5) is about to be introduced into the cap and in **Figure 46** is in position. In **Figure 46** the distending fluid (6) is being introduced; usually about 40–50 ml are needed. Viewing through the eyepiece (7) can take place after the fibre optic light source (8) is connected.

46

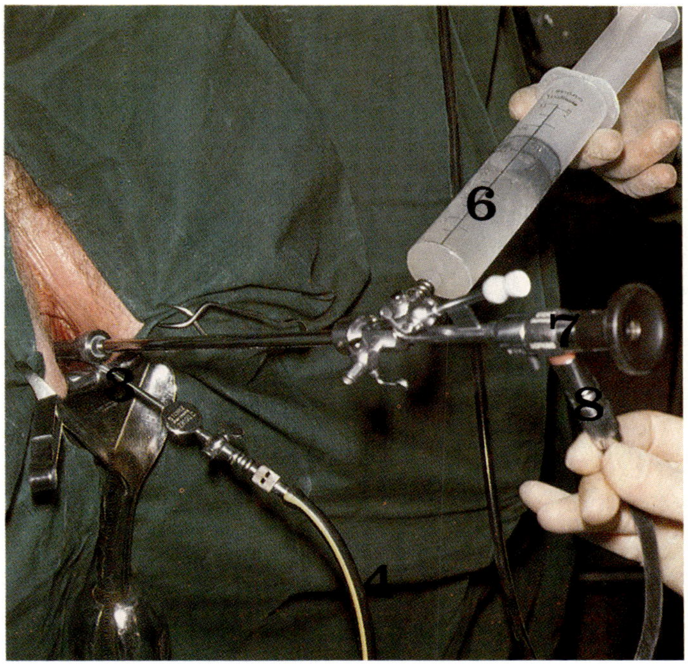

47

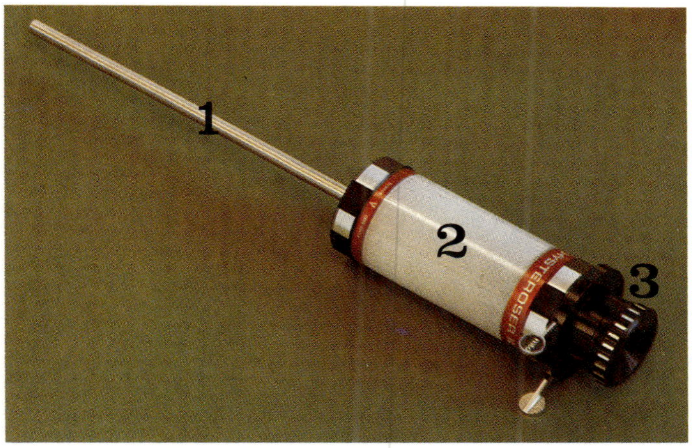

47 Contact hysteroscope (MTO, Paris)
The instrument consists of a transparent rod (1) of either glass or silica of 200 mm length protected by a stainless steel tube which transmits light collected in the light recovery jacket (2). Natural or artificial light is utilised by this jacket and transmitted by multiple thin coated lenses and mirrors to the object being viewed. The light is then projected back through ground optical glass to the eyepiece where the magnification is 1.6×. An optical magnifying device that gives an additional 2× magnification is attached to the eyepiece of this model (3).

The device is inserted into the dilated endocervix; dilatation to 7 mm for the 6 mm device (corresponding to Hegar 7/8 or 21 French) and 9 mm for the 8 mm device. The uterus is sounded and a single tooth tenaculum grasps the anterior cervical lip. Barbot (1980) recommends moving the device successively upon the two walls, the two edges and the fundus of the cavity in order to explore it totally (field by field sweeping technique). The examination should take about 10 minutes.

48 a b c d

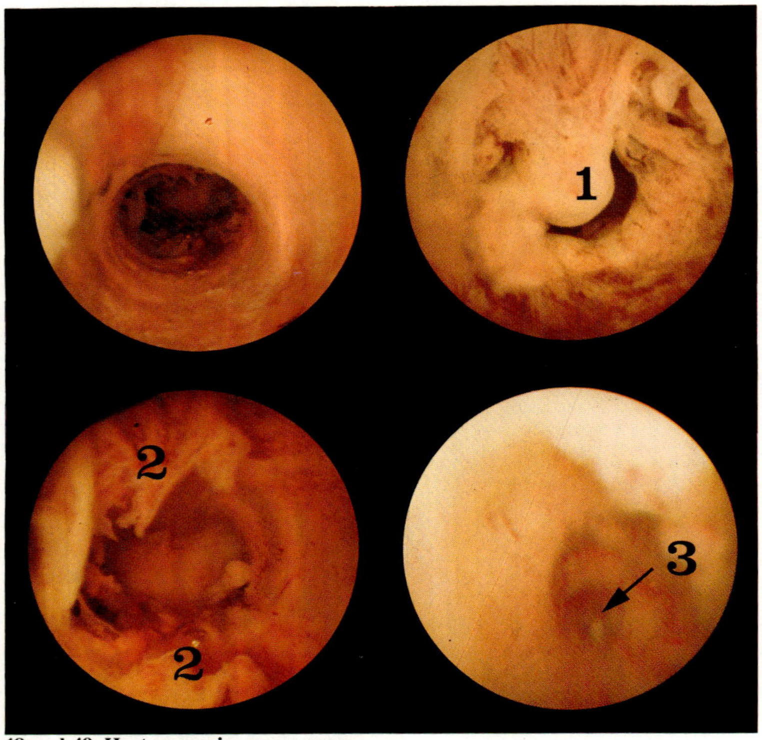

48 and 49 Hysteroscopic appearances
In **Figure 48**, four views within the endometrial cavity have been obtained using a distension medium (dextran 70, 32 per cent w/v). In **a** the circular endocervical canal at the level of the internal os is seen while in **b** a polyp (1) is seen protruding into the canal. In **c** the hysteroscope has entered the uterine cavity and the endometrium (2) in the secretory phase is prominent. Inspection of the fundus by sweeping from left to right shows the ostium of the left fallopian tube (3 and arrowed in **d**).

49 a b c d

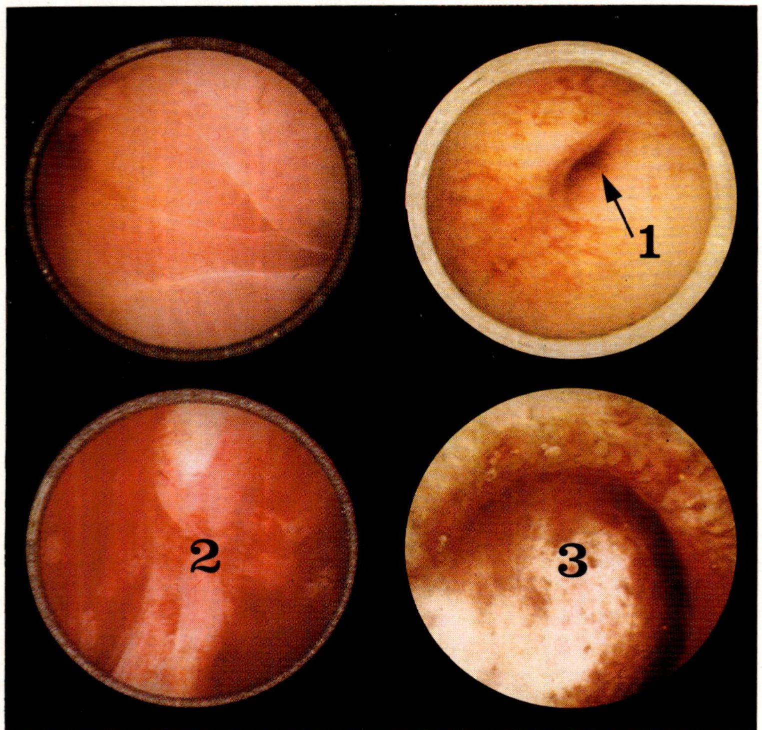

In **Figure 49** the contact hysteroscope is used without distending medium. In **a** the rose-white proliferative endometrium of the lower uterine cavity is easily seen while in **b** the ostium of the right fallopian tube is prominent (1) and arrowed. In **c** an intrauterine synechia or adhesion (2) stretches between the anterior and posterior uterine walls. In **d** a submucous fibroid (3) with its typical yellow/orange colour protrudes into the endometrial cavity, obliterating most of its area.

Indications for hysteroscopy

Hysteroscopy is indicated in women with recurrent *first trimester miscarriages* in whom a submucous fibroid or polyp is suspected. Hysteroscopy as a *routine procedure* at the time of laparoscopy has been suggested, especially in the woman suffering from ovulatory infertility. Its employment prior to operations for *uterine abnormalities* is advocated by some so that the relative size of the cavity and the location of the tubal ostia can be determined. Intrauterine adhesions in association with pelvic adhesions are increasingly noted especially in *secondary infertility* and are a further reason for using the method.

Recent studies have shown that the overall detection rate of presumably significant abnormalities was markedly increased by the addition of hysteroscopy to the routine laparoscopic examination. Cummings and Taylor (1980) performed both techniques in 162 women with ovulatory infertility. They found significant pelvic abnormalities in 49 per cent of those laparoscoped and in 66 per cent of those submitted to laparoscopy and hysteroscopy. The commonest lesions found at hysteroscopy were intrauterine adhesions (in 35), polyps (in 26) and submucous fibroids (in 5 women); these findings occurring in 30 per cent of those with primary and 55 per cent of those with secondary infertility. Rosenfeld (1979) in a similar study found 8 per cent of those with primary and 33 per cent of those with secondary infertility to have an obvious hysteroscopic abnormality; many also had laparoscopically detected pathology. The majority of the intrauterine lesions were either adhesions or polypi. The exact role of these seemingly common intrauterine adhesions, polypi and small submucous fibroids in the causation of infertility is still very uncertain but Oelsner et al (1974) improved the reproductive performance of 41 women with a history of recurrent abortions after treatment of their intrauterine adhesions.

The technique has an extremely low failure rate (<4 per cent) and the complications (2–3 per cent) are of a minor nature. Barbot et al (1980) using a contact hysteroscope had only 2 complications (small easily detected uterine perforations) in over 1000 cases. Its ease and safety has made hysteroscopy increasingly popular. But its exact place in gynaecology and especially in infertility management has yet to be assessed.

3: Anatomy and instruments

(i) Developmental anatomy of genital tract

Congenital abnormalities of the genital tract sometimes make conception impossible; more usually they do not and as long as an obstruction within the tract is not complete the sperm is frequently able to fertilise the ovum. The question of whether or not such defects cause subfertility is difficult because few series of any size are reported in the literature and while it has always been taught that surgery is meddlesome there is increasing evidence that it has a useful application in some cases. Apart from the effect on conception the capacity to carry a pregnancy may be adversely influenced by congenital defects such as septate uterus and cervical incompetence. These problems are considered in relation to individual operations; in this chapter the principal steps in the development of the lower urogenital tract are revised so that the anatomical abnormalities are recognised and understood when they are encountered.

Development of the Mullerian duct

It will be recalled that the Mullerian duct develops a few weeks later than the Wolffian duct – from the same lateral aspect of the urogenital ridge and subsequently forms the fallopian tube and one half of the uterus and the upper part of the vagina on each side. The upper end of each Mullerian duct is open to the coelomic cavity. The distal end migrates caudally across the anterior or ventral surface of the Wolffian duct to meet its fellow in the midline and they continue distally to join the urogenital sinus posteriorly at Muller's tubercle (**Figure 1**). The two ducts subsequently fuse centrally and vacuolation then occurs in a cephalad direction to provide a central uterine tube which later becomes the uterus and cervix (**Figure 2**). Muller's tubercle is the advance point of the Mullerian mesodermal columns and is at a level which closely corresponds with that of the cervix. Where the Mullerian ducts reach the urogenital sinus a thickened

1 and 2 Formation of female genital tract
The genital tract develops from the Mullerian ducts slightly later and then concurrently with the urinary tract derived from the Wolffian duct system. **Figure 1** shows the situation at 8 weeks development when the Mullerian ducts impinge on the urogenital sinus at Muller's tubercle. **Figure 2** represents the situation 3–4 weeks later with the genital tract essentially complete.

1

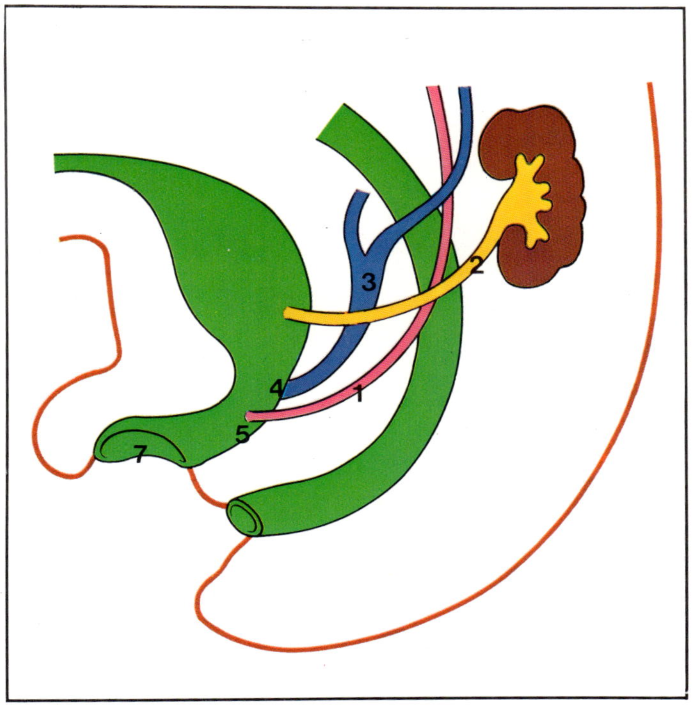

2

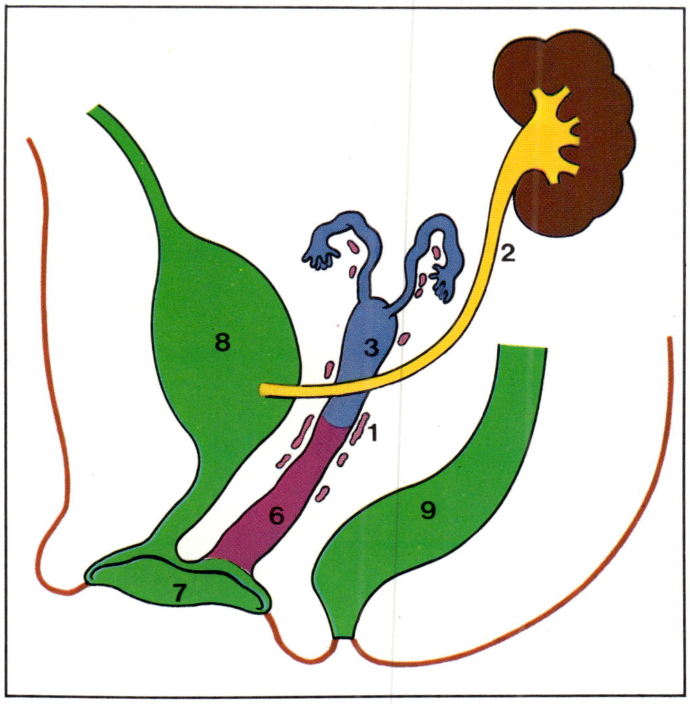

1 Wolffian (mesonephric) ducts or remnants of these structures
2 Urinary tract
3 Mullerian ducts and uterine tube
4 Muller's tubercle
5 Site of sino-vaginal bulbs
6 Vagina
7 Urogenital sinus
8 Bladder
9 Rectum.

3

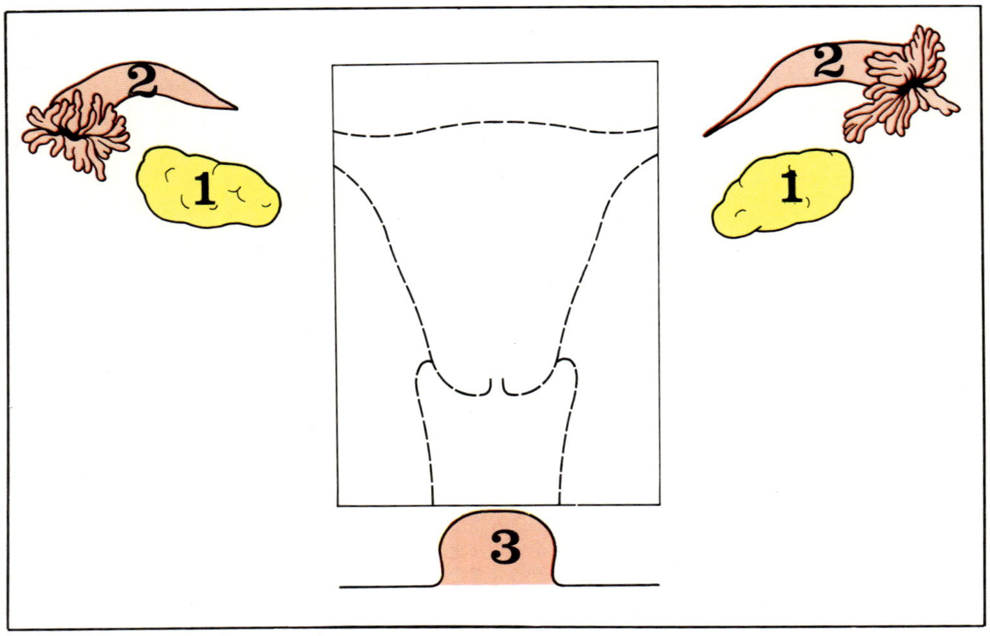

3 Complete failure of Mullerian ducts to develop or canalise
The structures within the inner rectangle do not develop. The ovaries develop normally, the fimbrial ends of the tubes are vestigial and the vaginal fossa is very shallow. The structures are numbered thus:
1 Ovary
2 Fimbrial ends of fallopian tube
3 Vaginal fossa.

4

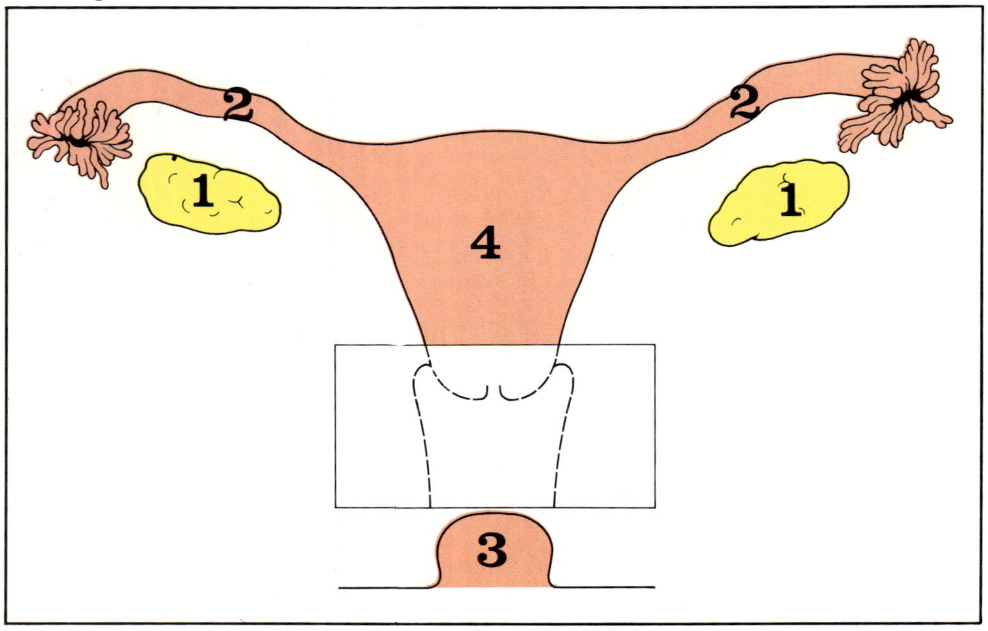

4 Partial failure of Mullerian ducts to develop or canalise
The extent of this aberration varies. In general the cervix and upper two-thirds of the vagina are missing. The ovaries (1), corpus uteri (4), fallopian tubes (2) are present and the vaginal fossa (3) is deeper in this case.

plate of endodermal tissue – the vaginal plate – extends to two more distal points on the posterior wall of the urogenital sinus and are known as the sino-vaginal bulbs. The exact sequence of subsequent events is not clear but it is generally thought that mesoderm from Muller's tubercle advances to meet endoderm of the sino-vaginal bulbs within the vaginal plate while at the same time the mesodermal mass elongates in a cephalad direction. The vaginal plate continues to grow and displace the Muller's tubercle upwards while laying down a mass of tissue between it and the urogenital sinus. This specific area eventually becomes the vagina which develops as a distal continuation of the uterine tube.

Complete failure of the Mullerian ducts either to develop or canalise means that the uterus, fallopian tubes and part of the vagina are absent (**Figure 3**) and the patient is sterile. There is an incomplete stage with poor or absent development of the Mullerian duct distally (**Figure 4**) and this is also likely to cause complete sterility. Complete absence of one Mullerian duct would result in a unicornuate uterus but this is rare and a hypoplasia of the distal part of one Mullerian duct is more likely. In such cases the fallopian tube is present on the affected side although the condition is usually diagnosed clinically as unicornuate uterus. Fertility is not apparently greatly influenced by this latter defect.

The vast majority of congenital defects are due to imperfect fusion of the Mullerian ducts and the more commonly encountered examples are shown in **Figures 5–9**. In uterus bicornis bicollis with septate vagina (**Figure 5**) the two ducts remain completely separate, while at the other end of the scale the only evidence of incomplete fusion is seen in uterus subseptus or septus (**Figure 8**). It is frequently difficult to establish clinically that there is a defect. Deformities occur in all possible combinations

5
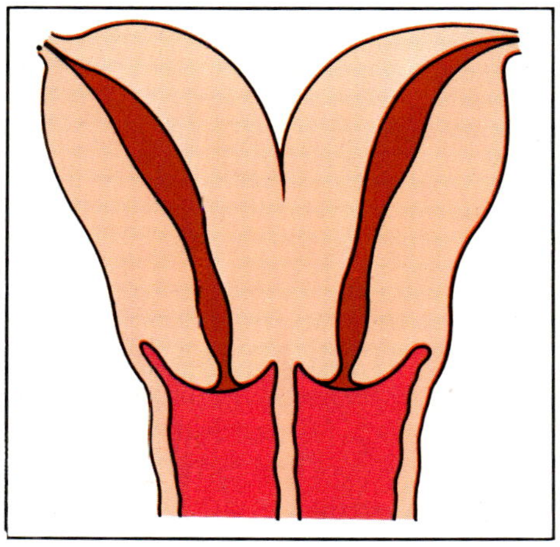
6
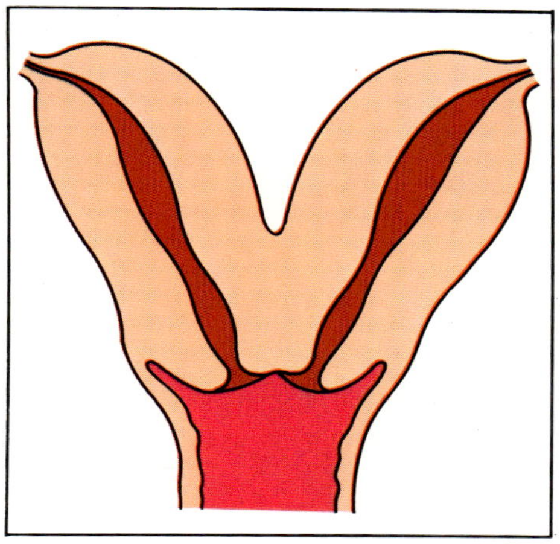
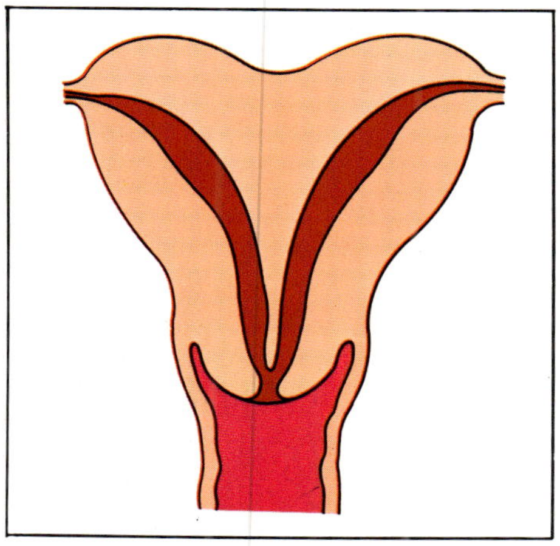
7

Congenital defects due to imperfect fusion of Mullerian ducts

5 Uterus bicornis bicollis with septate vagina.

6 Uterus bicornis, uni/bicollis with normal vagina.

7 Cordiform uterus unicollis with deep septum.

8
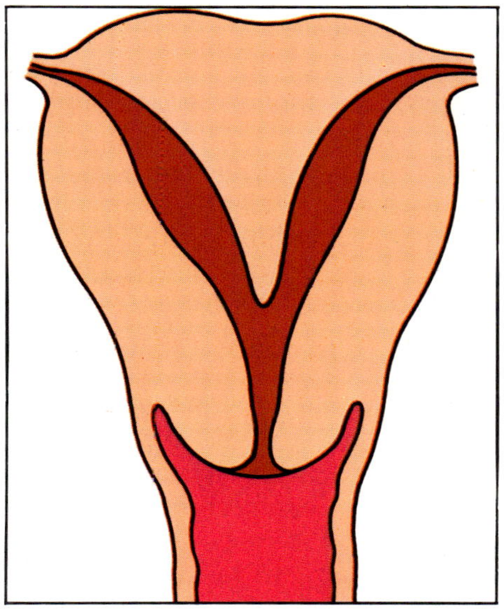
9
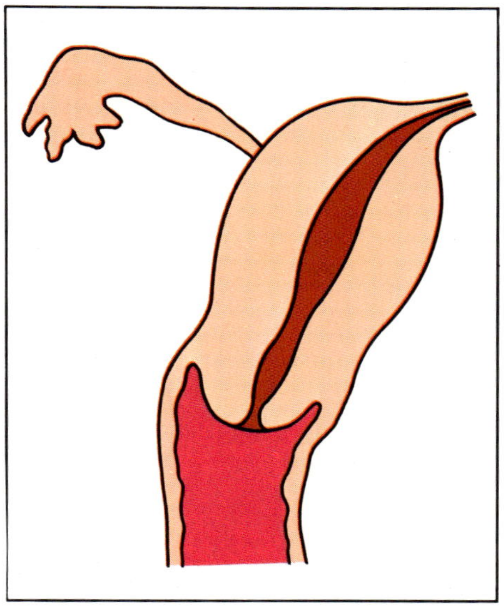

8 Normal outline uterus with less deep septum.

9 Uterus bicornis unicollis with one rudimentary horn.

(from maldevelopment in one or both ducts). A diverticulum of one or other duct may give rise to very complex appearances and if distal development is deficient unilaterally there may be no communication between the upper genital tract and the vagina on that side. The effect of fusion failure defects on fertility is difficult to assess but is probably minimal and it is worthy of note that some fertile women also possess some of these abnormalities. Surgical treatment is generally contraindicated although it should be remembered that uterus bicornis and uterus septus are sometimes responsible for recurrent abortion and may require surgical treatment. The appropriate procedures are described in Chapter 7.

Vaginal development

The vagina is derived partly from the distal uterine tube and partly from the vaginal plate although the contribution from each is in debate. In regard to congenital abnormalities it is clear that vacuolation takes place within two columns of the vaginal plate and is followed by fusion of the resultant two ducts as occurs in the uterine tube. Abnormalities in the lower genital tract are therefore of the same type as those already seen and double or septate vagina is the most common vaginal defect. There may be indications for surgical division of the dividing membrane and such a procedure is described on page 46.

The distal end of the vagina is closed by a membrane which separates it from the urogenital sinus until late in fetal development. The membrane may sometimes persist as a transverse lower vaginal septum associated with infertility and cryptomenorrhoea. In such circumstances it obviously has to be divided surgically (see Volume 4, page 21). The hymen sometimes remains imperforate or very tight and affects fertility by preventing penile penetration. The precise embryological origin of the hymen is uncertain but knowledge on this point would not in any case influence treatment which is either by stretching or surgical division. Questions about the origin of the vaginal epithelium were referred to in Volume 4, page 10. Those relative to present considerations are again academic.

Hormonal influence on fetal development

In the investigation of infertility the clinician should be on the alert for evidence of unusual hormonal influence. This may be present in a degree of vulvar maldevelopment indicating an excess of androgens. It will be recalled that the external genitalia of the fetus develop towards a male or female configuration from the ninth week of development onwards and in direct response to hormone action. Excess androgens arising from an adreno-genital syndrome in the female fetus or progestogens ingested (in pregnancy testing) by the mother in pregnancy can lead to a male phallic development, a penile type urethra and scrotal appearance of the labia which may be adherent to each other (Dewhurst 1970).

(ii) Surgical anatomy of genital tract

The surgery of infertility is confined to an area which is easily accessible both vaginally and abdominally and the availability of hysterosalpingography and laparoscopy ensures that the surgeon knows the situation he will encounter with considerable accuracy.

Pelvic operations for infertility involve the body of the uterus, the ovaries and the tubes and except for large uterine fibroids, sizeable ovarian cysts or previous severe pelvic infection there is no enlargement or distortion of these organs. Surrounding structures such as bladder, ureters, bowel and large blood vessels are not normally in dangerous relationship and are usually excluded or isolated from the operative field immediately the abdomen is opened.

Unnecessary disturbance of the blood supply to uterus, ovary and especially fallopian tube is the one factor which will cause immediate problems and will also have an adverse effect on results. Occlusive clamps are used to interrupt the blood supply in uterine operations but despite meticulous suturing considerable bleeding may follow removal of the clamps and can lead to subsequent haematomata and abscess formation. In operating on the body of the uterus it is very important that the blood supply be fully understood.

The ovary is less of a problem because the vessels enter at the hilum with a simple fan-wise distribution to the gland: they are easily visible and can be picked up with the diathermy forceps or underrun with a stitch during the operation.

The blood supply to the fallopian tube has several sources and forms fine anastomoses in the mesosalpinx so that the terminal branches to the tube are thin-walled and easily damaged. While the use of fine instruments and local blood control by vasoconstrictors are of great importance it is essential that the surgeon recognise the direction and source of the blood flow. With this knowledge much can be done to avoid a vascular operative field which can only hinder precise work and may result in subsequent haematomata or peritoneal bleeding and adhesion.

Uterine blood supply

The uterine artery crosses over the ureter in the base of the broad ligament and approaches the uterus at the level of the cervical internal os. After giving off its cervical branch it ascends along the lateral aspect of the uterus between the layers of the broad ligament and it assumes a tortuous or coiled attitude so that it can enlarge with the uterus in pregnancy. This main uterine artery gives off transverse uterine vessels at all levels of the uterus up to and including the fundus. These branches divide into anterior and posterior coronary branches which supply the anterior and posterior muscle mass of the uterus respectively. They anastomose with their fellows of the opposite side in the midline. The main uterine artery meets the ovarian artery in the region of the cornu of the uterus allowing the ovarian artery to make a contribution to uterine blood supply and the uterine artery to the ovarian. The arteries to the uterus are shown diagrammatically in **Figure 11** and the radiographs (**Figures 10A and 10B**) show the rich vascular supply and the anastomosis with the ovarian artery.

With such a dense blood supply the surgeon must seek the least vascular areas when making an incision and the choice generally lies between a vertical incision centrally in what will probably be the least vascular area or a horizontal incision which will hopefully fall between the segmental blood supply from the coronary arteries. Such is the muscular configuration of the uterus that the latter is nearly always preferred and the lower on the uterine body it can be placed the better. In myomectomy the incision should be horizontal, as near the midline of the uterus as possible, and no longer than is necessary to enucleate the fibroid. The lateral aspect of the uterus with its main vessel should be avoided.

The venous return from the uterus is mainly via the pampiniform plexus of veins in the broad ligament, the uterine and the ovarian veins.

Ovarian blood supply

The ovarian artery arises from the aorta and runs caudally and retroperitoneally to the pelvis where it enters the infundibulo-pelvic ligament. One branch runs to the hilum of the ovary through the mesovarium while the other continues as a loop which runs parallel to and supplies the fallopian tube before anastomosing with the uterine artery at the cornu of the uterus.

Surgery of the ovary not involving the hilum can therefore be practically bloodless and the concentration of the arteries in one small area makes vascular control very easy. It should be remembered that the anastomosis between the uterine and ovarian vessels is a free one as can be seen from pelvic arteriograms where the uterine vessel clearly gives a major ovarian supply (see **Figures 10A and 10B**). That the converse is true is evident if the uterine arteries are occluded without also clamping the ovarian pedicles.

10 a

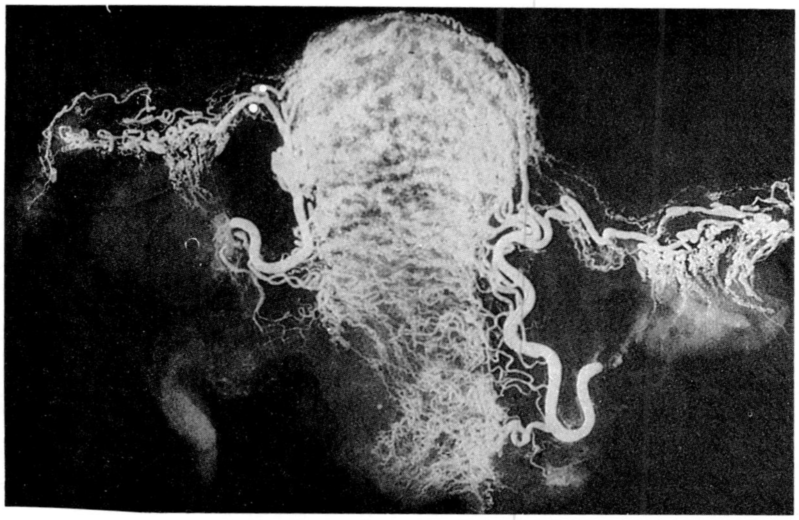

10 b

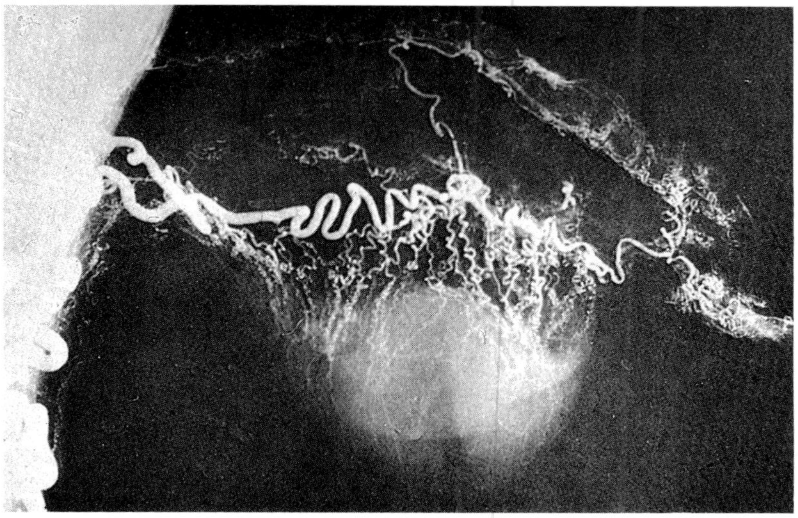

10a A radiograph of the uterus and ovaries showing the uterine arteries injected with radio-opaque material
The right uterine artery was damaged and displaced during hysterectomy but the descending cervical branch is well seen on the left side. Note the characteristic spiral shape of the coronary arteries in the myometrium and of the arterioles in the ovary. The ovarian arteries were *not* injected and the radiograph indicates the free anastomosis between the uterine and ovarian vessels.

10b The blood supply to the ovary and fallopian tube as revealed by a uterine arteriogram
The ovarian artery was not injected but is shown filled from its connexion with the terminal part of the uterine artery. The spiral arterioles entering the ovary through the mesovarium are well shown, and also branches to the fallopian tube with a continuous vessel running just below and parallel to it.

(**10a** and **10b** have been reproduced with kind permission from *Principles of Gynaecology*, 4th Edition, 1975, by Sir Norman Jeffcoate, published by Butterworths, London.)

11

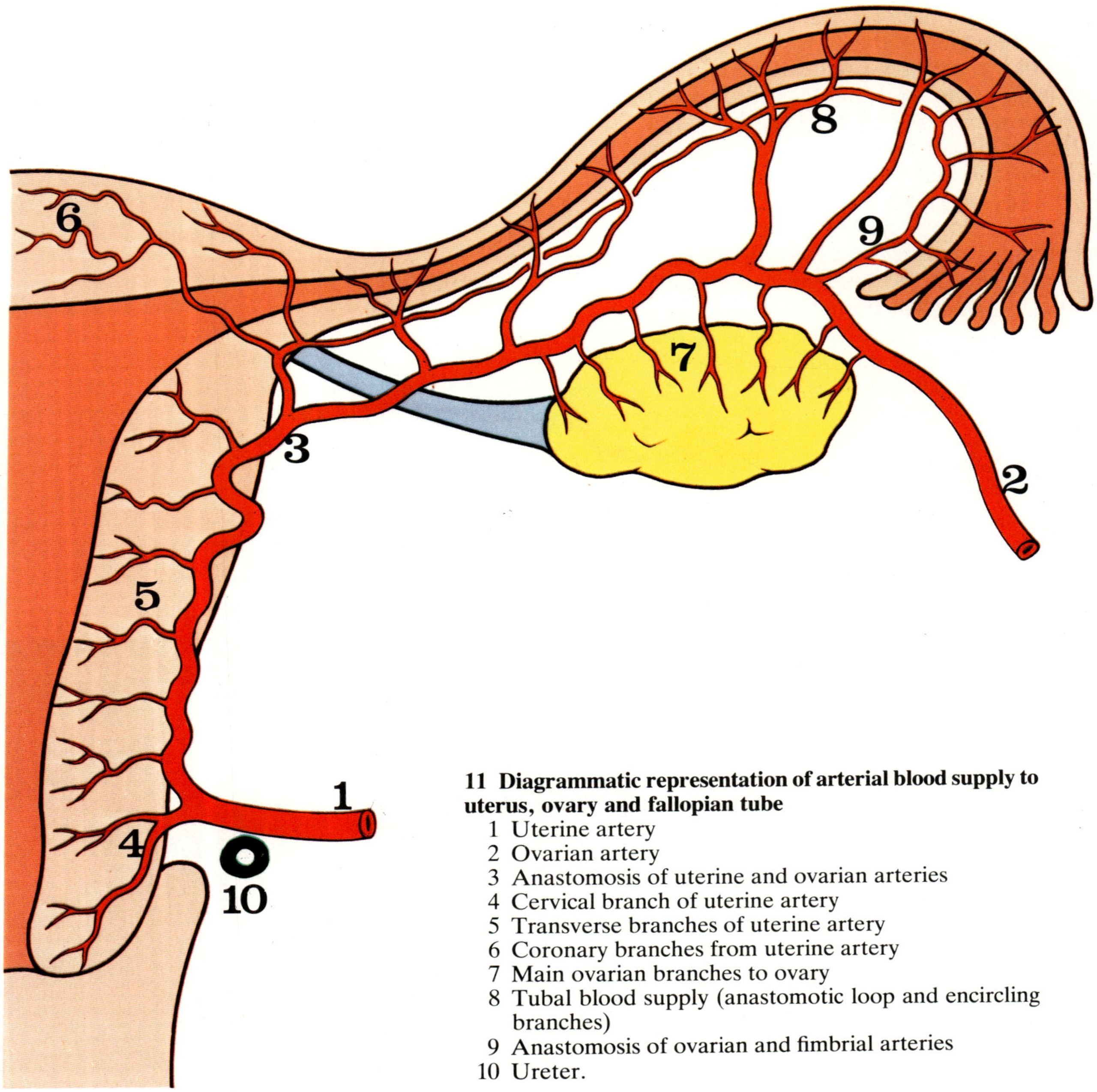

11 Diagrammatic representation of arterial blood supply to uterus, ovary and fallopian tube
1 Uterine artery
2 Ovarian artery
3 Anastomosis of uterine and ovarian arteries
4 Cervical branch of uterine artery
5 Transverse branches of uterine artery
6 Coronary branches from uterine artery
7 Main ovarian branches to ovary
8 Tubal blood supply (anastomotic loop and encircling branches)
9 Anastomosis of ovarian and fimbrial arteries
10 Ureter.

Tubal blood supply

The division of the ovarian artery which runs parallel to the fallopian tube and anastomoses with the uterine artery gives off a series of branches which encircle the tube. The blood supply from these two vessels is an exceedingly rich one and there is little fear of tubal necrosis if surgical principles are observed. A greater problem is post-operative oozing of blood which may cause adhesions or tubal blockage. The principal point to remember is that the utero-ovarian anastomotic loop lies close to the tube in the mesosalpinx and it is important to avoid making incisions or using needles in that area without being able to see clearly what is being done. Once bleeding starts it is difficult to control, the tissues quickly become soft and discoloured and adequate vision is lost.

The fimbrial and ovarian anastomosis which runs in the fimbrio-ovarian ligament is very easily damaged when dissecting the tube from the ovary during the division of adhesions and salpingostomy. This anastomosis is very clearly shown in the arteriogram **10B** on page 41.

(iii) Surgical instruments

It has been the custom at the beginning of each volume of the Atlas to show a set of surgical instruments suitable for the operations about to be described. With the exception of the tubal procedures no special equipment is required for the infertility operations described in this volume, and a standard abdominal and/or vaginal set will meet all requirements. If the reader wishes to have guidance on choosing instruments he is referred to the vaginal set illustrated on page 42 of Volume 1 and page 14 of Volume 2 of the Atlas.

Success in tubal surgery depends greatly on having suitable equipment and this includes small light instruments with which to handle the delicate structures. The average gynaecologist performing tubal surgery by methods short of a full microtechnique would require the type of equipment shown in **Figure 12**. The artery and dissecting forceps, scissors and diathermy equipment are those used in microsurgery; the Alliss' tissue forceps, glass rods and probes are also of that type. A small pointed scalpel might be preferred to the microscalpel on the grounds of familiarity and the same might apply to needle holders, but that would depend on the degree of magnification used during the operation.

The surgeon embarking on full-scale microsurgical procedures will find a wide selection of purpose-built instruments on the instrument makers' shelves.

12

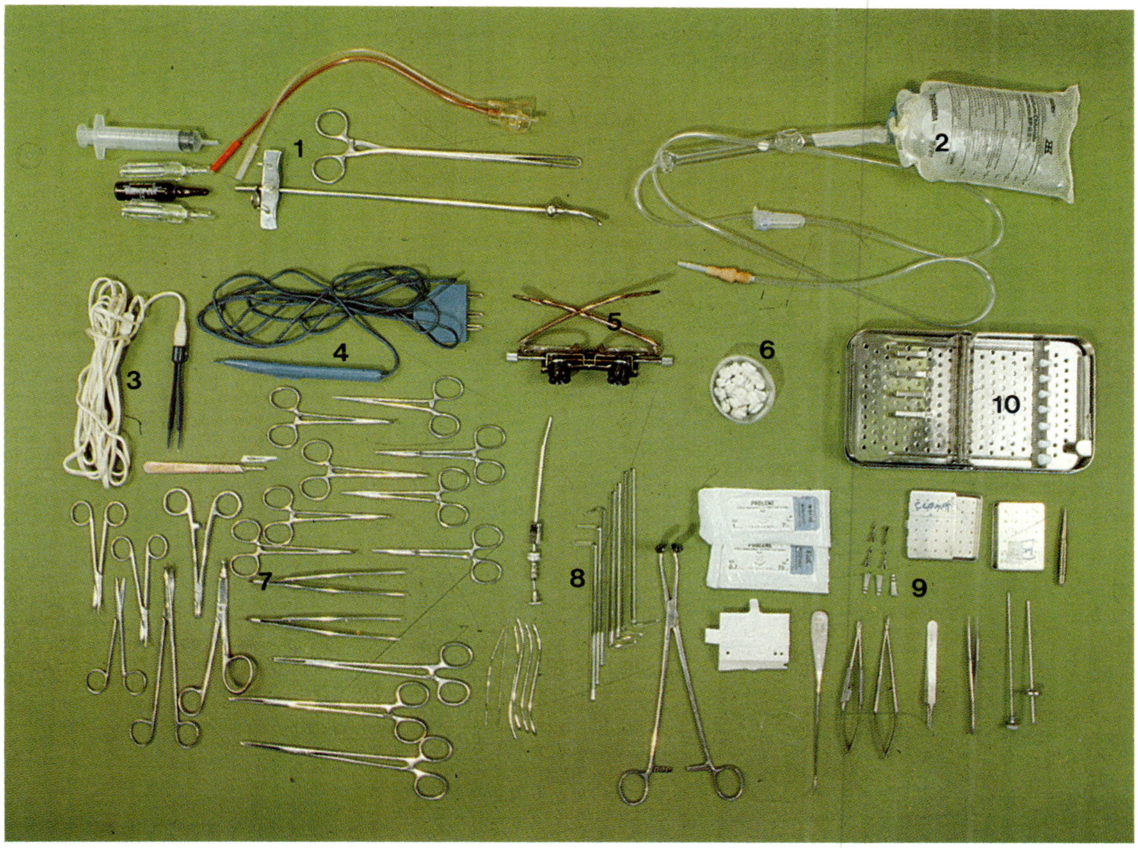

12 Instruments for tubal surgery

1 Hydrotubation instruments – Spackman cannula, tenaculum forceps, cervical cap, syringe and dye solution ampoules
2 Ringer-lactate solution
3 Bipolar diathermy
4 Insulated unipolar diathermy
5 Magnifying spectacles
6 Pledglets
7 Macroscopic (lightweight) instruments – scalpel, dissecting and tissue forceps, straight and curved scissors, needle holder
8 Instruments for tubal surgery generally – fine sucker, tubal dilators, fine probes and Siegler-Hellman clamp
9 Microsurgical instruments – needle holders, fine sutures, dissecting forceps, microclips, microscalpel, uterine trochar and cannula
10 Sterilising box for microsurgical instruments.

A uterine holding forceps or clamp is essential equipment in tubal surgery. Of the various types available the authors prefer the Shirodkar clamp. It is seen in use on page 162 of this volume.

4: Psychological factors in infertility surgery

In the initial investigation of infertility it is generally unwise to form immediate impressions of the patient's psychological state; the infertile woman should be seen as a rational individual with a specific medical problem. The authors make this point because there is at present a great deal of emphasis on the mental attitude of the patient and the new subjects of psychogenic infertility and psychopathology of infertility are in vogue. Such aspects are obviously enormously important in a total study of the subject; what must be ensured is that the investigation of these aspects awaits a full clinical assessment of both partners' physical and reproductive capacity.

The situation in relation to women being considered for surgical treatment is a delicate one. They have continued with tedious investigations while their friends have apparently conceived with the utmost facility and the normally expressed sympathy has only accentuated their feeling of failure. Investigations are often inconclusive with no single factor seen as a likely cause of the infertility and the now despondent patient is informed that the normal range of tests and treatment has been completed. At this stage attention invariably reverts to any abnormality of structure or pathology that may have been noted or suspected during investigation. Uterine fibroids, smaller ovarian cysts, retroverted uterus and early pelvic endometriosis are examples. There is no definitive indication for an operation although the patient desperately hopes that it might somehow break the impasse and she and her husband have come to believe that only surgery will solve the problem. The presence of such a couple in one's consulting room is both disconcerting and demands that the surgeon take matters firmly in hand without delay. The possibility of surgical operations being done without adequate indication and perhaps with little prospect of success makes the situation a serious one. This section of Volume 5 is written with the express purpose of identifying the dangers and ensuring that the interests of both patient and doctor are safeguarded.

The advice is set out in the form of a ten point 'code of practice' or protocol which the authors have been accustomed to use and which is offered as a guide to less experienced readers.

1 Clinical record available
In cases previously seen by colleagues the surgeon should always ask for permission to write and obtain the clinical history to date, with full details of the investigation results. Patients should not be subjected to repetition of surgical procedures unnecessarily.

2 Infertility investigations completed on both partners
Every case must be fully investigated clinically, radiologically and endocrinologically before considering surgical treatment. Operations for infertility should not be done unless there is evidence that the male partner is fertile.

3 Non-surgical treatment exhausted
Unless the indication for operation is an absolute one, non-surgical treatment should be exhausted before resorting to surgery.

4 Full discussion of proposed treatment
The clinical situation and the reasons for considering or proposing surgery should be fully discussed with the patient and her husband preoperatively.

5 Requests for operation by the patient
The request for operation should always come from the patient herself, even to the extent of the surgeon asking if that is her wish. Where the success rate of a proposed procedure is low this becomes particularly important.

6 Second opinion encouraged
Any suggestion by the patient that she might have a second medical opinion at this stage should be actively encouraged.

7 Full facilities available
The surgeon should not agree to operate unless he is satisfied that the facilities and available expertise (assistants, nursing etc.), are available.

8 Laparoscopy and HSG complete
The abdomen should not be opened unless hysterosalpingography and laparoscopy have been done.

9 Full discussion of prognosis
Prognosis is always difficult and while the surgeon has no option other than to quote published results these must be qualified by firmly stated 'caveats'. It must be pointed out that no two cases are alike, that the published results are likely to be better than average and that the number of cases in any series is too small to be significant. A 20 per cent success rate may seem reasonable to the patient until it is pointed out that the failure rate is therefore 80 per cent and/or there is only one chance in five of success. The question of ectopic pregnancy and possible abortion must also be taken into account.

10 When to stop
Treatment should be stopped or suspended when everything reasonably possible has been done. The patient is asked to try to forget her problem for a spell and await the results of what has been done. She is also counselled against seeking further investigations and treatment at the hands of still more specialists.

5: Operations on the vagina

Vaginal abnormalities are only occasionally the sole cause of infertility; more frequently it is difficult to decide whether they are indeed causal factors. There are two principal groups:

1 Local or general narrowing of vaginal canal making penile penetration incomplete or impossible.
- (i) tight hymen
- (ii) narrowing of vagina either from persistence of a congenital septum or as a result of a gynaecological operation.

2 Vaginal conditions which impede access of spermatozoa to cervical canal.
- (i) large vestigial vaginal cysts
- (ii) longitudinal vaginal septum.

A tight or rigid hymen is easily treated by dividing it radially at several points under general anaesthesia and taking the opportunity to dilate the canal digitally at the same time. Congenital septa and postoperative narrowing both demand surgical treatment. The former require individualised incision and dilatation according to vaginal level: procedures for correction of the latter are described elsewhere in the Atlas (Volume 1, page 201 and Volume 4, page 81).

One further group of patients in whom vaginal narrowing may cause a problem are those suffering from vaginismus. This is not a surgical problem except where dilatation under anaesthesia is carried out and a large dilator is left *in situ*. The patient then has the evidence of her own eyes that the vaginal capacity is adequate and this is used as part of a predominantly psychiatric approach.

In the second group of cases one sometimes finds that a large and usually lax cyst occupies and distends the whole vagina with upward displacement of the cervix towards the opposite side and such a case is described and illustrated in Volume 4 of the Atlas (page 34). The principal steps in the procedure are repeated here. It is not normally considered necessary to divide a longitudinal vaginal septum unless it is impeding delivery of the presenting part and this was mentioned previously in Volume 4 (page 25). The condition is usually revealed in hysterosalpingographic investigation of infertility. The septum may be complete so that there are two separate vaginae with two cervices. In such circumstances removal of the septum provides a more capacious vaginal vault and makes spermatazoa available to both cervices. In the unicollis situation the cervix may open into the non-used vagina and there is therefore considerable advantage in dividing the septum.

Excision of congenital lower vaginal septum (imperforate hymen)

1

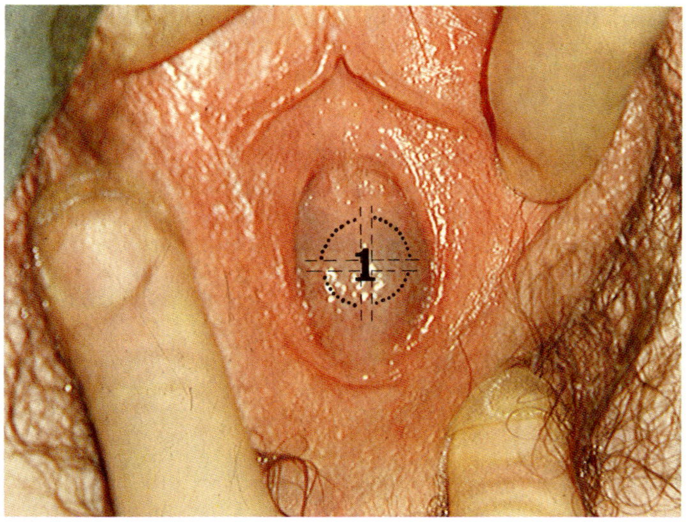

1 Clinical appearance seen vaginally: site of incision
The intact membrane (1) is bulging and dark blue in colour so that the menstrual fluid of the cryptomenorrhoea is under considerable pressure. This is consistent with the abdominal finding of uterine enlargement to 20 weeks pregnancy size. The general vulvar appearance and hair distribution suggest full development of secondary sex characteristics which is usual in these cases. The membrane is first incised by two bisecting incisions each 2.5 cm long at right angles to each other. The double broken lines indicate their placement. Each of the resultant four skin tags will subsequently be removed along the dotted lines to open up the introitus.

2

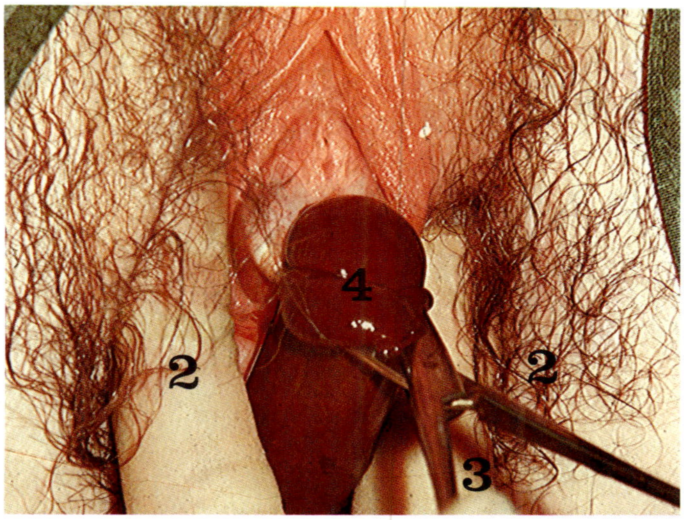

2 Release of menstrual fluid
The patient is in the lithotomy position and the bladder has been decompressed over 48 hours preoperatively. The labia are displaced laterally by the fingers of the left hand (2) and following the cruciate incision a forceps (3) is introduced and opened to facilitate the drainage of pent-up menstrual fluid (4) from the vagina and upper genital tract. When the flow has ceased the ends of the four tags of membrane are removed along the lines indicated in **Figure 1**. It is very unusual for there to be any bleeding and no dressing is required.

A fuller account of this operation is given in Volume 4 of the Atlas, pages 21–24.

Division of longitudinal vaginal septum

3

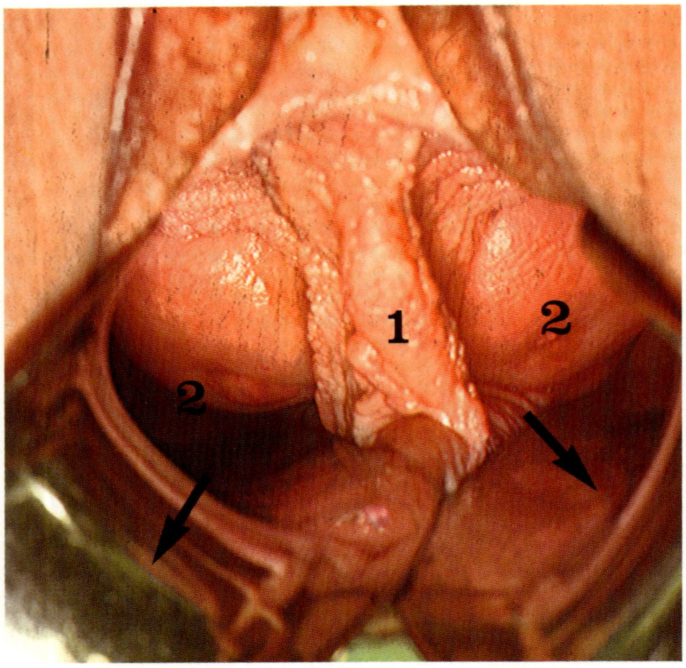

4

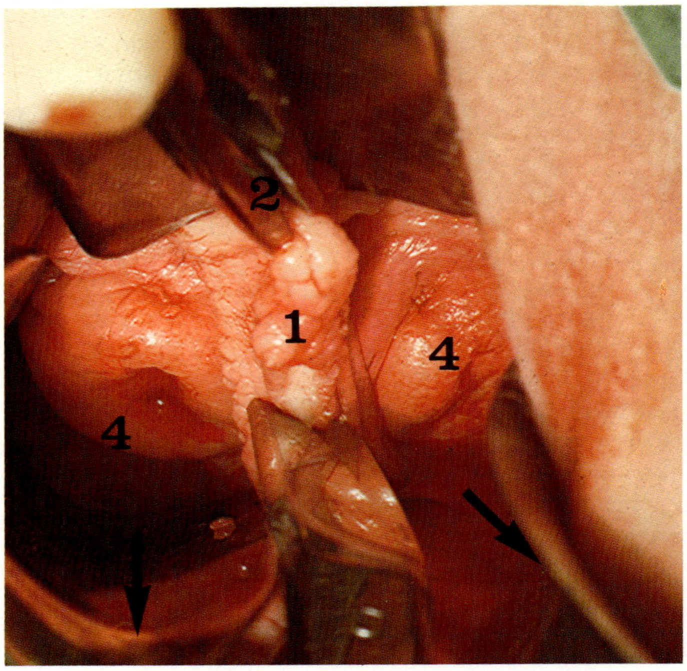

3 Clinical appearance on speculum examination
Sims' specula gently retract the posterior vaginal wall in the direction of the arrows to show the lower edge of the longitudinal septum (1) which is about 1 cm thick. There is a vaginal cavity on each side (2) and (2).

5

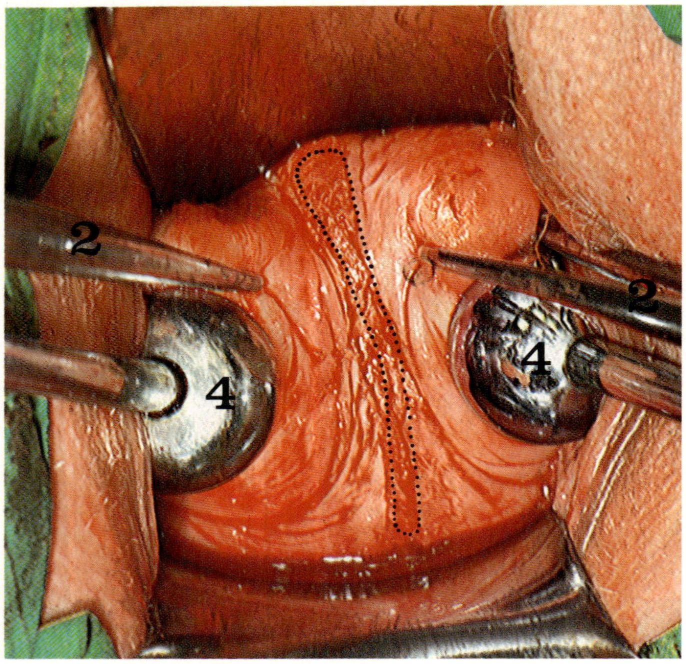

4 Division of longitudinal septum with scissors
With Sims' specula retracting the vaginae in the direction of the broad arrows the septum (1) is thrown into relief and is steadied by the dissecting forceps (2) while the angled scissors commence its division as near centrally as possible and in the axis of the vagina. The two vaginal cavities are numbered (4) and (4).

5 Division of septum completed
Division has been carried as high as possible between the cervices and the upper vagina is seen to be very capacious. The raw surface resulting from the incision of the septum is very narrow and is outlined by the dotted line between the retracting forceps (2) and (2). Spackman cervical cannulae (4) and (4) have been introduced into each of the cervices for demonstration purposes.

A fuller account of this operation is given in Volume 4 of the Atlas, pages 24–29.

Marsupialisation of large (Wolffian) vaginal cyst

A fuller account of this operation is given in Volume 4 of the Atlas, pages 34–40.

6

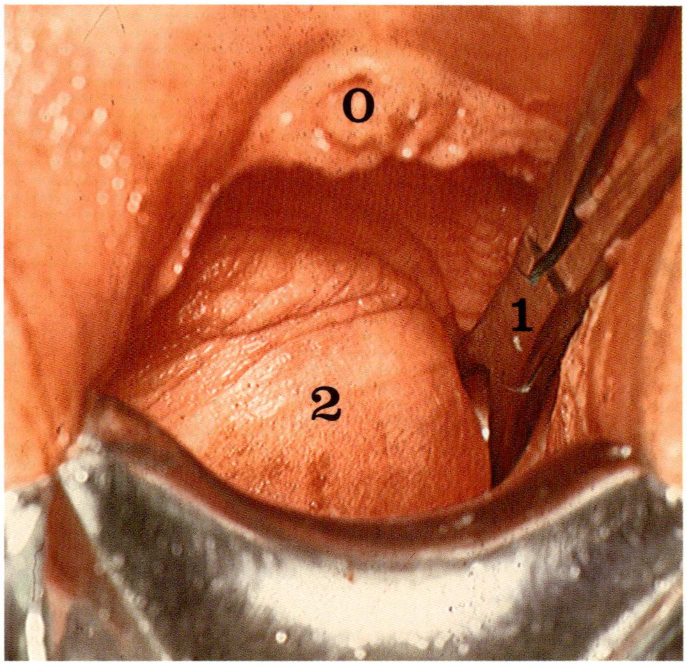

6 Clinical appearance of large right-sided vaginal cyst
The tissue forceps (1) is on the anterior lip of the cervix and the large cystic swelling (2) which occupies the right lateral fornix has all the appearances of a Wolffian remnant. The urethral orifice is numbered (0).

7

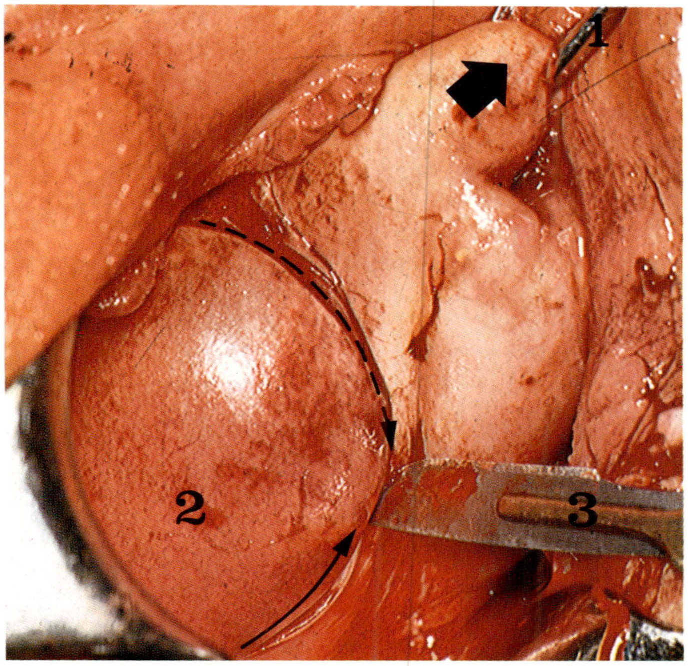

7 Outlining skin incision while cyst is intact
The cervix is drawn to the left (broad arrow) by the tissue forceps (1) to display the lower pole of the cyst (2). The line of incision will represent the stoma and is carefully delineated with the scalpel (3).

8

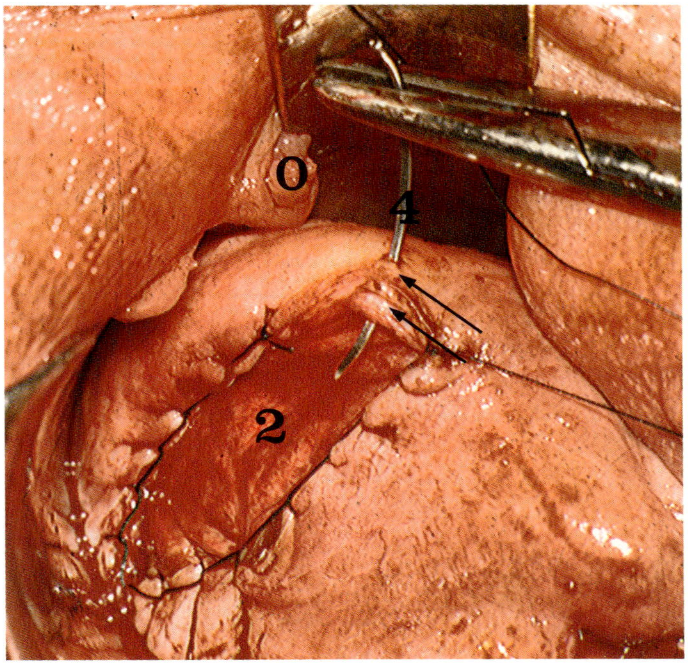

8 Suture of skin to cyst wall (marsupialisation)
The atraumatic needle (4) carrying a No. 00 PGA suture picks up the skin and the edge of the cyst wall in turn (fine arrows); the locked stitch approximation of these two layers is now almost complete. The cavity of the cyst is numbered (2) and the urethral orifice (0).

9

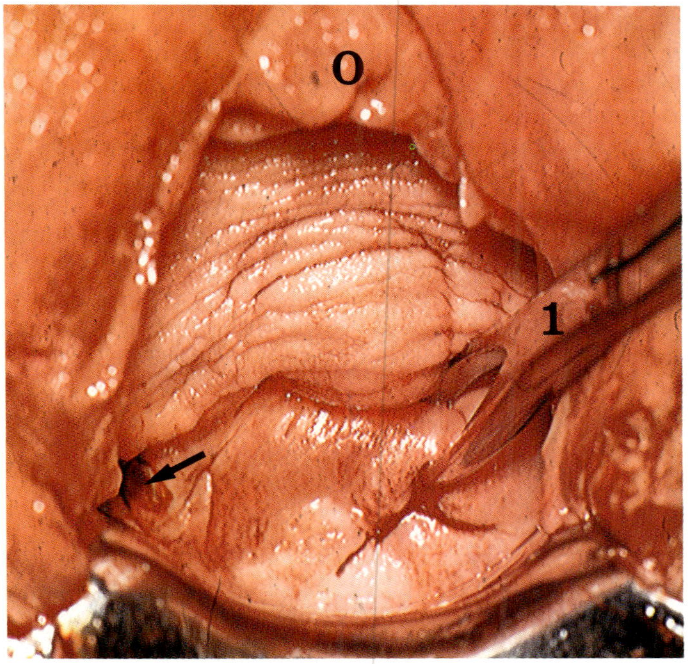

9 Appearance at completion of operation
With the collapse of the now empty cyst the cervix has returned to its normal position at the centre of the vaginal vault. The extreme medial edge of the marsupialisation stoma is just visible where arrowed. The other structures are numbered as previously.

6: Operations on the cervix

It would be surprising if abnormalities or lesions of the cervix did not have a bearing on fertility since the sperm is deposited in the posterior vaginal fornix and must negotiate the ectocervical surface and the cervical canal to reach the uterine cavity. The cervix also has an important function in the retention of the developing ovum within the uterus and muscular incompetence might be expected to lead to miscarriage in the second trimester of pregnancy. It is exceedingly difficult to obtain reliable evidence on the importance of any of these conditions and clinicians adopt widely differing stances in relation to cervical treatment in infertility. In attempting to find a middle and logical course the subject is dealt with under the following separate headings.

1: Inflammatory conditions of the cervix

Chronic cervicitis presenting with a large area of exophytic glandular epithelium on the ectocervix and producing a muco-purulent discharge may impede sperm motility and provide a hostile environment through alteration of the upper vaginal pH. Such lesions are of course treated when recognised and is believed by some to increase fertility. Obvious polypi within the cervical canal should be removed. Every gynaecologist of experience has anticipated with pleasure how swiftly the removal of a cervical polyp from a long married and childless patient will make her an elderly primipara. Excision of a cervical polyp is simple and once recognised the clinician may be tempted to grasp it in a sponge forceps and twist it off in the out-patient department or office. Such a policy is unwise on two counts. The cervical canal and the uterine cavity should both be explored with a curette to exclude further polypi at a higher level, and any gratitude the patient may feel for instant treatment will quickly be replaced by resentment if continuing vaginal bleeding necessitates her admission to hospital in the middle of the night.

2: Occlusion or narrowing of cervical canal

The authors do not believe that this is other than a very rare cause of infertility in nulliparae; its exclusion however is repeatedly cited as one of the principal reasons for 'doing a D & C' in infertility. Random procedures to confirm cervical patency, possibly uncover some intrauterine defect and provide a fresh new endometrium to encourage nidation are still too often being done. They have no place in modern management. The lumen of the cervix will be adequately checked during the routine infertility investigations (ie hysterosalpingography, laparoscopy or the occasional D & C).

3: Cervical incompetence

It is exceedingly difficult to be certain about the incidence and the precise implications of cervical incompetence. Obstetricians regularly see and sometimes observe throughout complete pregnancies a partially open cervix which later becomes fully effaced yet maintains the fetus safely in utero till term and beyond. On the other hand miscarriage in the second trimester due to cervical deficiency is a well recognised and documented clinical entity and where the cause is known it demands treatment. This type of incompetence may be present without a previous history of trauma of pregnancy so that some cases would seem to be congenital in origin. Others result from damage to the circular muscle structure in pregnancy or as a result of rapid dilatation of the cervix during a surgical operation. We have all watched with dismay a stubborn cervix 'give way' to an impatiently forced dilator while a gratified trainee is oblivious of the damage he has done. The possibility of the cervix suffering occult damage in a previous pregnancy is of course always present and in such cases retrospective study of the obstetric record may disclose overenthusiastic stimulation of uterine contractions or a very rapid second stage of labour.

Cone biopsy of the cervix is another cause of clinically occult incompetence. Over recent years and until the advent of colposcopically directed biopsy and local destructive methods for treating preinvasive cervical cancer the message was that cone biopsy should be both deep and extensive. Apart from the complications of bleeding and infection which followed this unnecessarily severe treatment, the internal os, which is the real area of incidence in cervical incompetence, was damaged and weakened (Jones et al 1979).

When healing and fibrosis are complete in these cases the cervix can look remarkably normal. Gross cervical incompetence related to an obviously torn and lacerated cervix is a form of untreated trauma demanding correction and is dealt with under a separate heading on page 53.

Treatment of cervical incompetence demands demonstration that it is indeed present. Prima facie evidence would take the form of repeated midtrimester miscarriage with expulsion of an intact sac without bleeding or noticeable warning and the diagnosis would not be acceptable unless a No. 7 or 8 Hegar dilator could be passed into the uterus with ease. Some clinicians would demand radiological evidence as when a viscid radio-opaque medium injected into the uterus escapes around the cannula to outline a wide and deficient cervix (see **Figure 1**). However, this technique does have a significant false positive rate as many cervices in the immediately premenstrual phase have a similar appearance.

Cerclage is the accepted treatment for the condition and a very large number of such operations are done during and sometimes between pregnancies. It is entirely likely that too many are done but there are no reliable statistics because the circumstances do not permit controlled trials (*Lancet* editorial 1977).

Shirodkar (1960) described encirclement of the supravaginal cervix at the level of the internal os during pregnancy and although a relatively minor operation it does entail a transverse incision and reflection of the bladder. McDonald (1980) uses a simpler and apparently no less effective method in which he inserts a simple purse-string suture around the cervix at the cervico-vaginal junction. The stitch is inserted deeply into the muscle in 4 or 5 bites and runs deep to the blood vessels laterally. The knot is placed anteriorly.

Results from cerclage operations

Shirodkar (1968) claimed 81 per cent fetal salvage rate after operative intervention for cervical incompetence and such a high rate may be obtainable where the operation is particularly indicated. If one admits the claims of less typical second trimester or even late first trimester abortions and cases of recurrent early labour for the operation, then the success rate drops very steeply.

McDonald has recently reviewed his own results employing his own and Shirodkar's methods in 269 cases. Using the former technique the live birth rate was 86.5 per cent; with the latter it was 72.9.

1a to d Cervico-hysterograms of the proposed incompetent cervix
Cervico-hysterograms showing extensive widening of the internal cervical os (arrowed), an appearance regarded by many clinicians as pathognomonic of cervical incompetence. All these women had at least two second trimester miscarriages. Prophylactic repair of the cervix in the interpregnancy period was undertaken in one of them (as discussed on page 50) and the insertion of a Shirodkar suture inserted at the 15th gestational week in two others resulted in the carriage of a live infant to term in each case. Reproduced from *The Cervix*, Jordan, J. and Singer, A. (1976), Saunders, London.

1a b c d

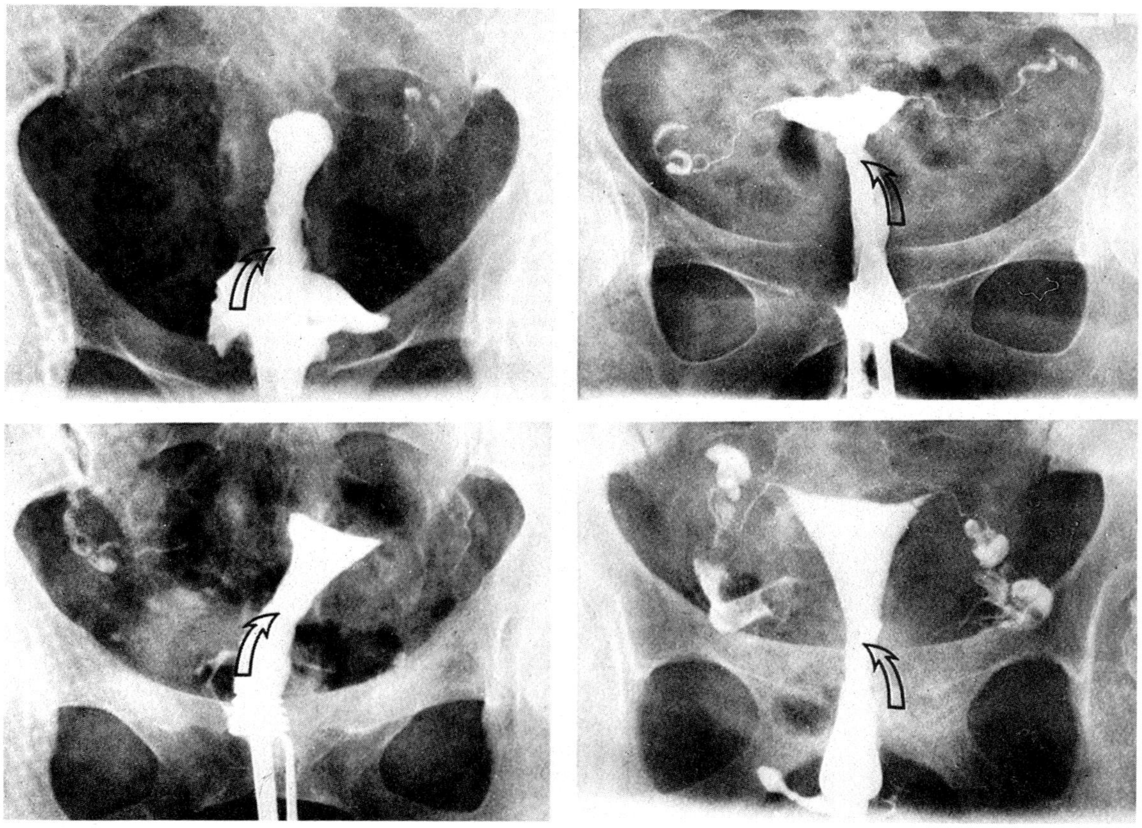

Insertion of Shirodkar suture

There are several methods of cerclage but that of Shirodkar is the most popular. The operation is not done before 12–14 weeks of pregnancy and the suture should preferably be in place before 20 weeks. It is a planned anticipatory procedure and if the cervix has already begun to dilate or if a bulging sac has to be pushed back into the uterus the chances of success are minimal. The operation should be done with extreme gentleness and the supporting suture should be at the level of the internal cervical os. It is carried out under light general or epidural anaesthesia and the patient is in the lithotomy position with the bladder previously emptied by catheter. The patient remains in hospital and at rest for at least 48 hours postoperatively. It is common practice to administer a beta mimetic agent postoperatively in an attempt to prevent the onset of premature labour.

2

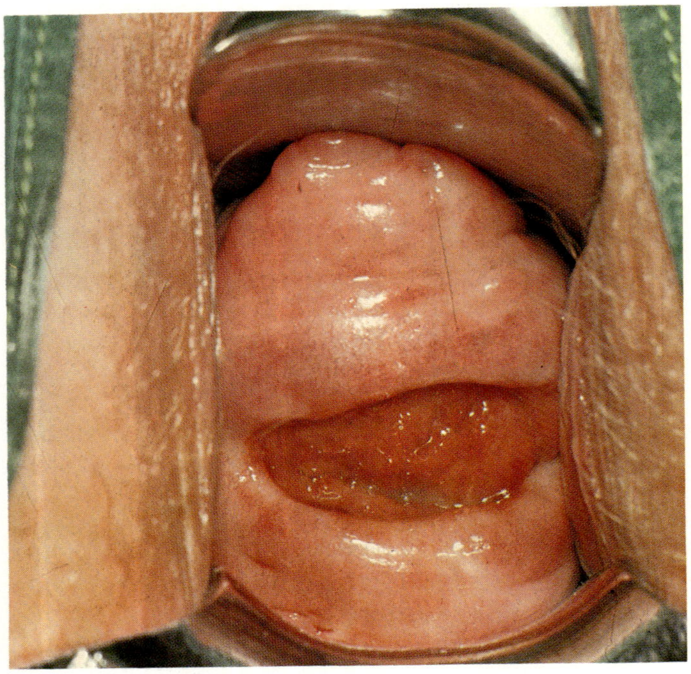

3

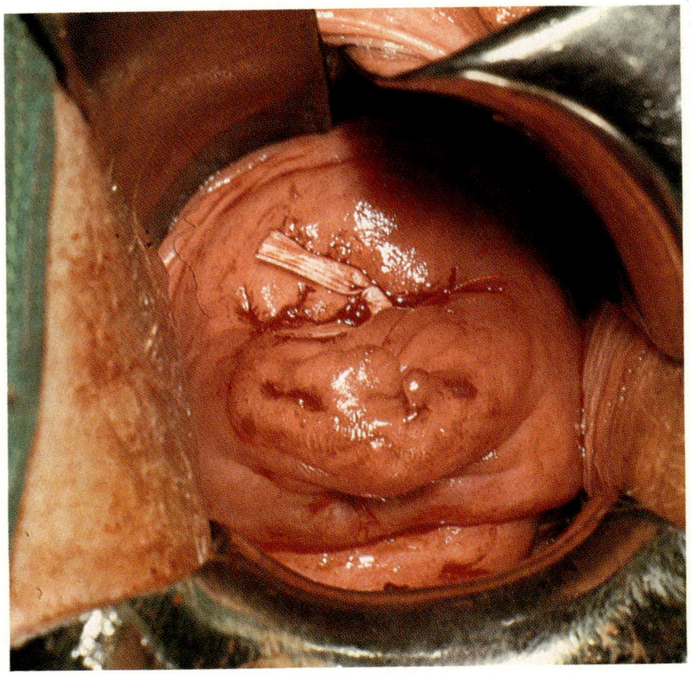

4

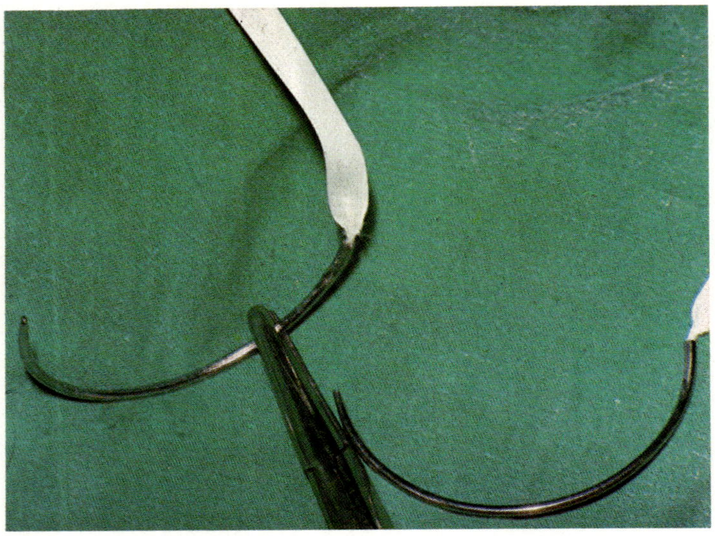

2 Clinical appearance of cervix at 14 weeks pregnancy in recurrent abortion case
The external os is slightly open but not obviously more than in many normal cases. The decision to operate is based on a history of three almost unheralded mid-trimester miscarriages and evidence of an incompetent cervix on clinical and radiological investigation carried out between pregnancies.

3 Appearance of cervix after insertion of Shirodkar suture
This photograph shows the suture *in situ*. It is firm but not too tight and as near the internal os as feasible. When the suture is tied it should lightly grasp a No. 6 Hegar dilator placed in the cervical canal. The stitch is buried in the cervical muscle except where tied off anteriorly; it is thus easily accessible for removal when labour ensues.

4 Suitable type of Shirodkar stitch
The needle on each end allows the stitch to be completed in two anteroposterior or postero-anterior semi-circles and that may be considered an advantage; the method described here requires only one needle. The needle is round-bodied in shape, strong and of half circle type. The tape is of braided nylon and can be tied securely in a reef knot.

5

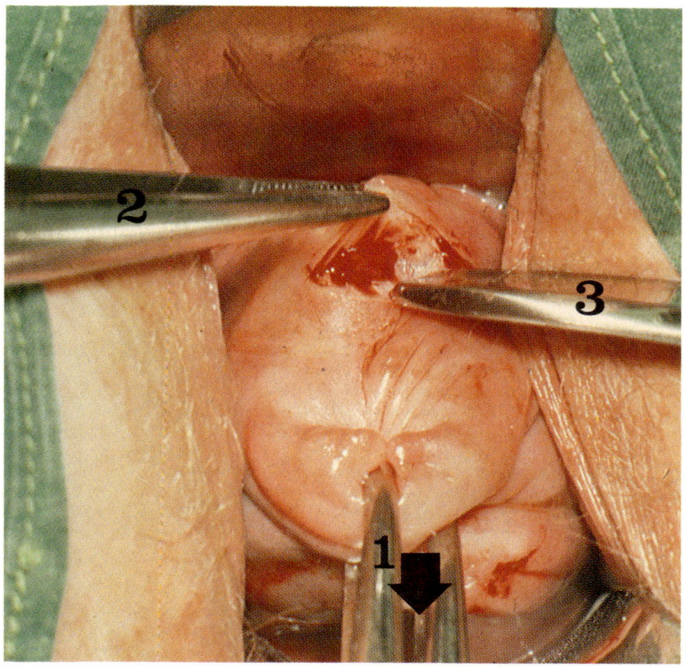

5 Incision of vaginal skin on anterior aspect of cervix
A tissue forceps (1) steadies the anterior lip of the cervix in the direction of the arrow and the dissecting forceps (2) elevates the skin where it becomes loose on the anterior aspect of the cervix, just about the level of the internal cervical os. Angled scissors (3) open up a 1 cm transverse incision at the estimated level of the internal os.

6

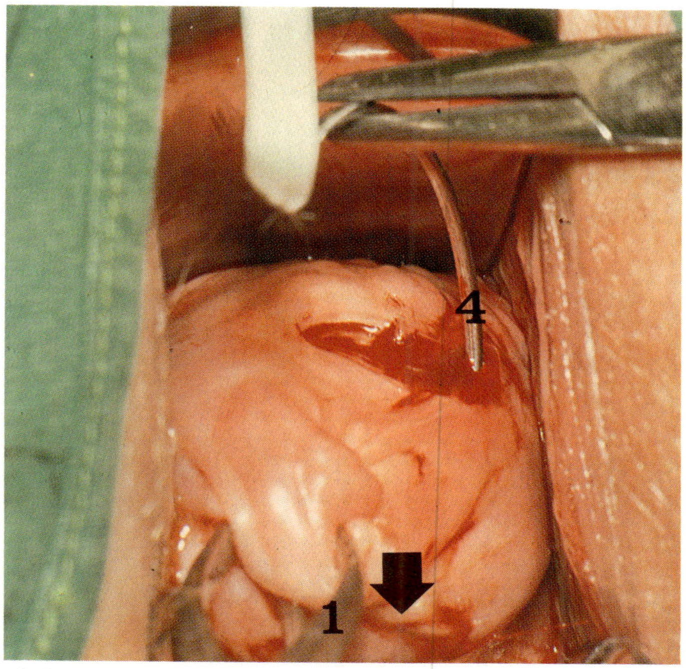

6 Commencing insertion of Shirodkar suture
Loose subcutaneous tissue at the site of incision could possibly contain a fold of bladder and is therefore pushed upwards off the anterior aspect of the cervix to leave it bare where the needle (4) is about to enter on its course through the muscle of the left side of the cervix.

7

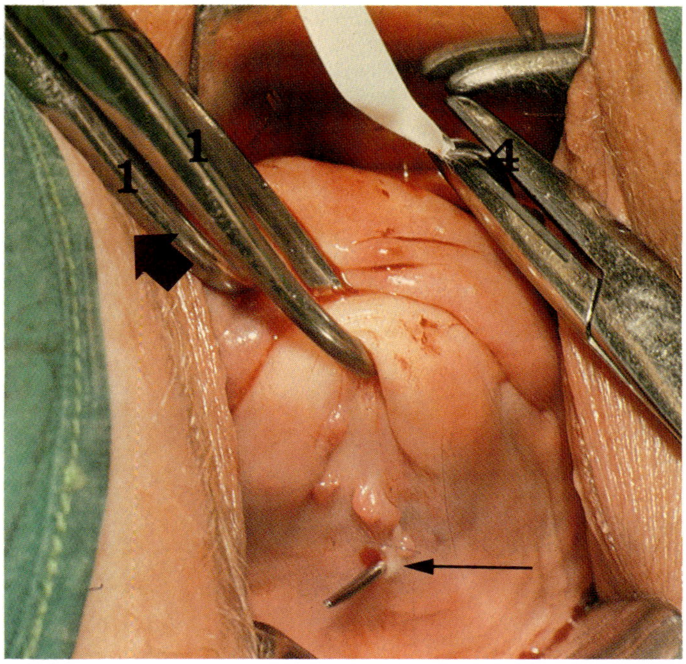

7 Needle traversing left side of cervix
The cervix is drawn to the right by the tissue forceps (1) and (1) in the direction of the broad arrow. The needle holder guides the needle gently and slowly through the centre of the muscular wall in a semi-circle at the estimated level of the internal os. It is aimed to emerge at the same level in the midline posteriorly and can be seen to do so (arrowed).

8

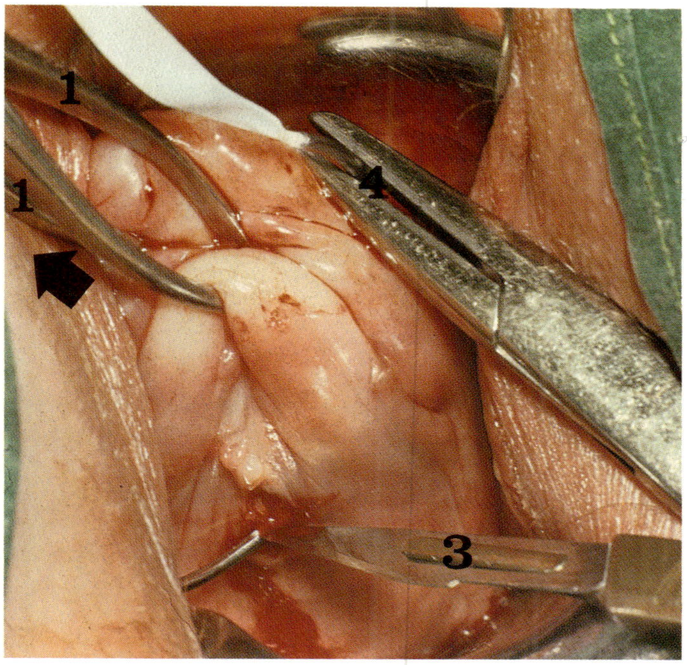

8 Small posterior skin incision for emerging needle
The round-bodied needle requires a small incision to emerge easily and that is made with the tip of the sharp pointed scalpel (3). The needle holder can now grasp the point and bring it through in the same semi-circular arc and in a controlled manner.

9

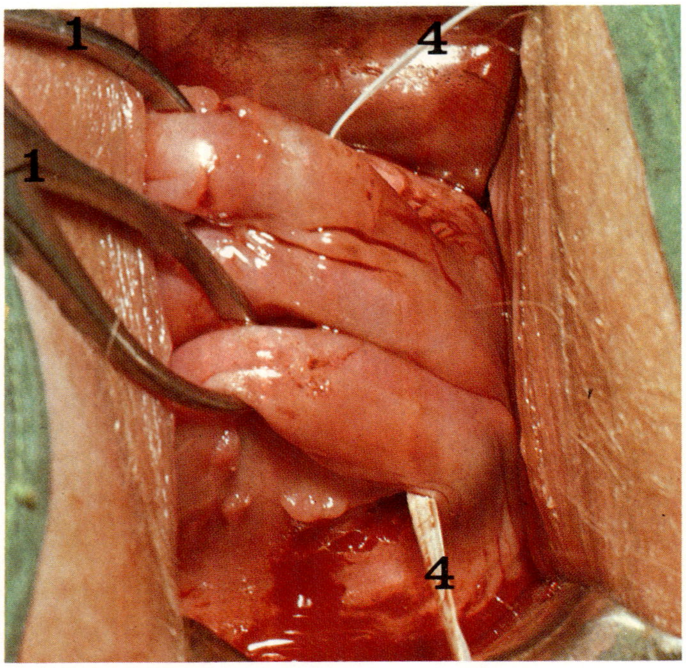

9 Suture inserted in left side of cervix
The photograph shows the suture placed at the correct level from anterior to posterior in the left side of the cervix.

10

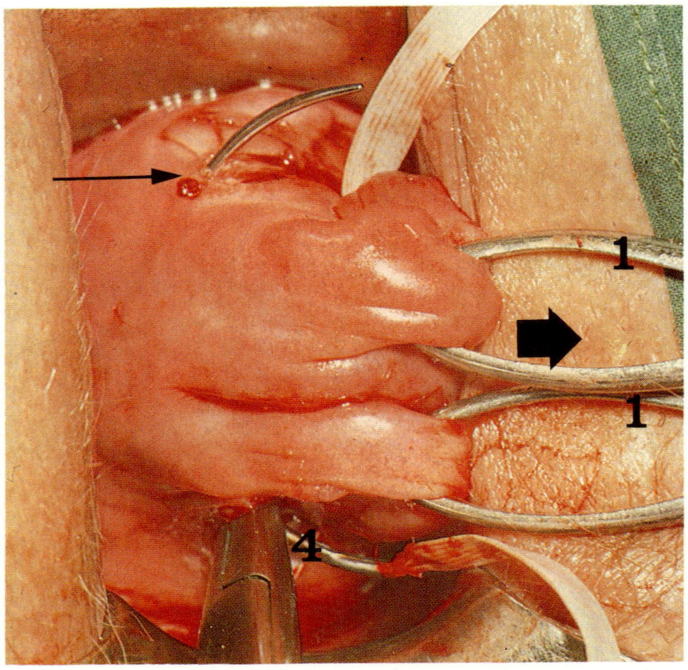

10 Needle traversing right side of cervix
The tissue forceps (1) and (1) draw the cervix to the left as arrowed and the needle traverses the right side of the cervix in a semi-circular arc from posterior to anterior. It enters at the small posterior incision and emerges at the larger anterior one (arrowed).

11

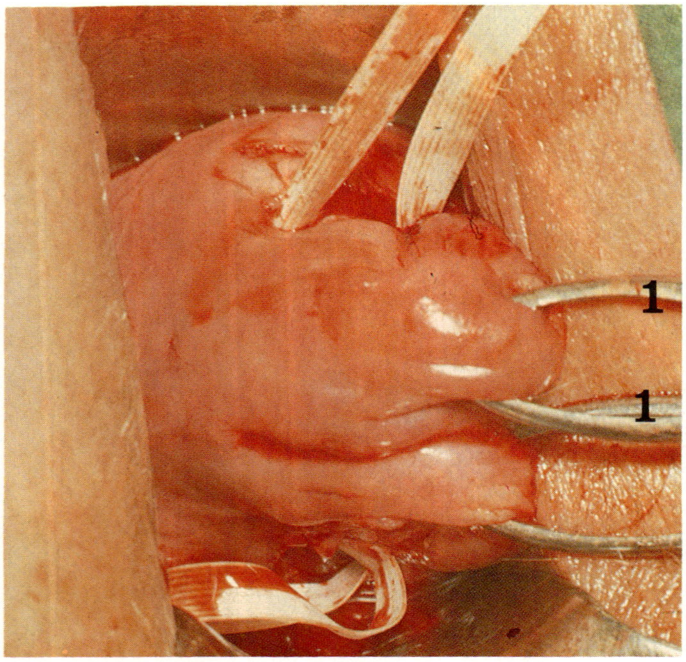

12

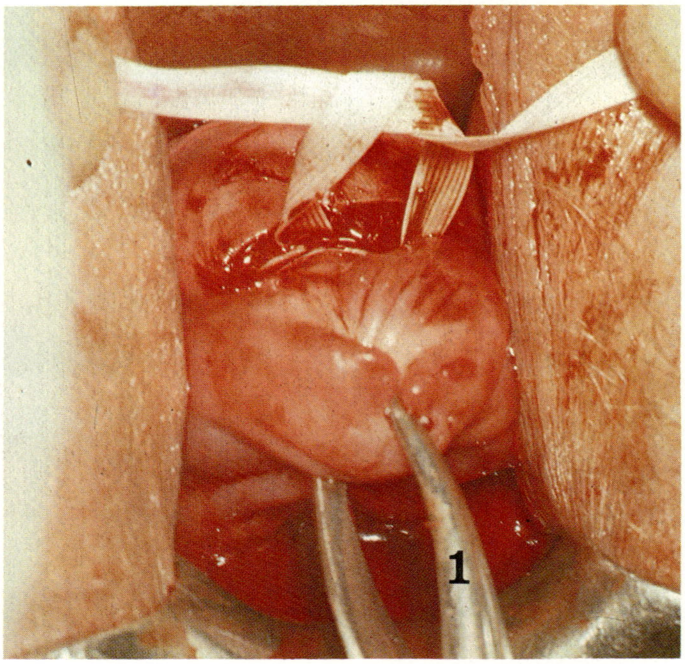

11 and 12 Placing of suture complete
The cervix is drawn to the left by the tissue forceps (1) and (1) in **Figure 11** to show the two halves of the stitch *in situ* and ready to be tightened and tied. The stitch has been tightened in **Figure 12** to give maximum support without endangering the blood supply to the cervix and a No. 6 Hegar's dilator is used to estimate tightness. The reef knot is then tied.

Trachelorrhaphy

This operation does not enjoy wide popularity with gynaecologists and some experienced clinicians deny that there is any place for it in the treatment of infertility. Such an attitude arises from uncertainty regarding the effects of muscle rupture on cervical competence and while it may be unwise to attempt a surgical narrowing of an allegedly incompetent cervix which looks normal, the treatment of a lacerated and patent cervix is a totally different proposition. These latter cases will no doubt decrease in number as the practice of obstetrics improves but there are three types of cervical damage which are still too frequently encountered. In the commonest form there is a lateral split on one side and the cervical canal is laid open as far as the internal os. In another type the split is bilateral resulting in an ectropion and effacement of the whole canal to give the appearance of a large 'erosion'. The third and least common is a deep split in the midline posteriorly. All are associated with excessive mucus secretion and vaginal discharge.

The authors believe that these cases of overt damage should be repaired and as illustrated in the following pages the procedure is seen to be a simple and in some respects almost a minor one. In principle a V-incision removes the epithelium from the edges at the site of the split or tear and the exposed raw muscle surfaces are carefully approximated with precisely placed sutures. The operation rids the patient of her vaginal discharge, appears to increase fertility and gives an added prospect of carrying the pregnancy to term.

The patient needs to exercise care and avoid possible trauma to the cervix during pregnancy; the surgeon has to realise that vaginal delivery may lead to the sutured area giving way and the operation might subsequently need to be repeated.

Surgical technique

13

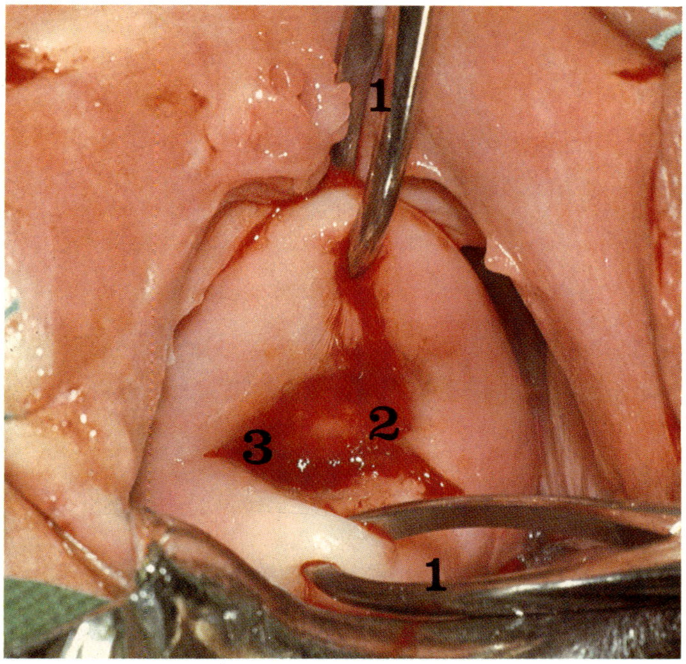

13 Appearance of cervix before operation
The anterior and posterior lips of the cervix are held in tissue forceps (1) and (1) to demonstrate the deep laceration (2) on the left side of the cervix and a lesser degree of tearing opposite it on the right side (3). The left sided defect extends to and includes the internal os. There is resultant ectropion and the cervix is much shortened.

14

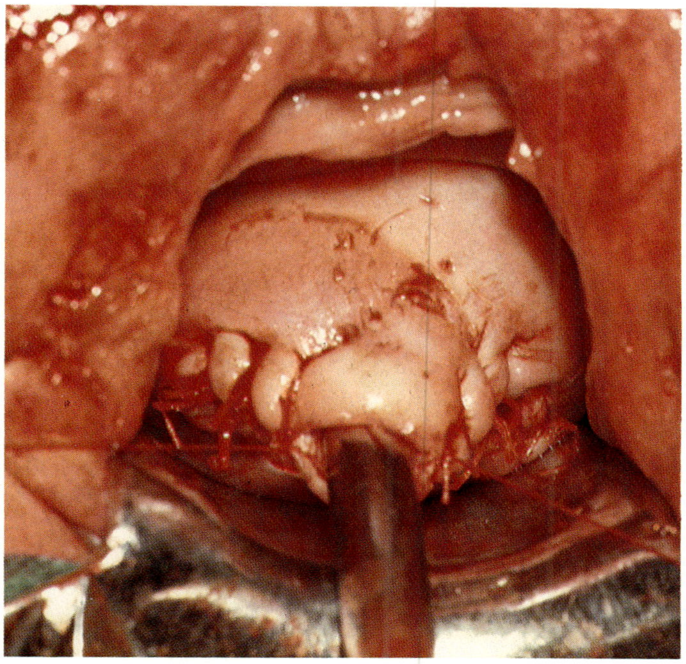

14 Appearance of cervix following trachelorrhaphy
A No. 8 Hegar dilator is firmly held in the reconstituted cervix. It has been repaired in full thickness after excision of the torn edges. There is now no ectropion and the cervix has been restored to normal length.

15
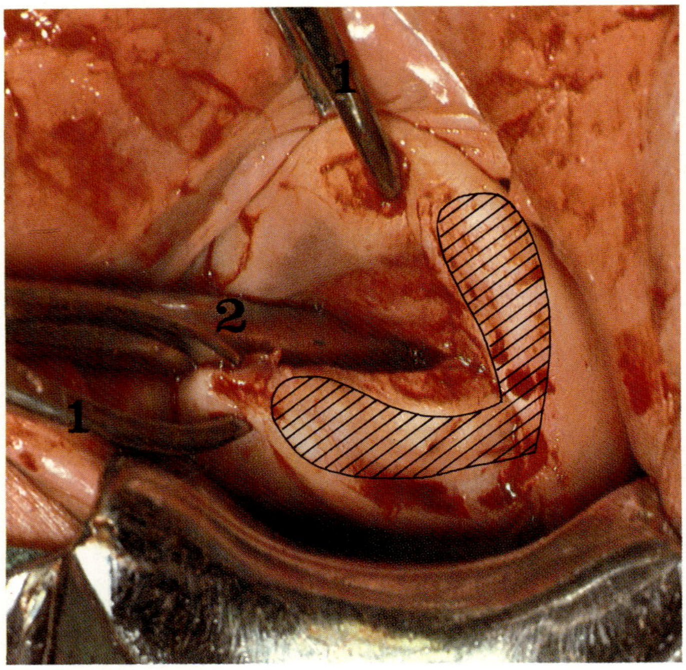

16
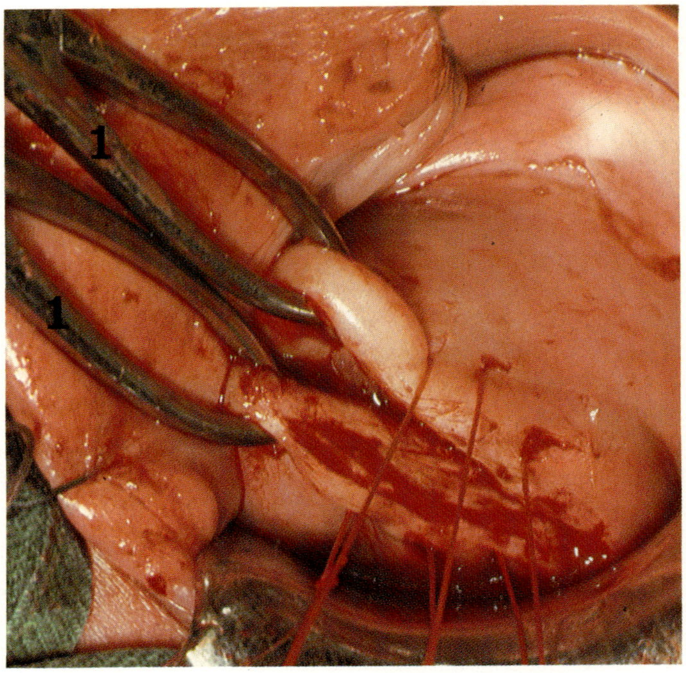

15 to 18 Principal steps in surgical repair
The cervix is held open by the tissue forceps (1) and (1) and a V-shaped incision is made through the full thickness of the cervical muscle in a direction corresponding to and parallel with the tear. A shaving of cervical tissue approximately 5 mm thick and which includes the epithelialised torn edge is removed on the left side to leave a deep V-shaped raw surface. A No. 8 Hegar dilator is placed in the uterus as a guide to the correct diameter of cervical lumen. It is numbered (2); the rawed area of the cervix is 'toned-in'. In **Figure 16** a series of full thickness matched sutures of No. 0 PGA are inserted along the edges of the V incision at

17
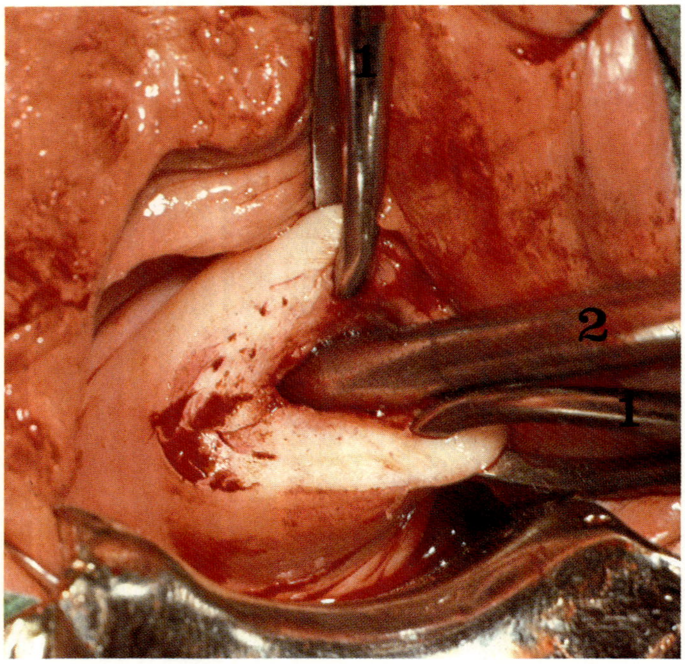

18
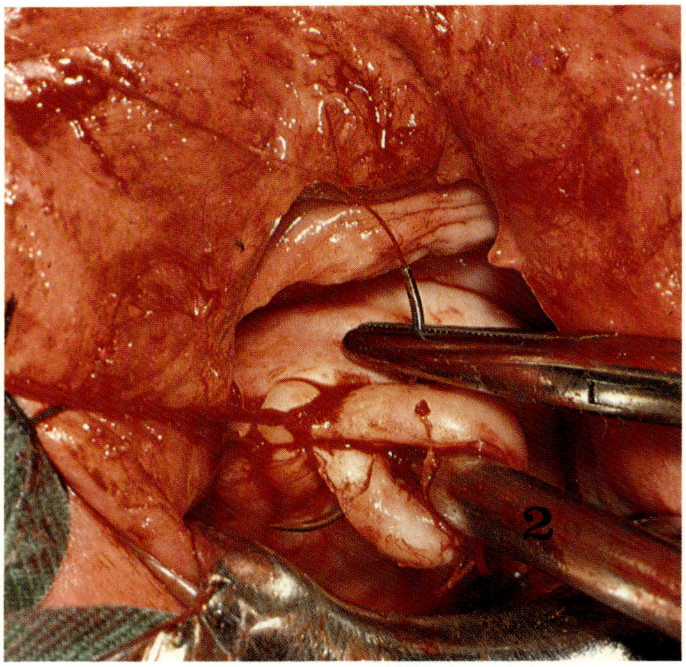

intervals of 1 cm. The stitches are then tied in turn beginning with the highest one which is placed immediately below the apex of the V. The process of making a clean raw edge for accurate suture is repeated on the right side in **Figure 17** and it is seen to be much less deep. In **Figure 18** a final fine suture of No. 00 PGA is being placed on the right side of the new external os and one is usually required on each side to give a neat effect. The dilator is then removed from the cervical canal. It is numbered (2) and the rawed area is 'toned-in'.

7: Operations on the uterus

1: Congenital abnormalities – double uterus

Some of the uterine abnormalities which may be encountered are referred to in Chapter 3; in only a small proportion of these would surgical treatment increase fertility and it has always been taught and accepted that operations are likely only to be meddlesome.

The condition of uterus didelphys is not associated with infertility but in certain other forms of double uterus repeated second trimester miscarriage is known to occur. Despite a general reluctance to use surgery experience has shown that it can overcome the problem in many of these cases and the authors have no hesitation in recommending surgical management when the necessary indications are present. With regard to that, the only true indication for operating on a double uterus is recurrent abortion in the late first trimester or early second trimester. Jones and Wheeless (1969) in a group of cases with untreated uterine duplication found that 43 per cent of 321 pregnancies resulted in abortion or premature delivery – an obviously high figure. The uterine abnormality is held to be responsible for varying degrees of menorrhagia, dysmenorrhoea, dyspareunia and primary infertility in addition to the miscarriages but these symptoms rarely provide even a relative indication for surgery. There is one point that should be remembered and that is the possibility of associated urinary tract anomalies and particularly renal agenesis. It is only prudent to have an I.V. urogram done in all cases being considered for surgery.

These abnormalities may well increase in frequency in the future as it is becoming obvious that a long-term effect of maternal ingestion of diethylstilboestrol is that of congenital uterine abnormalities in the offspring. The subject has recently been reviewed by Kaufman et al (1980).

Results of surgical treatment

It would be satisfying if one could provide convincing figures to support the advocacy of surgical treatment in such cases but there are few reports. The most helpful study we have found is again that of Jones and Wheeless (1969). A group of 53 patients had been studied for reproductive difficulties and had been found to have a double uterus. All of these were treated by hormones initially and 31 of them had at least one child following such therapy. The remaining 22 patients in this group had reconstructive uterine

1

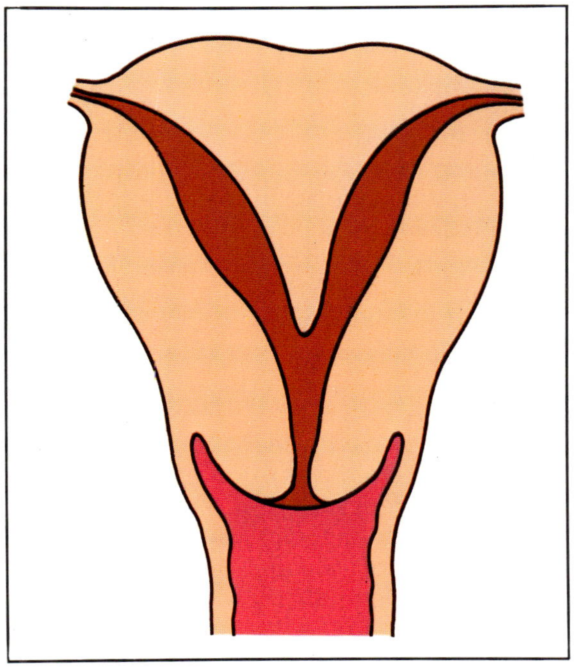

2

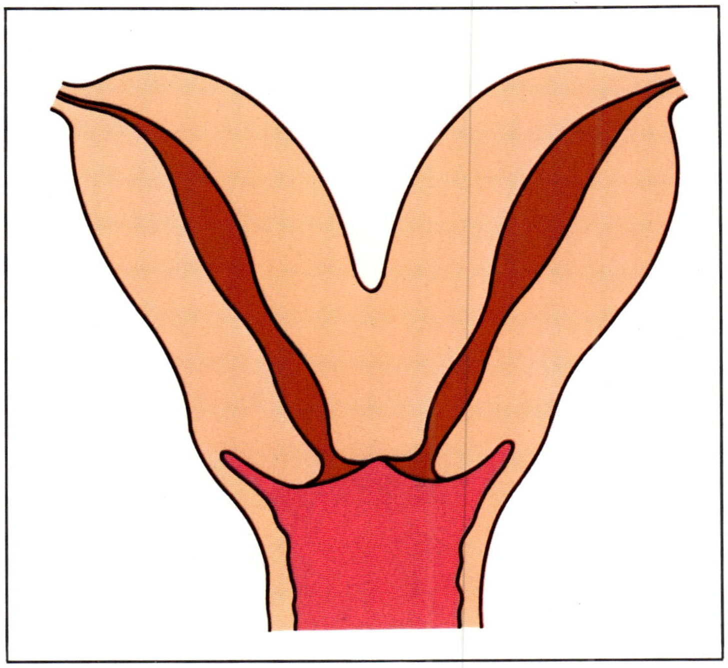

1 and 2 Types of double uterus considered for surgery
Figure 1 shows the standard appearance of a septate uterus which is suitable for a Jones type operation as outlined in **Figure 3** (page 56). **Figure 2** shows a bicornuate uterus which presents the frequently encountered and sometimes difficult question of whether it is actually unicornis or bicornis. Operation is contraindicated unless it can be clearly established that it is unicollis and preoperative investigation must be very precise on this point. The diagrammatic example shown here is borderline. **Figure 4** (page 56) shows a very obvious uterus bicornis unicollis for which the Strassman operation is ideal.

3

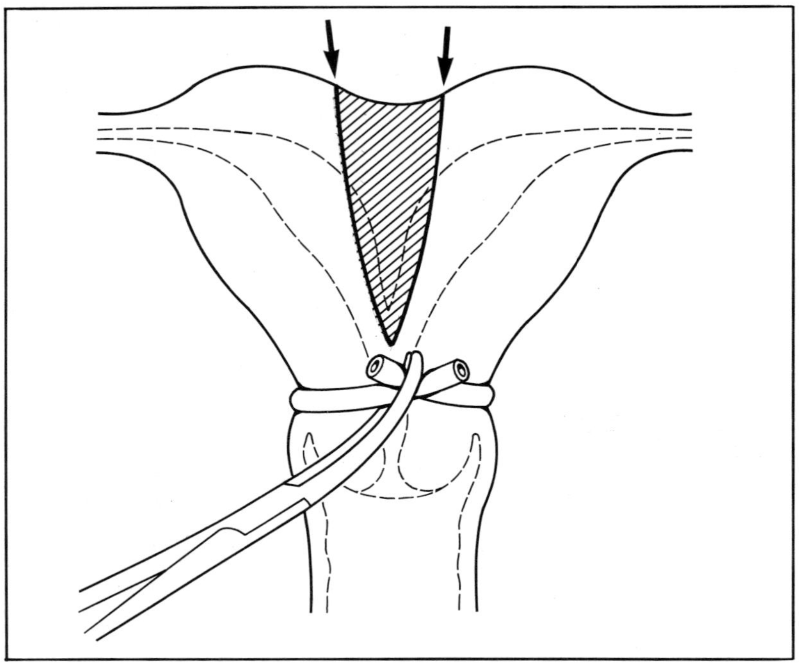

3 Diagram of plan for Jones operation

4

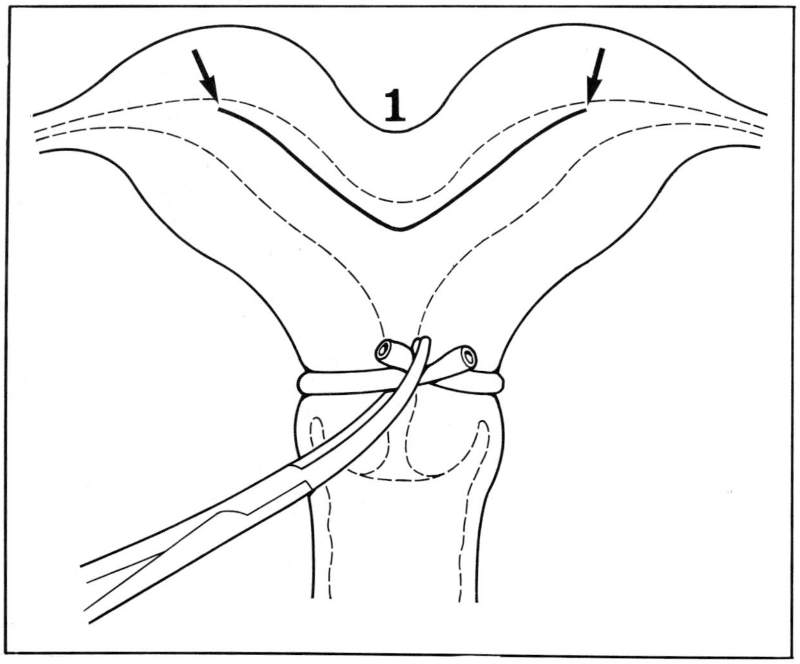

4 Diagram of plan for Strassman operation

surgery; 16 of them had a history of 3 or more miscarriages. The 22 had collectively 86 prior pregnancies of which none had gone to term. Following operation 16 of the 22 achieved a living child (73 per cent success rate) and there were altogether a total of 37 pregnancies of which 25 went to term, 3 were born prematurely and 9 miscarried. Further and more recent information is obviously required; for what it is worth the firm clinical impression of the authors and their colleagues is that these patients should have the benefit of operation.

Choice of operation

There are two types of double uterus which may require such surgery, the septate uterus (**Figure 1**) and the bicornuate uterus (**Figure 2**). In both instances the aim of the operation is to unify the two halves of the uterus by a plastic procedure and the general principles of the various operations are not very different. Strassman was the pioneer in this field although many believe that the operation he devised has now been superseded. The Jones procedure is the favourite one at the present time but there are many necessary modifications since each case presents particular and individual problems.

Figure 3 shows diagrammatically a toned-in narrow sector of uterine tissue which is removed with the septum in the Jones operation; the raw surfaces are thereafter approximated to reconstitute the uterus with an unimpeded cavity. **Figure 4** illustrates the unsuitability of such a strategy for a true double uterus. In the Strassman operation the intercornual sulcus ((1) in **Figure 4**) must be incised transversely (between arrows) so as to preserve all available uterine muscle tissue for the junction of the two narrow cavities. **Figure 5** is a diagrammatic impression of the uterine outline following operation with the vertical anteroposterior sagittal suture line indicating where the two halves are united. The completed appearance is usually more satisfying in the septate type; there tends to be some uterine distortion following operation on the more severe lesion.

In subsequent pages a Jones type of operation for a classical case of septate uterus is described and illustrated. An equally representative case of double uterus – bicornuate with two separate cavities and a single cervix – was particularly suitable for a Strassman operation and that procedure is also illustrated and described.

5

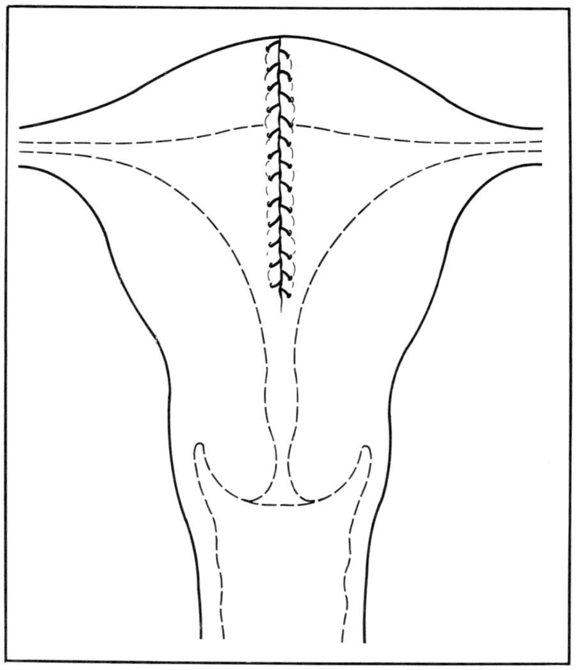

5 Diagram of uterine appearance following operation

Jones operation

Surgical technique

The necessary incisions into the muscle must encounter the rich coronary arterial blood supply to the uterus (see **Figure 9**) and even a limited amount of blood at the operation site interferes with the precise muscle suturing which has to be done.

Application of a rubber tourniquet around the uterus at the level of the isthmus satisfactorily occludes the uterine vessels and plastic covered bulldog clamps on the infundibulo-pelvic ligaments deprive the area of its alternative blood source (see **Figure 9**). A locally injected vasoconstrictor solution may be added to these measures. It should be used sparingly in the line of incision and will control small blood vessels in an amount that does not distort the uterine wall.

The initial steps of the operation are to fix the uterus in position and then outline a wedge-shaped excision over the fundus uteri; it is in the sagittal plane with its ends on the anterior and posterior uterine walls (**Figure 3**). It is placed centrally and includes the septum in the wedge or sector of uterine muscle to be excised. The uterine cavity is previously packed and distended with gauze soaked in methylene blue or other dye so that one cuts down onto a supporting and easily recognised cushion of gauze which delineates the uterine cavity on each side. The raw uterine muscle surfaces are bisected parallel to their serous edge by a scalpel cutting to a depth of 1.5 cm so that a combined muscle and endometrial layer can be approximated before suturing the remainder of the uterine wall thickness with a muscular and then a sero-muscular layer.

The operation is straightforward but there is one particular hazard. It is very easy to be left with insufficient muscle tissue medial to each cornu. This means that the new fundus will be too narrow and it particularly endangers the interstitial portion of the tubes which may be caught up in and occluded by the uterine muscle stitches. See **Figures 14–21** (pages 60–61) re correct placing of incisions.

Stage I: Vaginal preparation

6

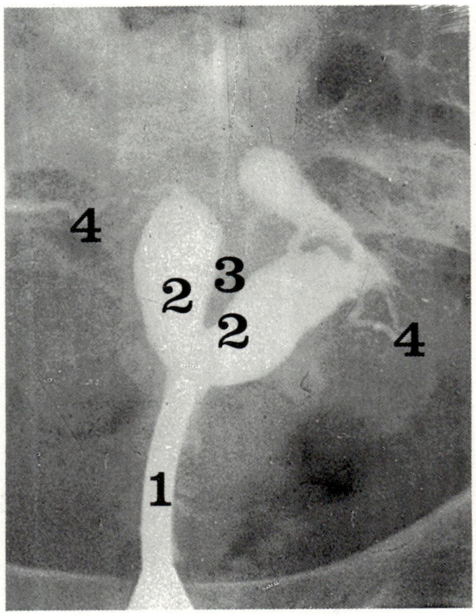

7

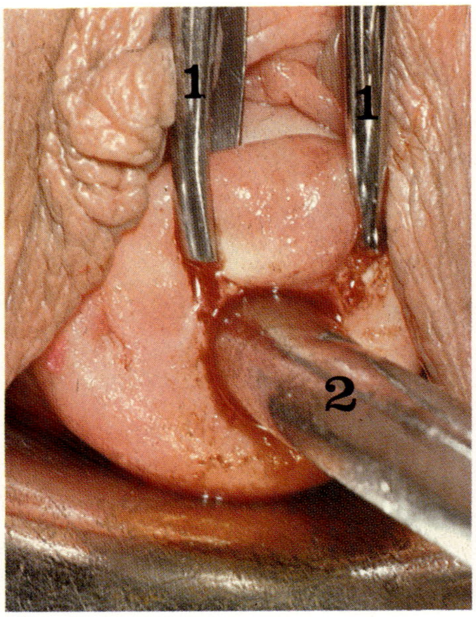

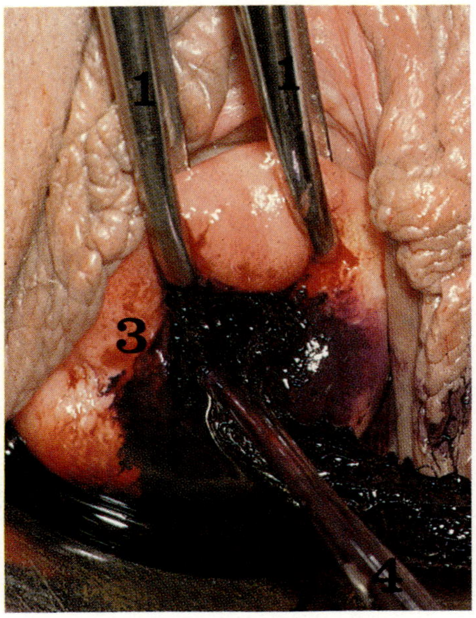

8

6 Hysterosalpingogram
The opaque medium instilled through the cannula in the cervical canal (1) outlines the cavity of the uterus (2) and shows the septum (3) in the anteroposterior view. The tubes (4) are patent and there is peritoneal spill.

7 and 8 Packing uterine cavity with dye-soaked gauze
With the patient in the lithotomy position the bladder is emptied by catheter. The anterior lip of the cervix is held in tissue forceps (1) and (1) and dilated to approximately 18 Hegar (2) as in **Figure 7**. The dilator is withdrawn and the uterine cavity packed tightly with ribbon gauze soaked in methylene blue or similar dye (3) and introduced with sinus forceps (4) as shown in **Figure 8**. This is done carefully and to maximum capacity to form a soft cushion of gauze on to which the uterine incisions are made.

9

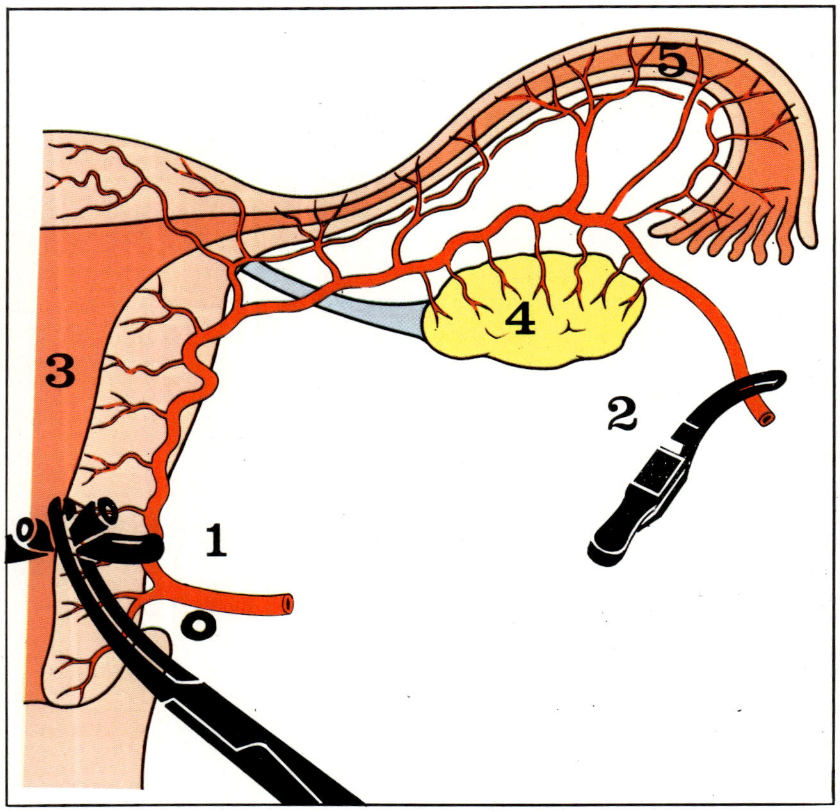

Stage II: Ensuring a bloodless field

A diagram of the uterine blood supply and the points at which the circulation can most effectively be interrupted are shown in **Figure 9**.

9 Plan for interruption of arterial blood supply to uterus
The tourniquet at isthmal level occludes the uterine artery (1) while the bulldog clamp on the infundibulo-pelvic ligament controls the ovarian artery (2). The uterus is numbered (3), the ovary (4) and the tube (5).

10

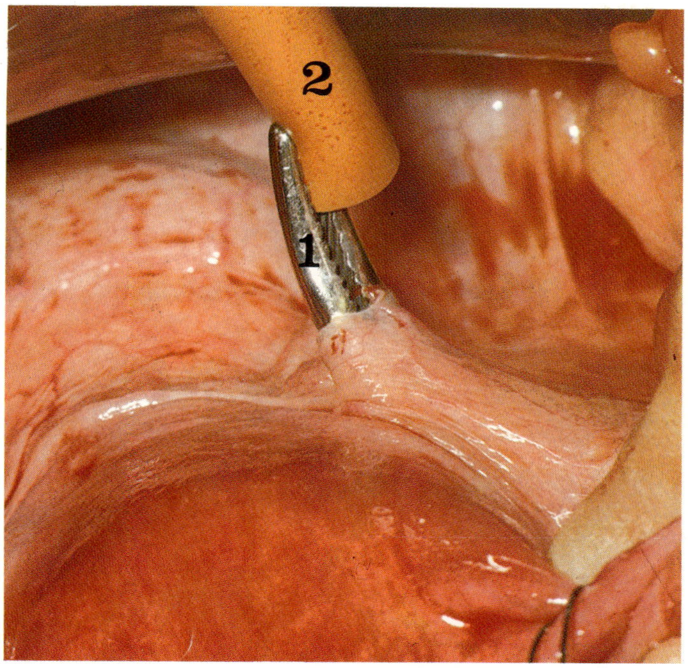

11

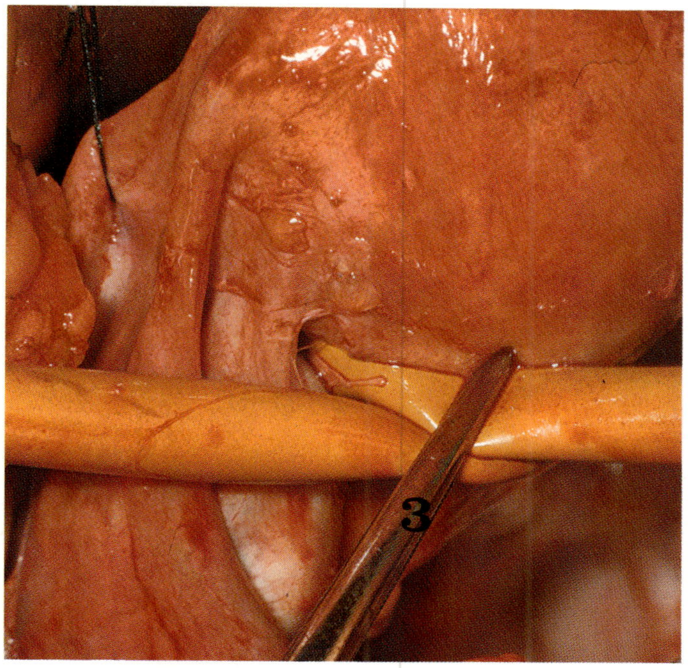

10 and 11 Applying tourniquet to uterine arteries
A rubber tourniquet is applied to the uterus at the level of the isthmus to compress the uterine vessels and in **Figure 10** a Miles Phillips' forceps (1) pierces the broad ligament postero-anteriorly at the isthmal level and grasps one end of a 12 mm rubber tube or tourniquet (2). The forceps is at a distance of 1.5 cm from the lateral aspect of the uterus to avoid damaging the uterine vessels. The same is done on the left side and the ends of the tourniquet are drawn tight to compress the uterine arteries. The two overlapping ends of the tourniquet are clamped together at that tension by the forceps (3) in **Figure 11**.

12

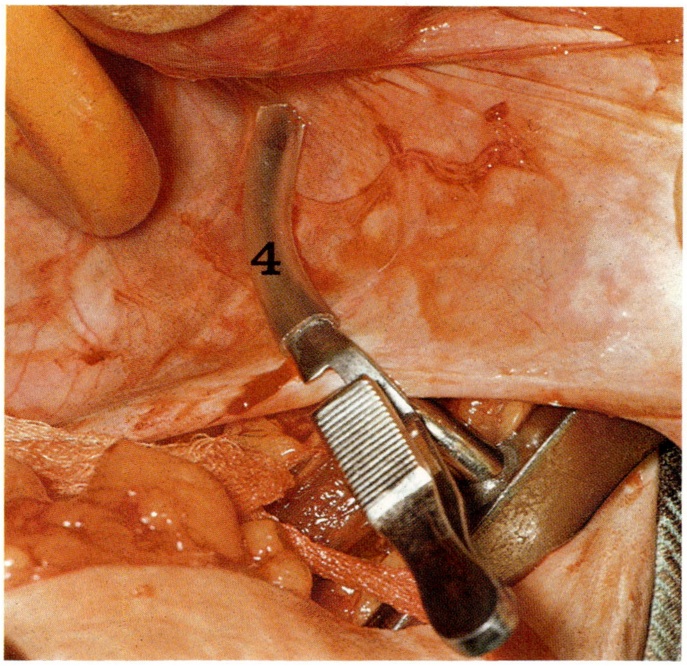

13

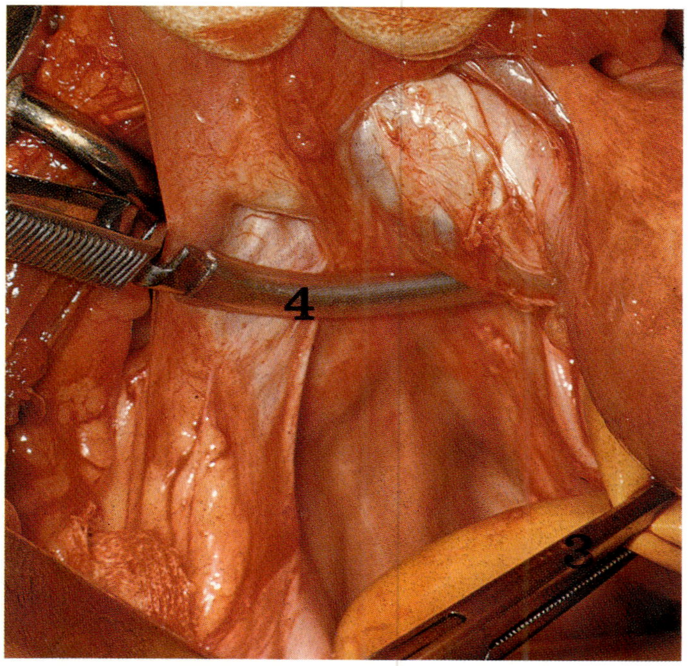

12 and 13 Applying clamps to ovarian arteries
Plastic-shod bulldog clamps are used to interrupt the ovarian arteries. In **Figure 12** a clamp (4) is applied to the free edge of the infundibulo-pelvic ligament and overlapping it by the full length of its 2.5 cm jaws. A similar clamp is being applied to the right infundibulo-pelvic fold in **Figure 13**.

In this case there were some fine periovarian adhesions present. Tubal patency was confirmed but division of the adhesions will be performed to improve potential ovum uptake.

Stage III: Fundal incision to excise uterine septum

14

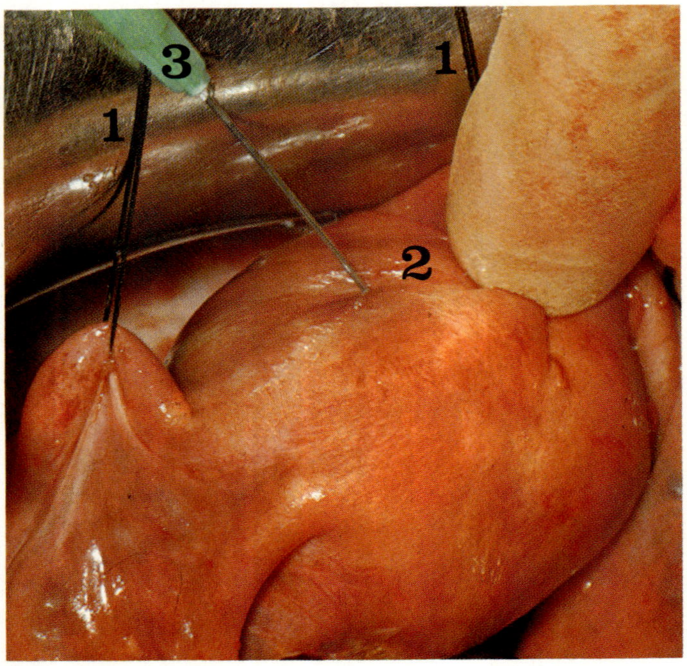

15

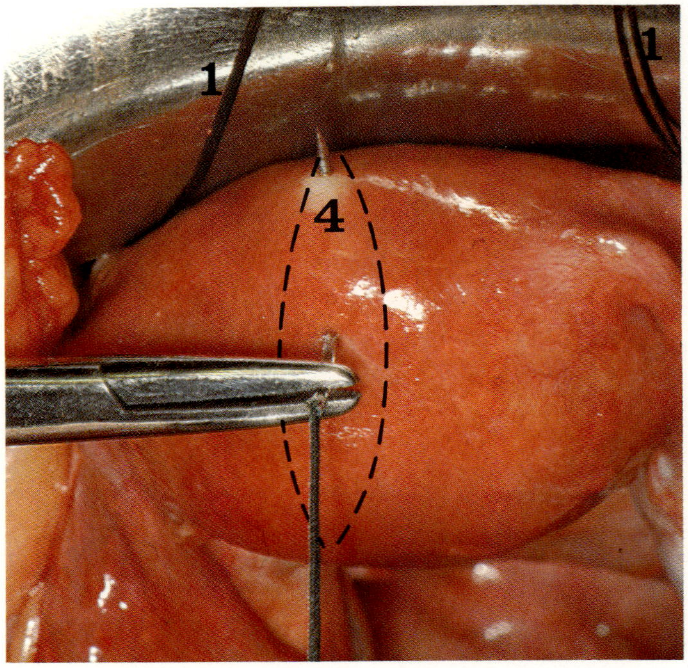

14 and 15
The uterus is held anteriorly by traction sutures on the attachments of the round ligaments (1) and (1) in **Figure 14** and an indentation (2) is seen on the uterine fundus indicating the site of the septum. A vasoconstrictive solution* is being injected (3) antero-posteriorly into the fundus to augment the other measures in ensuring a bloodless field. In **Figure 15** a stout mersilene suture (4) is placed antero-posteriorly at the centre of the indentation to elevate the sector of uterine wall which is to be removed. The broken lines indicate the placing of the subsequent excision.

16

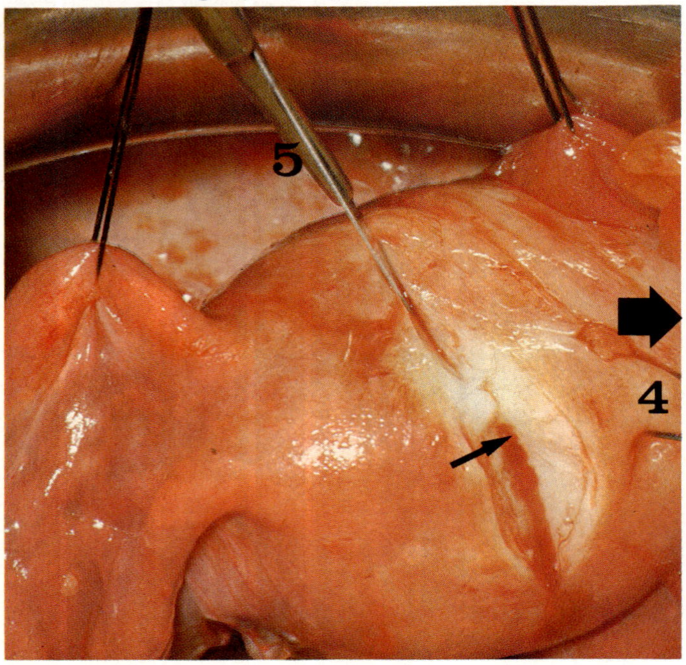

17

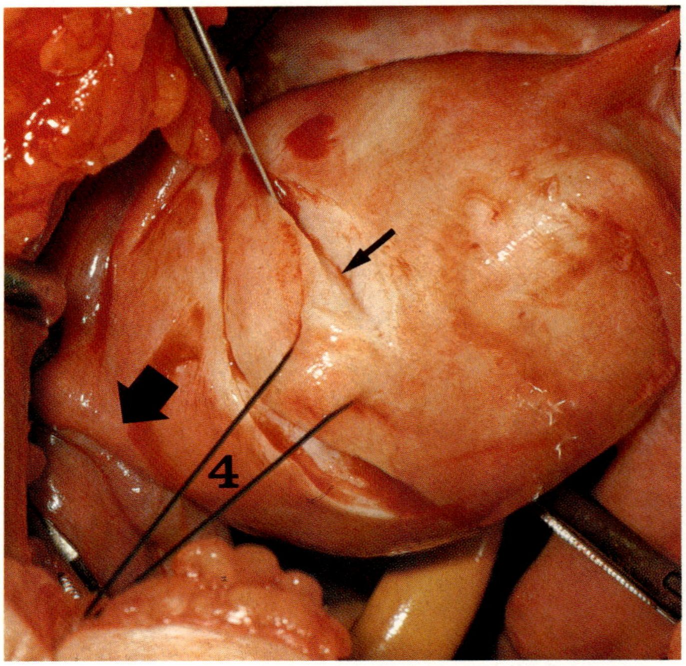

16 and 17
With the fundal stitch held to the right (broad arrow) the scalpel (5) makes a left-sided incision which slopes slightly inwards deep into the uterine wall in **Figure 16** (arrowed) and with the stitch held to the left in **Figure 17** a matching incision is made on the right side to the same depth (arrowed). The ends of the two incisions meet anteriorly and posteriorly on the uterine wall 2.5 cm from the fundus. The incisions have thus outlined a sector similar to that of an orange and it is anticipated that the septum will be included in that block of tissue since it must lie under the indentation at the fundus.

*Vasopressin 1 u per ml of normal saline.

Stage IV: Excision of fundal sector and uterine septum

18

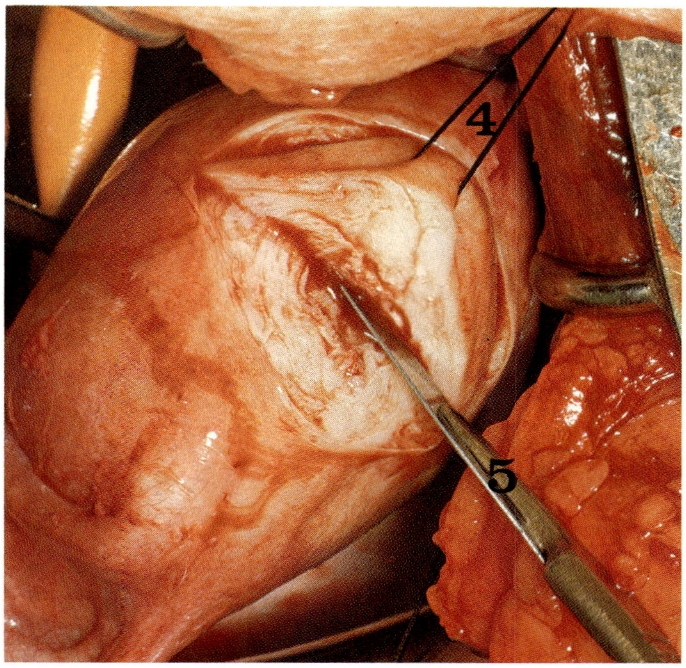

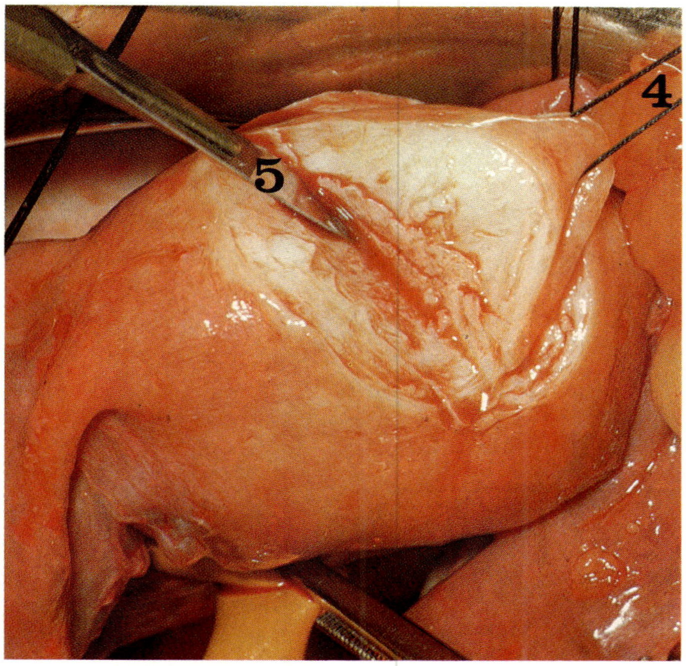

19

18 to 21

As the two incisions are deepened on to the gauze packing in **Figure 18** entry into the endometrial cavity is indicated by the escape of the dye into the wound. The muscle sector is drawn up by its supporting stitch (4) in the direction of the arrow on **Figure 19** and is finally freed by the scalpel (5). In **Figure 20** the central sector has been removed but there is an irregular area in the depth of the V incision towards the left side (6) which is clearly part of the septum. This is being shaved off with the scalpel in the area indicated by fine arrows. It is much better to limit the width of the sector and be prepared to remove part of the septum in this way than to take a wide sector and possibly endanger the cornual areas when reconstituting the fundus. **Figure 21** shows the fundal sector cleanly removed with flat raw muscle surfaces (7) and (7) and an elliptical opening into the fundus of the endometrial cavity.

20

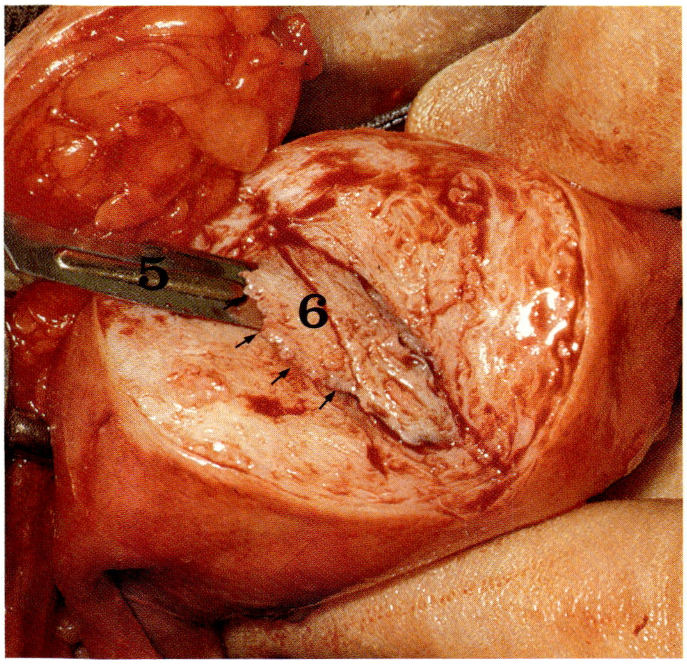

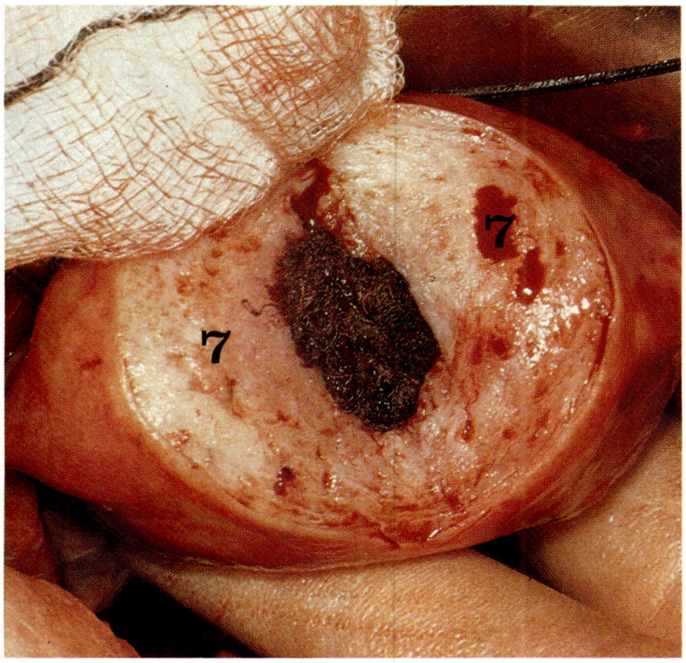

21

Stage V: Linear incision of uterine wall to allow of three-layer closure

22

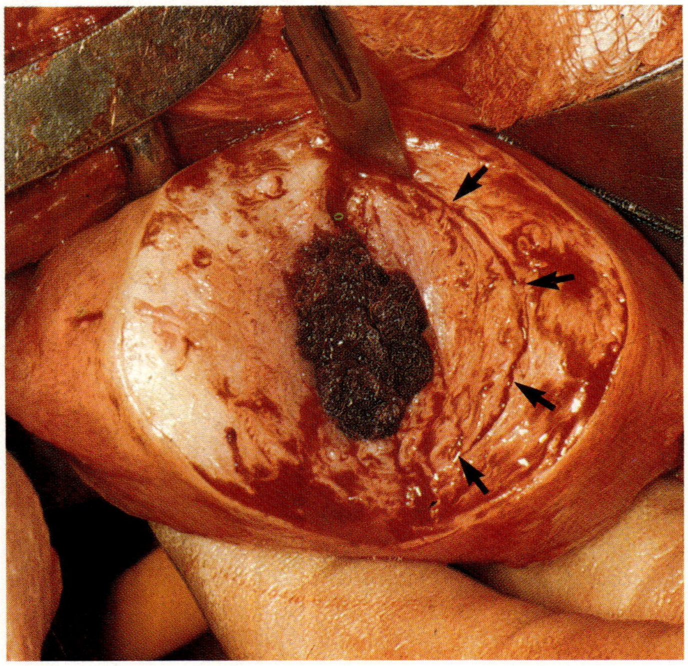

23

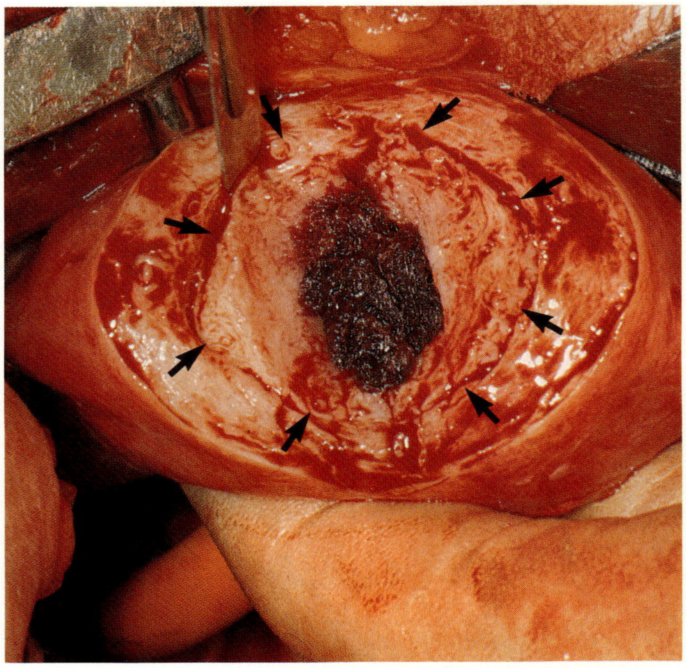

24

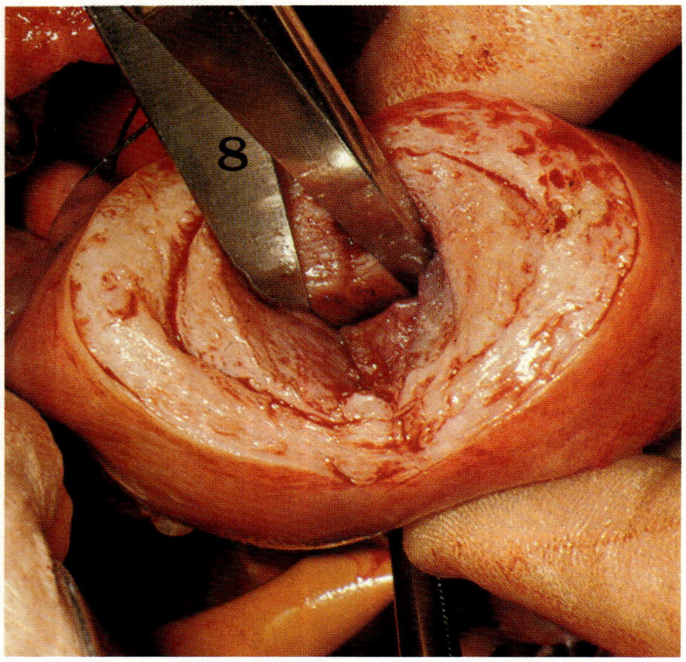

22 to 24
The myometrium is thick in this area so that a single layer closure would be imprecise and probably result in endometrial irregularity. A half-circle incision is therefore made on each side which bisects the raw muscle surfaces as it runs parallel to the serosal edge. The incision is to a depth of 1.5 cm and allows of a three-layer closure. The right-sided incision is seen and arrowed in **Figure 22**; the circle has been completed in **Figure 23**. **Figure 24** shows the uterus ready for closure immediately the gauze pack is withdrawn vaginally. The blades of the curved scissors (8) are opened to display the entry to the endometrial cavity.

Stage VI: Three-layer closure of uterine fundus

25

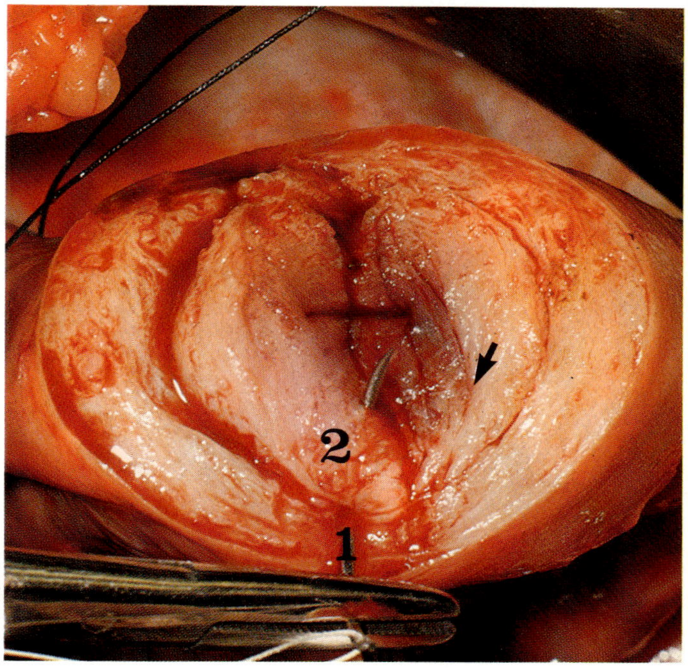

26

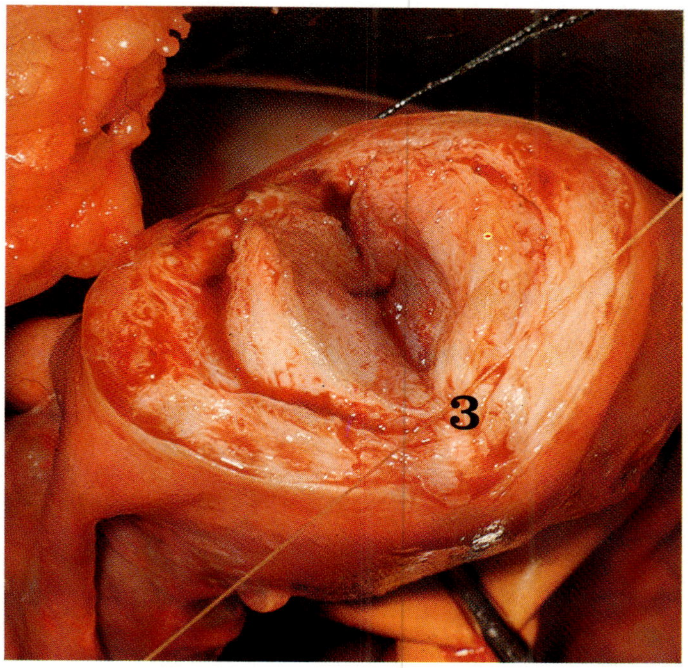

25 to 28 Suture of musculo-endometrial layer of the uterine wall

In **Figure 25** the round-bodied needle (1) carrying a No. 00 PGA suture picks up musculo-endometrial layer (2) on the left side. Only the muscle element is included in the stitch so that the endometrial surface of the uterus remains smooth and untraumatised where the epithelium is approximated. The corresponding edge is picked up on the right side where arrowed and the anchor stitch is shown tied off in **Figure 26** (3). A similar anchor stitch at the other end of the wound is numbered (4) in **Figure 27** and the original suture (3) proceeds as a continuous one which avoids endometrial inclusion. This continuous suture is complete and is being tied off in **Figure 28**.

27

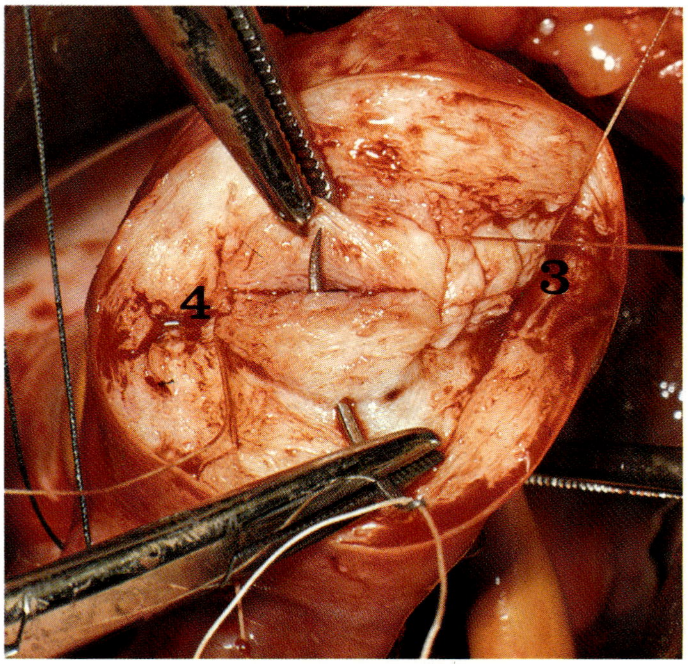

28

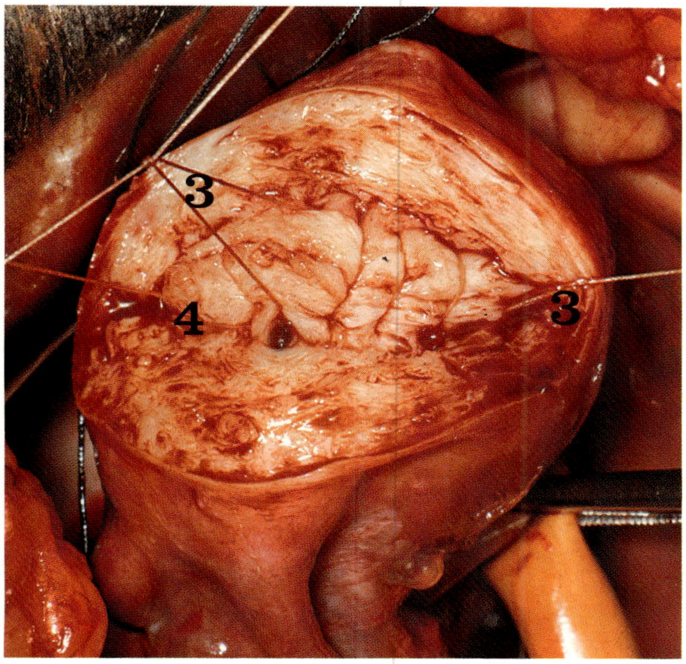

29

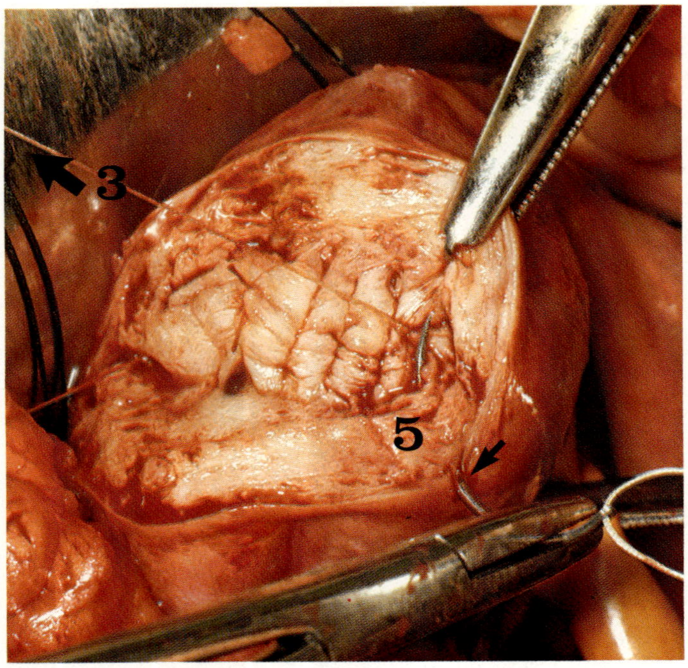

30

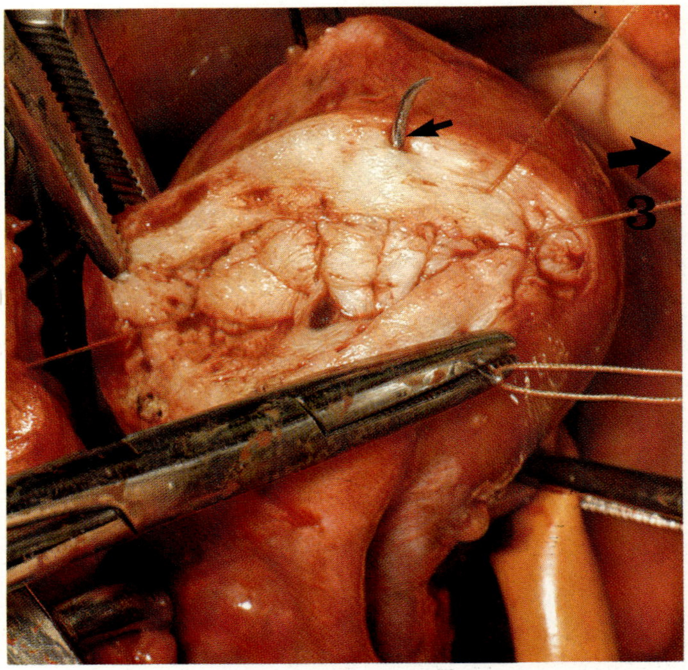

31

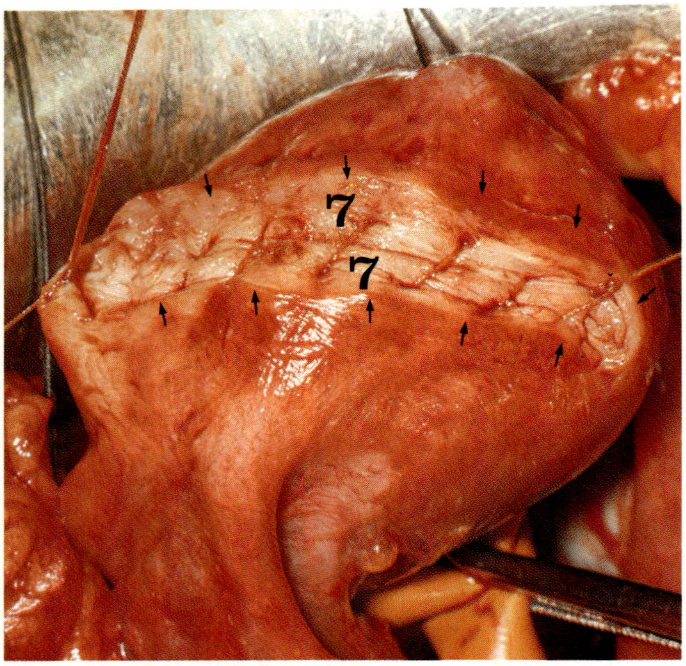

29 to 31 Suture of main muscular layer of uterine wall
The outer half of the bisected uterine wall is now closed by a continuous No. 00 PGA suture. In **Figure 29** the anchor stitch of the first layer (3) is put on the stretch to display the placing of the first stitch in the second layer. The needle omits the sero-muscular surface area to a depth of about 5 mm (where arrowed) but takes a firm bite of the muscle layer (5) and emerges in the incision space between the two layers. The needle then enters the opposite space and goes on to pick up a corresponding bite of muscle on that side. In **Figure 30** the method of continuous closure is clearly seen with a sero-muscular depth of about 5 mm omitted from the suture (arrowed). The result of this is seen in **Figure 31** where the second or muscle layer suture is complete but the sero-muscular edge is gaping and requires a further or third layer closure. The still unsutured muscle surface is numbered 7 and the peritoneal edge is indicated by fine arrows.

32

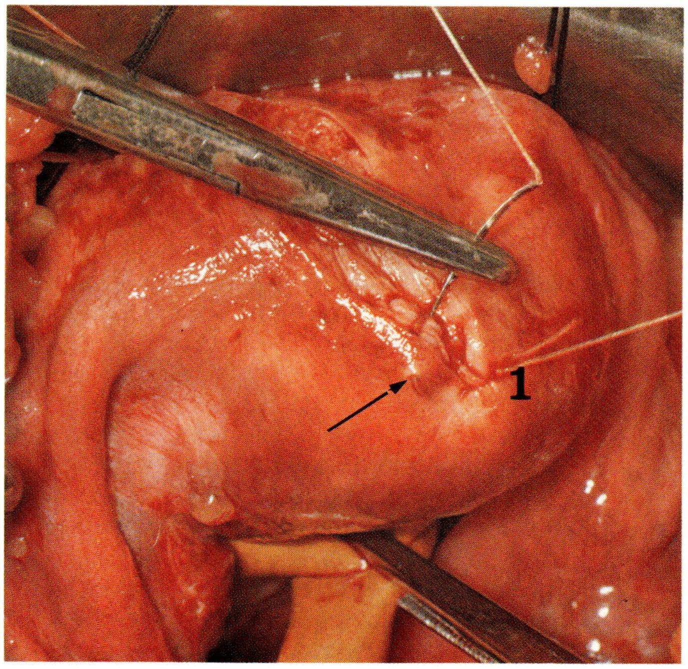

33

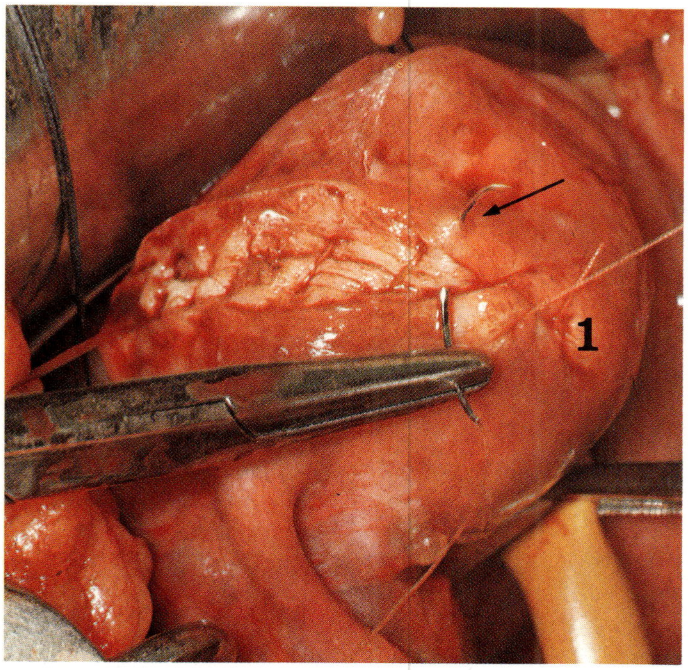

34

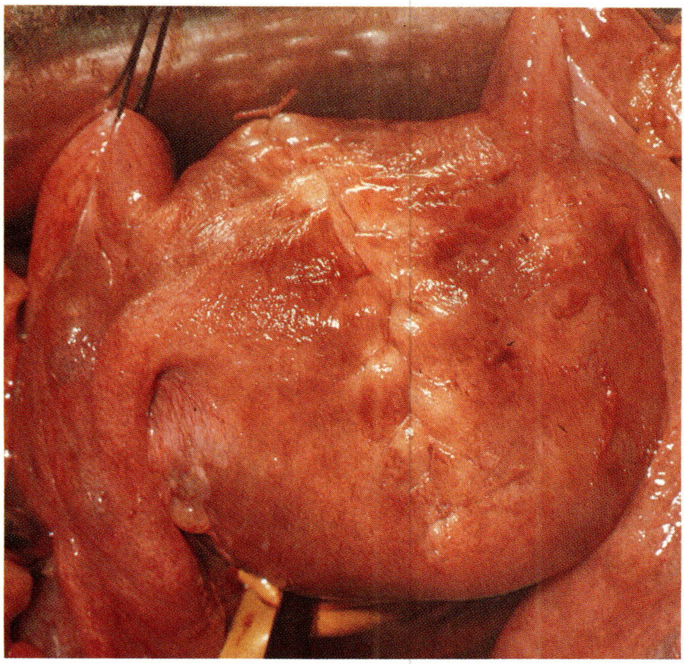

32 to 34 Suture of sero-muscular layer of uterine wall
An inverting type of suture is used to firmly approximate the edges while at the same time inverting them over the suture to give a completely peritonised surface which will not adhere to adjacent structures. In **Figure 32** an anchor stitch has been placed at (1). The needle carrying the No. 00 PGA suture picks up the left sero-muscular edge from within outwards at full depth and emerges 5 mm from the peritoneal edge (arrowed). In **Figure 33** the needle changes direction and transfixes the corresponding right-sided edge from within outwards in the same fashion. When the suture is tightened the edge is rolled together with peritoneum against peritoneum. This stitch is continued across the fundus and the end result is seen in **Figure 34**.

The operation is now complete and the uterus has lost its fundal indentation but retained its shape without appreciable narrowing between the cornua. The uterine tourniquet and ovarian vessel clamps are now removed and any bleeding point on the line of suture controlled by a very fine mattress stitch.

Strassman operation

Surgical technique

There is a general impression that the Strassman operation has been replaced by the various modifications of the Jones procedure but there are occasions when it still appears to be the most suitable operation. Strassman claimed that the operation was indicated in cases of bicornuate uterus accompanied by menorrhagia, sterility, dyspareunia, premature labour or habitual abortion. Modern opinion would consider that only the last of these is an admissible indication and would doubt if a bicornuate or uterus didelphys is ever the cause of infertility.

In the case described here, the patient had a history of recurrent abortion and operation appeared to be indicated. The anatomical features of the abnormality suggested that the Strassman operation was the most suitable procedure.

The line of the incision in the inter-cornual sulcus has already been indicated diagrammatically on **Figure 4**. No muscle wall tissue should be sacrificed because it is all required to construct an adequately sized uterus. The uterine blood supply is controlled as in the Jones operation. The uterus is steadied as previously and a deep transverse incision made on to the firm column of dyed gauze packing in each uterine horn. The surgeon may encounter a vesico-rectal fold of fascia running antero-posteriorly between the two uteri and that would be included in the incision. It is unlikely however that the operation would be indicated in a case of such severity. When both endometrial cavities have been entered and the packing removed any remaining lower segment division is divided with scissors. The raw cut surface of each uterus is bisected with the scalpel parallel to the serous edge and to a depth of 1.5 cm as in the Jones operation. The cut muscle edges are then joined in three layers as previously.

The patient in the case described below had had three mid-trimester miscarriages and has carried two pregnancies successfully to term since the operation.

35

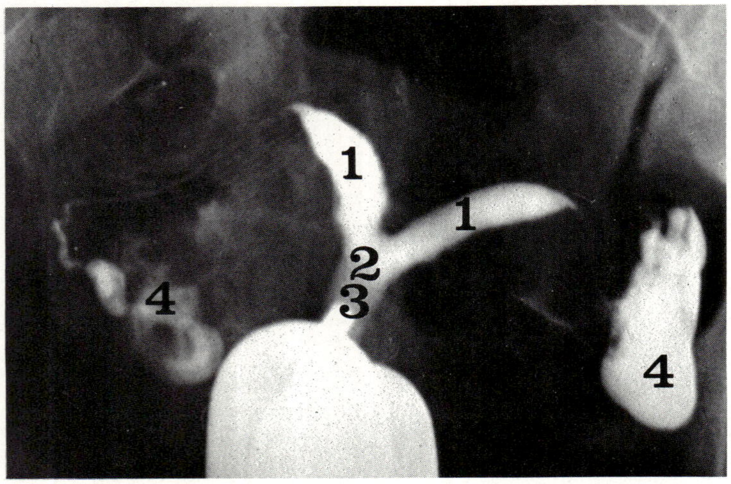

36

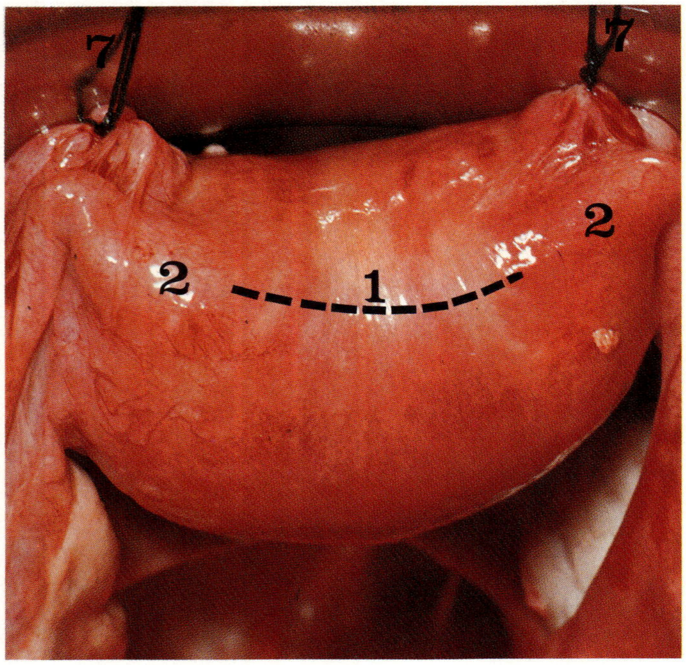

35 Hysterosalpingogram
The x-ray shows appearances typical of a bicornuate uterus. There are two endometrial cavities (1) and (1) and a single lower uterine segment (2) and cervical canal (3). Both tubes are patent with peritoneal spill seen on both sides (4) and (4).

36 Clinical appearance preoperatively; planning of fundal incision
The uterus is held forward to display the fundus by traction mersilene sutures (7) and (7) through the inner ends of the round ligaments. The abnormality is well marked in this instance but not severe; the fundus of the uterus (1) is very wide with central dipping and the cornua (2) and (2) are narrow. There is no sign of a recto-vesical fold and the uterus is unicollis. The transverse fundal incision to open into the two cavities is indicated by the broken line. Note particularly that it is no longer than absolutely necessary and keeps well clear of the cornua and the interstitial portion of the tube. Diagrams sometimes show a too generous incision which can result in dangers to the interstitial tube when splitting the muscle and suturing the uterus.

Stage I: Incision of uterine fundus

37

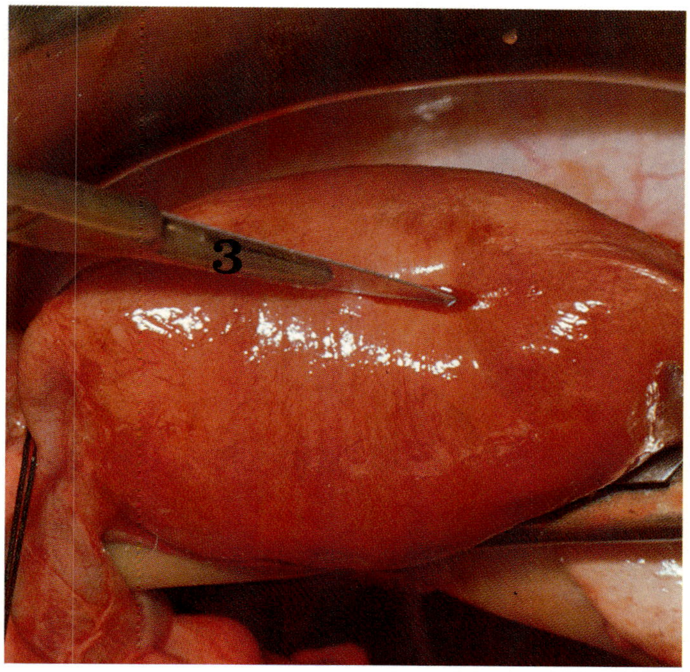

38

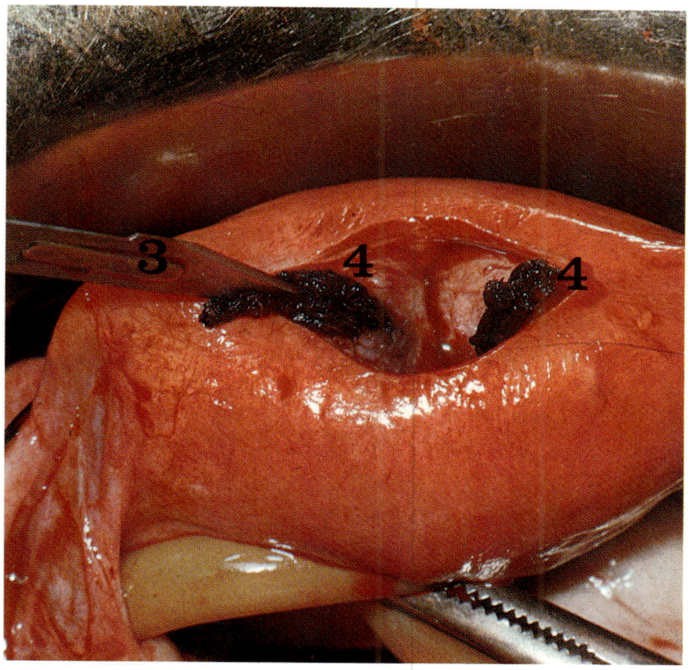

37 and 38
In **Figure 37** the scalpel (3) incises the fundus of the uterus transversely where planned. The surgeon cuts down boldly on to the gauze cushion in the cavities and these are revealed in **Figure 38** with the dye outlining each very clearly (4) and (4).

Stage II: Incision of remaining interuterine division

39

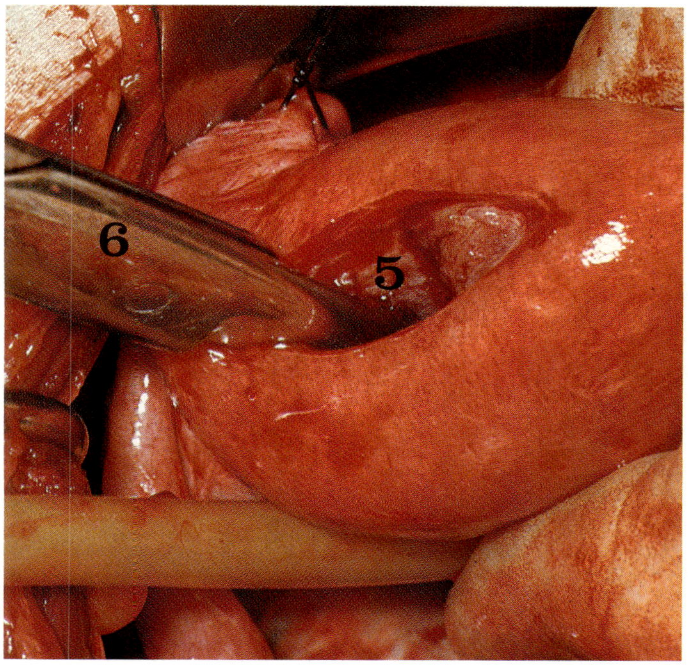

40

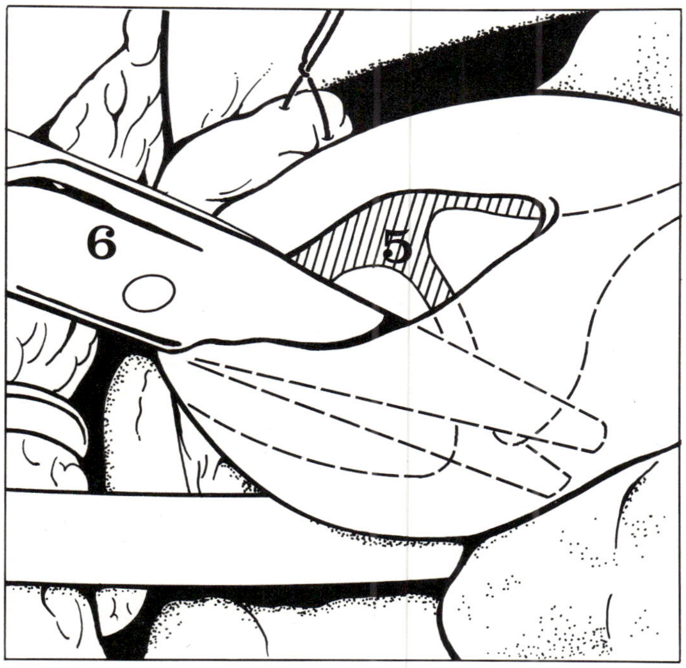

39 and 40
The area (5) is a muscle division rather than a septum and it is necessary to incise it centrally and without loss of tissue as far down as the common lower uterine segment. This is shown being done with the scissors (6) in **Figure 39** and the diagram in **Figure 40** indicates how the two halves fall away from each other to let the new cavity balloon outwards both anteriorly and posteriorly to assume a wider and more normal uterine configuration.

Stage III: Linear incision of uterine wall to allow of three layer closure

41

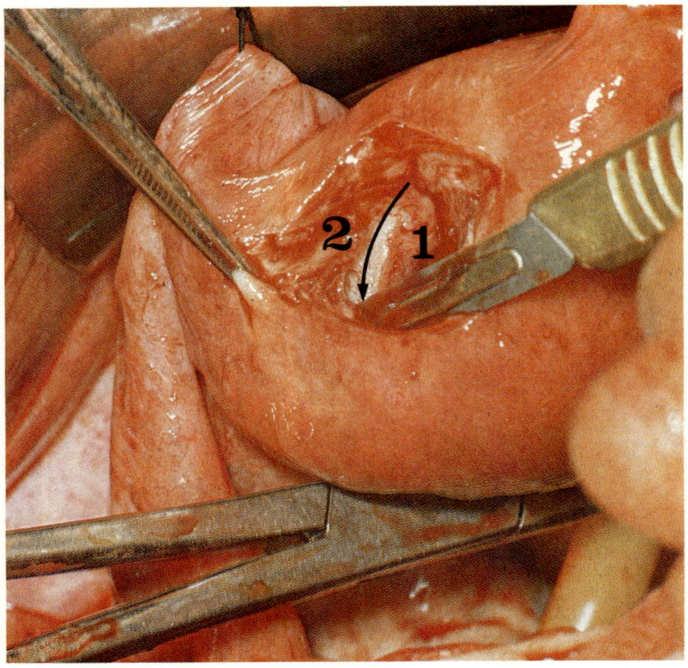

42

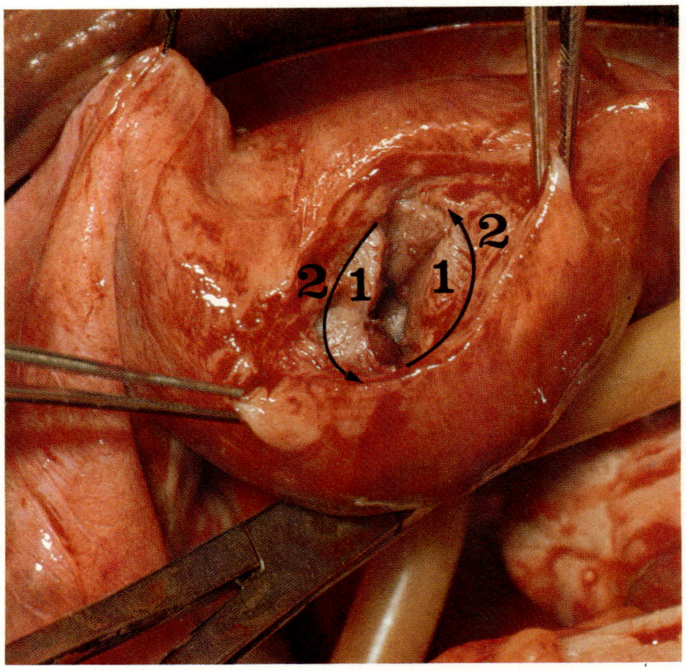

41 and 42
The raw uterine muscle surface is bisected circularly to a depth of 1.5 cm in a line running parallel to the cut peritoneal edge as described on page 62. The scalpel is making the incision in **Figure 41** and the two layers of muscle have been fashioned in **Figure 42**. The lines of the incision are indicated by fine arrows; the deeper musculo-endometrial layer is numbered (1), the main muscle thickness (2).

Stage IV: Three-layer closure of uterus

43

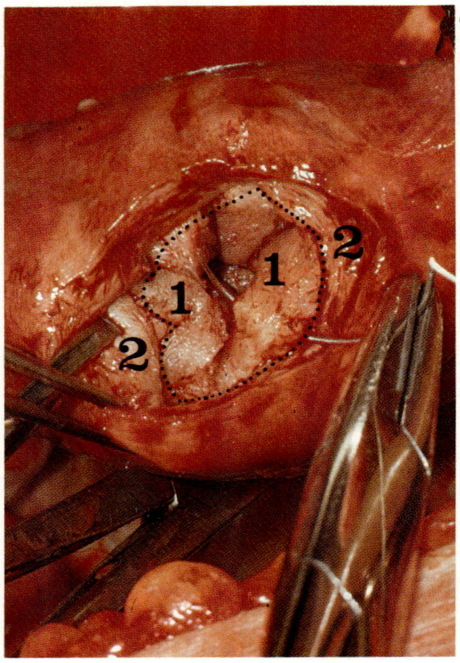

44

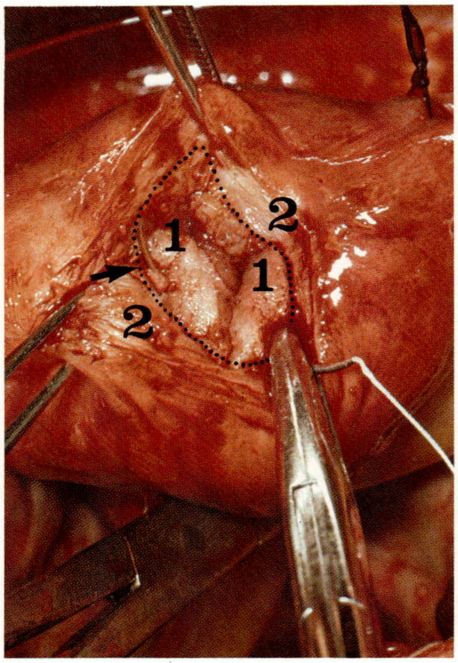

45

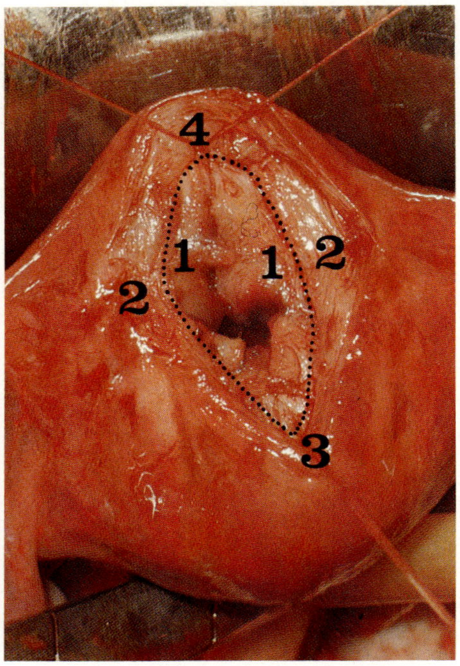

43 to 45
The first bite taken by the needle in suturing the musculo-endometrial layer is shown in **Figure 43**, and as previously noted only muscle tissue is included so that there is no involvement of the endometrium. In **Figure 44** the needle picks up the corresponding shoulder of muscle on the left side in the same fashion to complete the stitch in the posterior angle of the wound. In **Figure 45** the leaves of the deeper layer of muscle (1) are positioned ready for suture between the posterior (4) and the anterior (3) anchor stitches. The dotted line follows the incision which provides for the 3-layer closure.

47

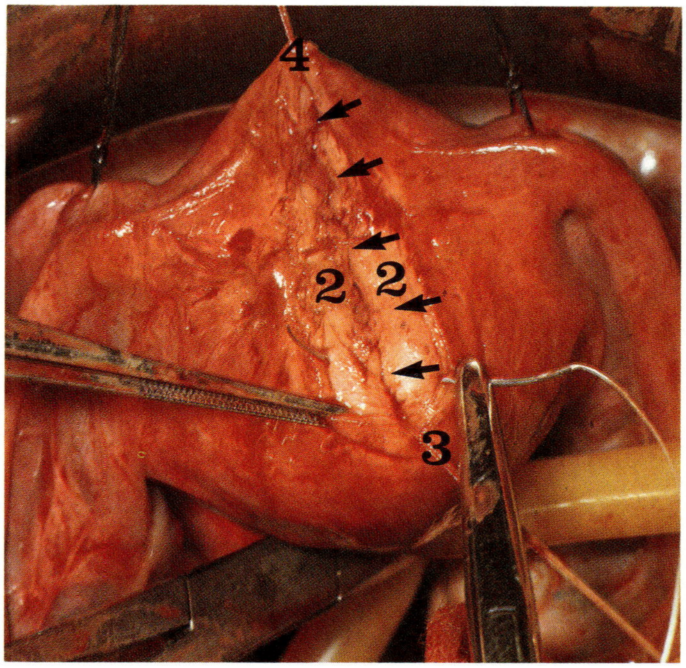

46

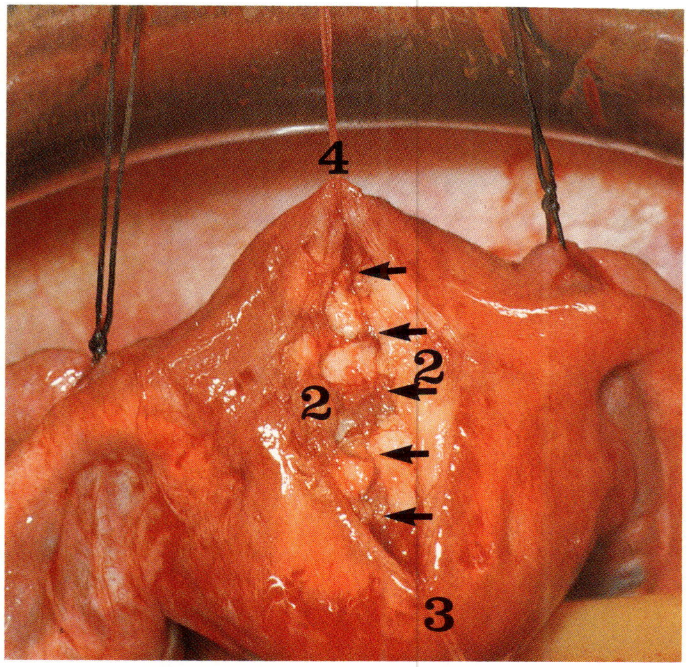

46 and 47
Note that although **Figure 46** is on the right side of the page it shows a stage of the operation which precedes that in **Figure 47**. In **46** the leaves of the deep layer of uterine muscle have been approximated by a series of sutures (arrowed). **Figure 47** shows the main muscle layer partially closed and as noted previously the needle leaves a muscle depth of 5 mm at the serous edge to be included with the peritoneal stitch. The sutures placed and about to be placed in this layer are indicated by arrows.

48

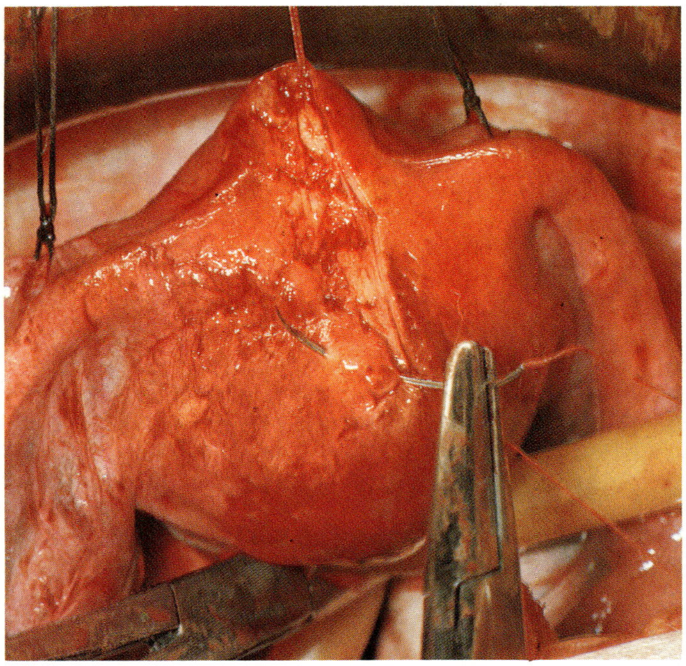

49

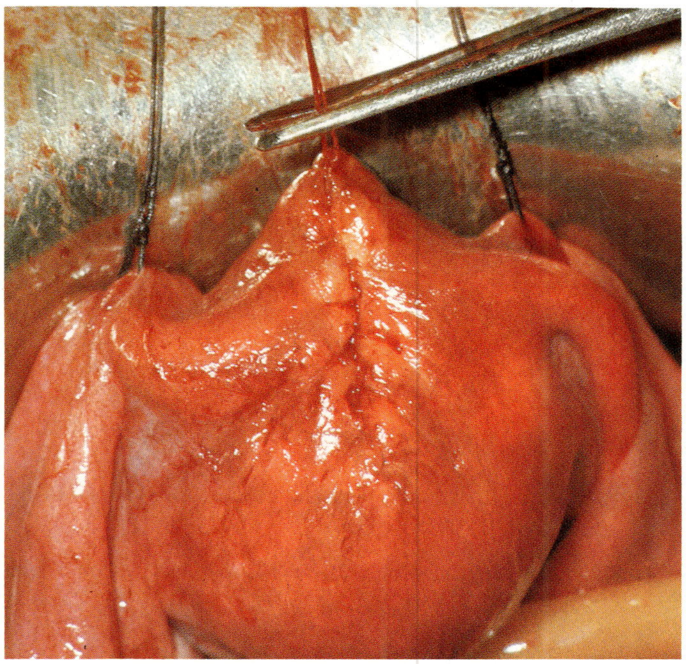

48 and 49
Closure of the sero-muscular layer is carried out as described for the Jones operation (page 65). The inverting stitch is seen progressing along the wound in **Figure 48** and the tied end is being cut in **Figure 49**.

2: Uterine fibroids

Barter and Parks (1958) reported fibroids in 5 per cent of infertile cases and thought them to be partially responsible for lack of conception. In a series of 481 women operated on for fibroids 42 per cent had never conceived and 18 per cent had only one child. Many fertile women however have fibroids of a size which are easily recognised clinically and many more have smaller undetected ones. Jones and Rock (1980) consider that when no other factor can be identified in a patient with infertility myomectomy offers the possibility of conception in about 50 per cent of patients. At the Johns Hopkins Hospital, of 67 patients having abdominal myomectomy 51 per cent conceived and 42 per cent had a term pregnancy (Babaknia et al 1978).

Operation is particularly indicated in the following circumstances:

1 Submucous fibroids likely to interfere with implantation: often associated with menorrhagia.

2 Intracervical fibroids.

3 Fibroids accompanied by other pelvic pathology (e.g. endometriosis or chronic pelvic infection).

4 Very large fibroids: frequent cause of pain and red degeneration, or obstruct labour.

5 Continuing infertility in the presence of known sizeable fibroids.

Myomectomy

Preoperative investigation and assessment must be complete and it is essential to know that the husband is fertile and ovulation normal; investigation should also have shown the cervix and ovaries normal and the tubes patent. Hysterosalpingography is therefore mandatory and laparoscopy should be used if possible.

Uterine external appearances can be deceptive as instanced in **Figure 50** and its legend, while care in interpreting hysterography is important in diagnosing a submucous fibroid (see **Figure 51** and its legend).

Myomectomy is done abdominally under general anaesthesia and uterine haemostasis is usually secured either by tourniquet around the uterine isthmus or by a Bonney's clamp; the ovarian vessels are controlled separately.

50

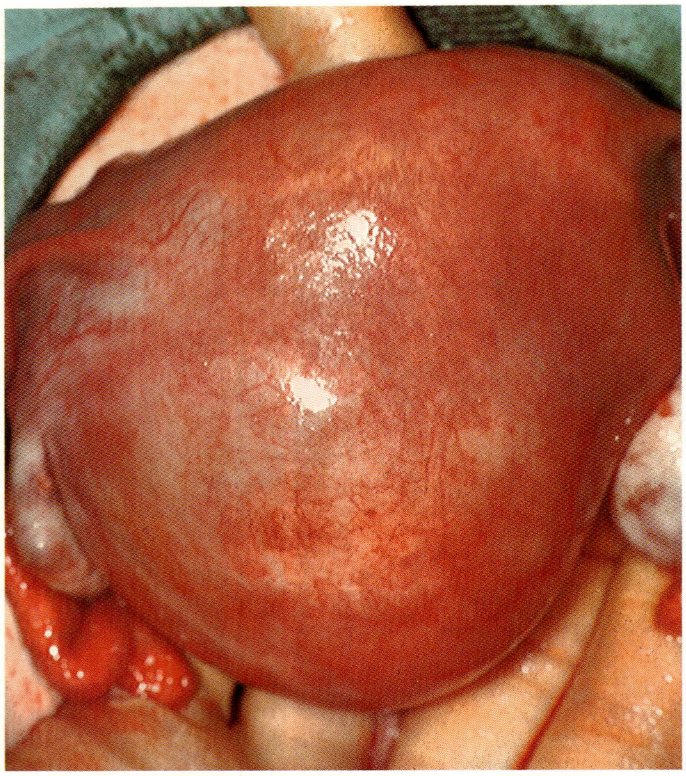

51

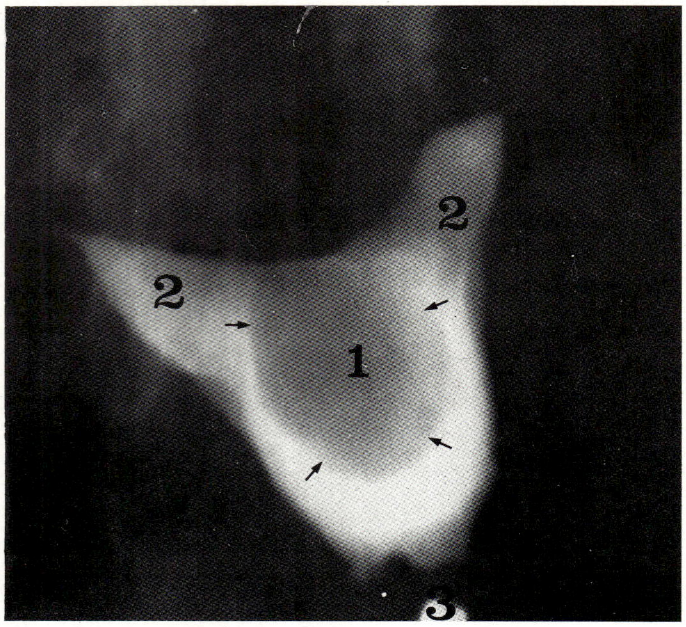

50 Fibroid causing menorrhagia and infertility
A large posterior wall fibroid in an infertile patient who suffered from menorrhagia. At myomectomy a smaller fibroid lay immediately underneath it and projected into the uterine cavity as a vascular submucous tumour. The smaller fibroid was responsible for both the menorrhagia and the infertility.

51 Hysterogram
The photograph was taken during radiographic screening with the patient in a moderate head-down position to encourage slow dispersal of the opaque medium within the uterine cavity. A large intrauterine fibroid polyp (1) arising from the fundus is outlined (arrowed). Within seconds the cornua (2) and the whole uterine cavity became opaque with nothing to suggest the presence of a fibroid. The opaque medium is being introduced through the cervix (3).

Stage I: Incision and enucleation of fibroid

52

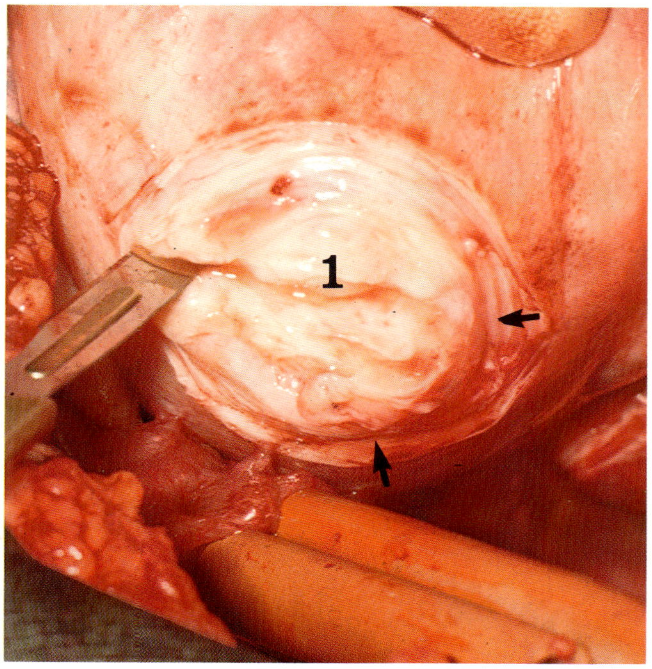

53

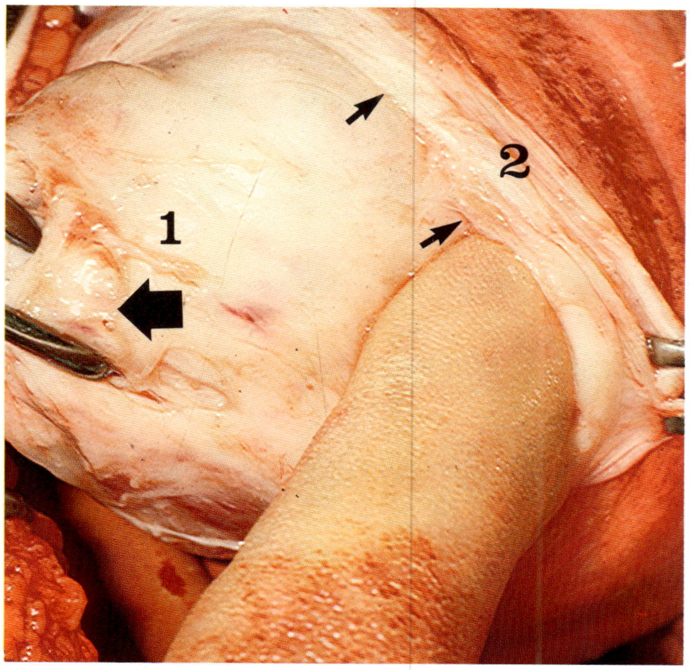

52 and 53
The incision is of minimal length to remove the fibroid (1) and is made boldly to extend into the tumour as shown in **Figure 52**. This serves to display the capsule of the tumour (arrowed). In **Figure 53** a plane of separation (arrowed) between the fibroid and its capsule (2) is opened up by the surgeon's forefinger which enucleates the fibroid.

Stage II: Opening into endometrial cavity

54

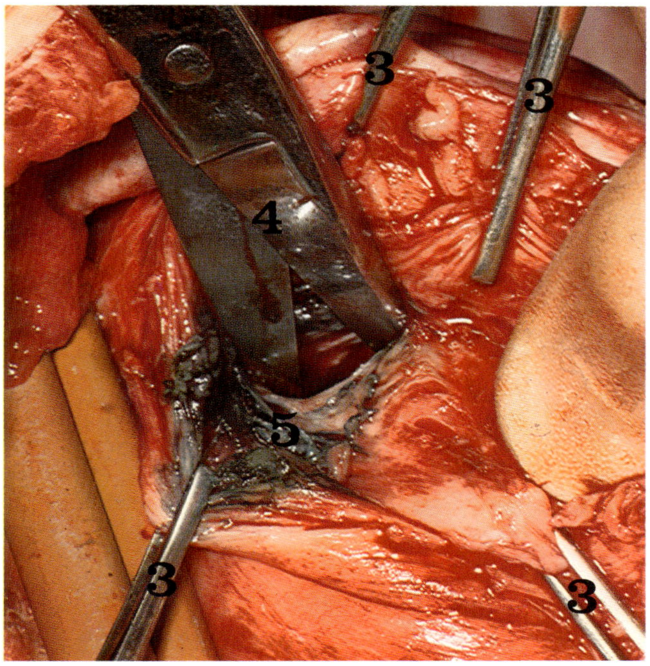

55

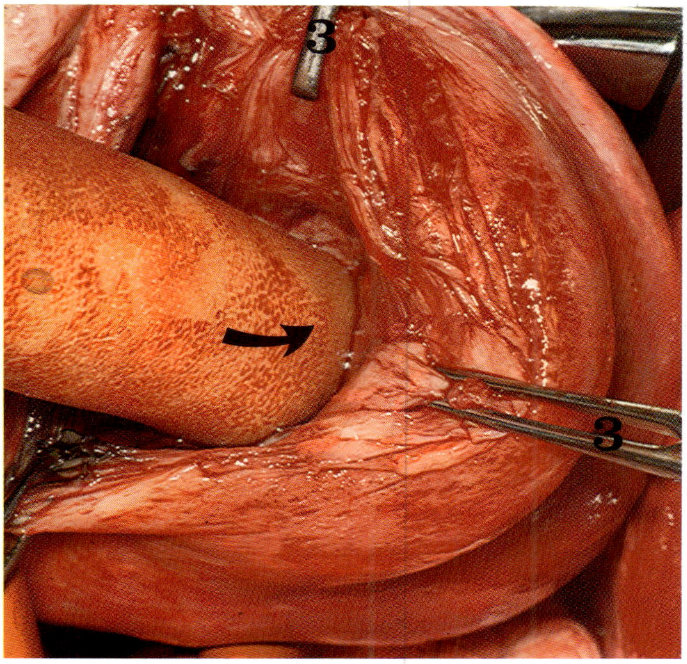

54 and 55
The authors consider it essential to open through from emptied fibroid cavities of any size into the endometrial space. This allows exploration of the uterus for submucous fibroids obtruding into it but the main reason is to allow drainage of blood from the cavity postoperatively. The blood drains through the cervix into the vagina and this safety-valve mechanism avoids the postoperative haematomata and abscesses which previously bedevilled the operation. In **Figure 54** the cavity of the enucleated fibroid is held open by tissue forceps (3) while the blades of the scissors (4) have opened the endometrial cavity as shown by the escape of methylene blue dye (5). In **Figure 55** the surgeon's finger explores the uterine cavity through the fibroid cavity (arrowed).

Stage III: Closure and covering of fibroid cavity

56

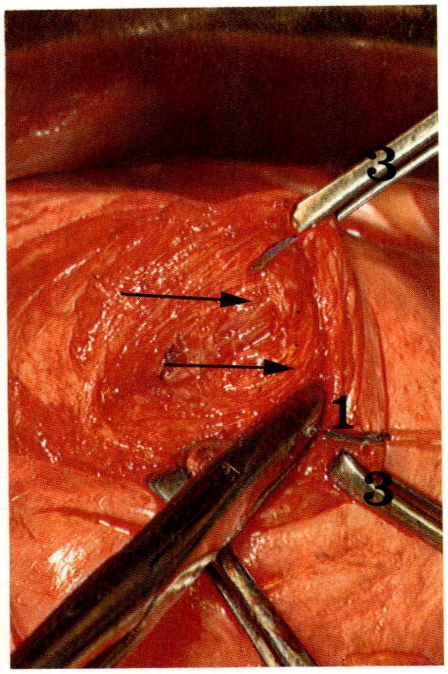

57

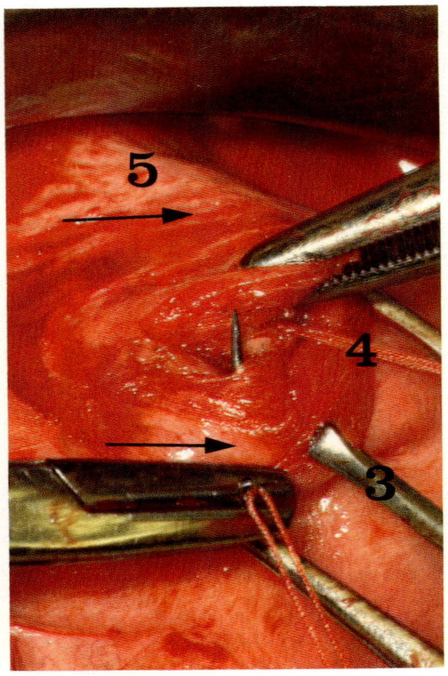

58

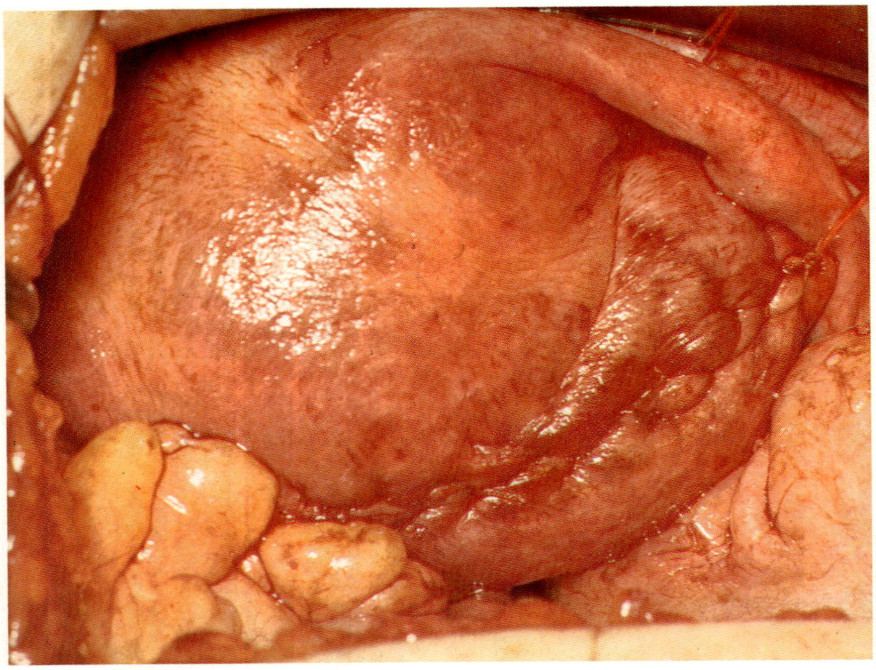

56 to 58
The cavity is closed in two layers and then covered by loose peritoneum or the sero-muscular stitch described on page 65. **Figure 56** shows the placement of the first stitch of the deepest layer while the tissue forceps (3) keeps the cavity everted. The needle (1) picks up a firm shoulder of muscle on each side (where arrowed) but does not include the endometrium so that the stitch remains outside the uterine cavity. The layer is completed with the requisite number of interrupted No. 00 PGA sutures. A second layer of interrupted sutures is then inserted and in **Figure 57** the final stitch in this layer is still uncut (4). The area of operation in this instance is the utero-vesical pouch so that there is available lax peritoneum (5) and this is picked up by the needle where arrowed to form the anchor stitch of a continuous peritoneal suture. It is always good practice to use loose peritoneum to cover the uterine incision if that is possible; it greatly lessens the risk of adhesions. **Figure 58** relates to myomectomy of a large posterior fibroid where there was no available free peritoneum to cover the incision. The continuous infolding stitch described on page 65 was used and gives a smooth and satisfactory end result.

A fuller account of myomectomy is given in Volume 2 of the Atlas, pages 165–181.

8: Operations on the ovary

Infertility surgery of the ovary is largely concerned with the effects of endometriosis and this chapter is mainly given over to the surgical management of that condition. There are few indications for removal of small benign ovarian cysts and the authors do not consider that there are any longer valid indications for wedge resection of the ovary in sclero-cystic disease. The management of large and potentially dangerous cysts is described elsewhere in the Atlas series (Volume 2, pages 191–201, and Volume 3, pages 243–291).

Ovarian and pelvic endometriosis

Endometriosis is exceedingly common in women and particularly during the second half of their reproductive life. Thus Williams and Pratt (1977) found it present in 50 per cent of gynaecological laparotomies. The disease is associated with infertility: Cohen (1976) found it at laparoscopy in 23 per cent of infertile patients and 25 per cent of primary infertility cases investigated at the Johns Hopkins Hospital had endometriosis (Jones and Rock 1980).

The natural history of the condition and its general management have both been exhaustively studied but it is important to recall why endometriosis leads to infertility. The predominant symptoms of pelvic pain and dyspareunia discourage coitus and reduce fertility, ovarian cortical involvement results in anovulation and the recurring haemorrhage with fibrosis in ovarian

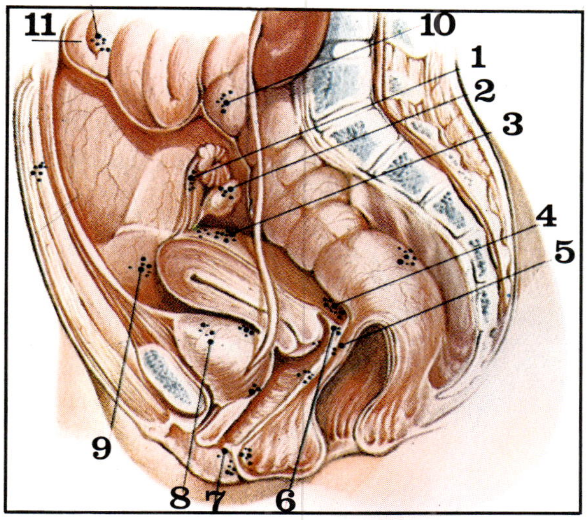

1

1 Structures which may be involved by endometriosis in infertility cases
(1) fallopian tube, (2) ovary, (3) uterus, (4) pouch of Douglas, (5) recto-vaginal septum, (6) posterior vaginal fornix, (7) perineum, (8) bladder, (9) parietal peritoneum, (10) small intestine, (11) umbilicus.

2

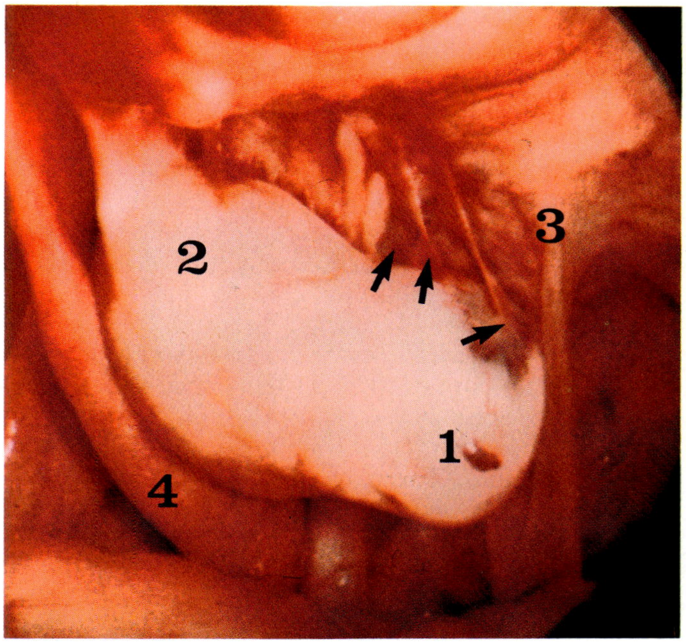

3

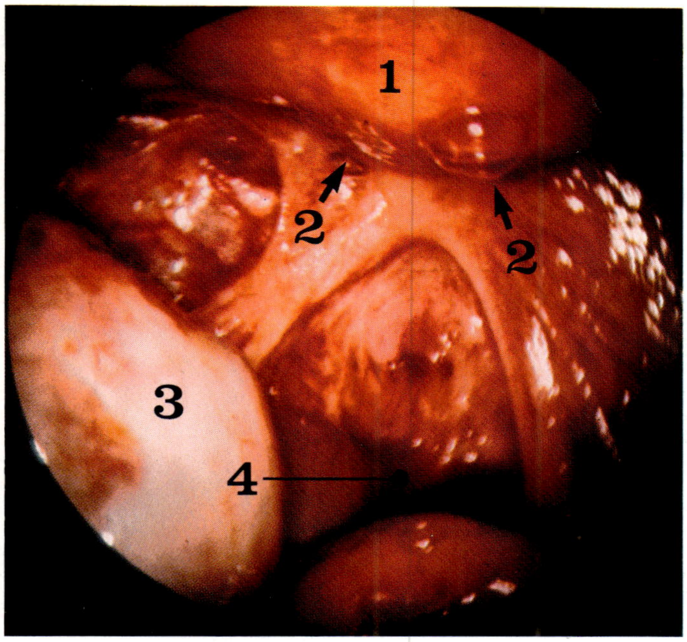

2 and 3 Laparoscopic appearances of pelvic endometriosis
Figure 2 shows an endometriomatous cyst (1) at the lower pole of the left ovary (2). It is drawn towards the uterus by adhesions where arrowed and also at the attachment of the left utero-sacral ligament (3). The left tube is numbered (4). In **Figure 3** the uterus (1) is drawn into retroversion by adhesions in an area of endometriosis (arrowed) just above the attachments of the utero-sacral ligaments (2). The left ovary (3) is enlarged and is incorporated in a pelvic haematocele. There is old blood free in the pouch of Douglas (4).

and cul-de-sac lesions leads to adhesions with tubal kinking, fimbrial blockage, pelvic haematocele and eventually a frozen pelvis. Early and minimal endometriotic changes accompanied by resistant infertility are more difficult to explain and Meldrum et al (1977) present evidence which suggests that ectopic endometrium releases prostaglandins which might impair tubal motility and ovum transport.

Endometriosis diagnosed during infertility investigations is often of a degree where primary surgery would be inappropriate. The tendency is to resort to immediate specific therapy with the antigonadotrophin drug, Danazol. Jones and Rock (1980) however, recommend that patients with minimal endometriosis and without significant symptoms other than infertility should simply be observed over a period of time, and Garcia and David (1977) had a mean pregnancy rate of 65 per cent in 17 patients so observed. Hormone therapy with the oral contraceptive steroids may be employed to induce a pseudopregnancy but there are widely differing opinions as to its safety, acceptability and effectiveness. One of the chief disadvantages is that it is time consuming and to a 35 year old woman with infertility time is a very scarce commodity.

4 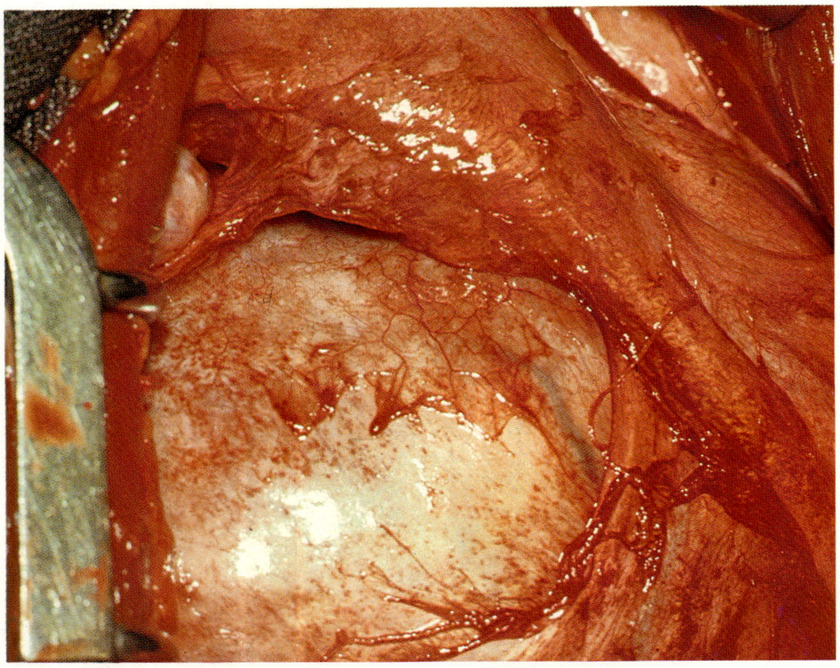

4 Severe degree of endometriosis with pelvic haematocele

5 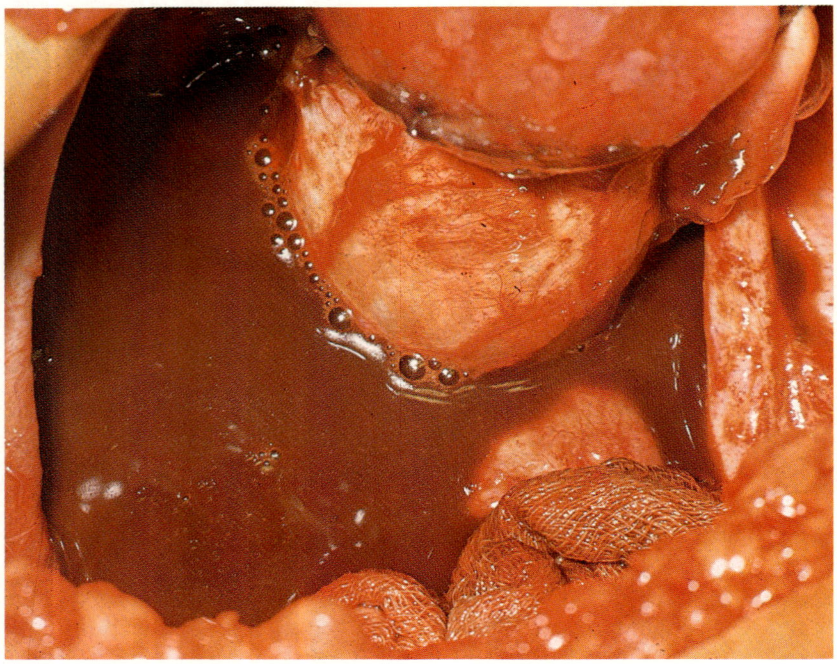

5 Appearances when haematocele is disturbed

Surgical treatment is most likely to succeed in early cases and Kistner and Patton (1975) pointed out that women over 35 years of age with severe endometriosis or who had previous surgery for the condition had a poor prognosis; the same applied to those with a long history. To ensure early diagnosis Cooke (1978) emphasises the importance of laparoscopic examination in young women with secondary dysmenorrhoea especially if they are infertile. Where pseudo pregnancy has been induced or where Danazol has been given as a first line therapy he recommends that it be followed up by a 'second look' laparoscopic examination.

Surgical treatment

The procedures most likely to improve the prognosis are limited in type and scope. Excision of an endometriomatous plaque from the surface of the ovary or an endometriomatous cyst from its cortex is easy and usually rewarding. Periovarian and peritubal adhesions of lesser degree are dealt with by a salpingolysis type of operation such as is subsequently described in Chapter 8. When both ovaries are involved and adherent to a retroverted uterus in the pouch of Douglas there is little prospect of achieving much and even less if there is a pelvic haematocoele. Old blood or chocolate brown fluid escapes into the pelvis immediately the ovaries are mobilised (**Figures 4** and **5**) and the condition clearly involves advanced pathology.

The surgical approach in conservative pelvic surgery for endometriosis is illustrated in Volume 2 of the Atlas, pages 210–213. The pelvic structures are carefully defined and this may entail gentle separation of the ovaries from the posterior leaf of the broad ligament. These cases are often complex and the hallowed surgical principle of removing all visible endometriosis need not always be observed. It is sometimes preferable to leave the pelvis dry and untraumatised even if some endometriomatous spots are visible on the rectum or utero-sacral attachments. Many of these areas will undergo spontaneous regression or yield to a limited course of specific drug therapy.

Surgical treatment of ovarian endometriomata

Excision of endometriomatous cyst

6

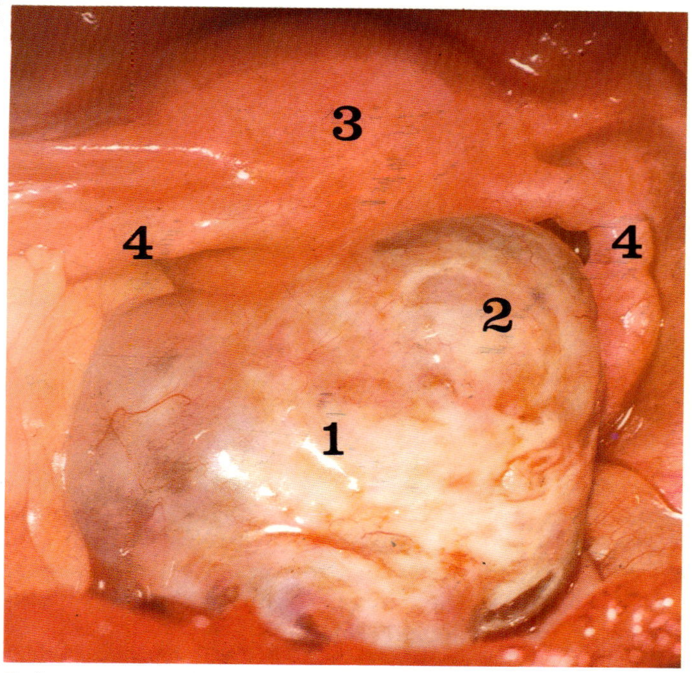

6 Appearance of ovary at laparotomy
The right ovary (1) has been elevated from the pouch of Douglas and contains a chocolate cyst (2). The uterus is numbered (3) and the tubes (4) and (4). The left ovary was also involved and contained a small endometriomatous cyst.

7

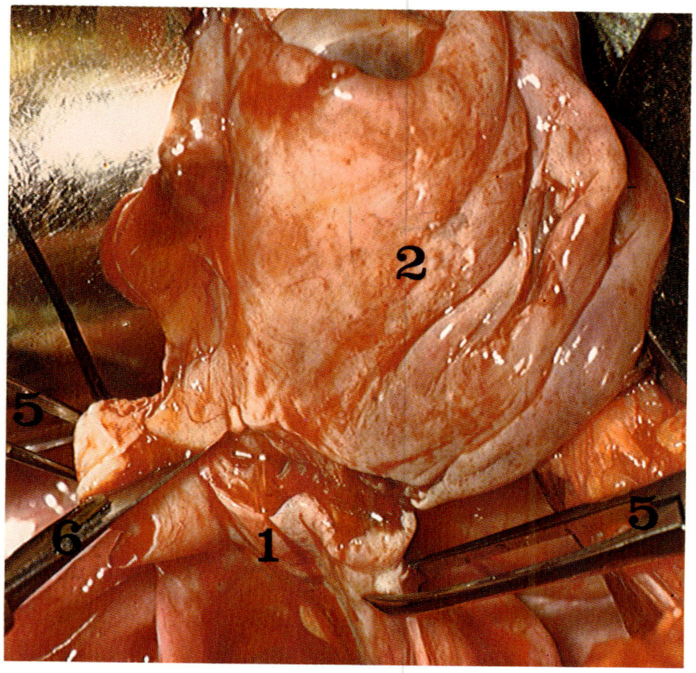

7 Excision of cyst from ovary
The main part of the ovary (1) is supported by the tissue forceps (5) while the scalpel (6) detaches an intact chocolate cyst (2) with its covering of ovarian tissue. Unless they are very small they invariably rupture.

8

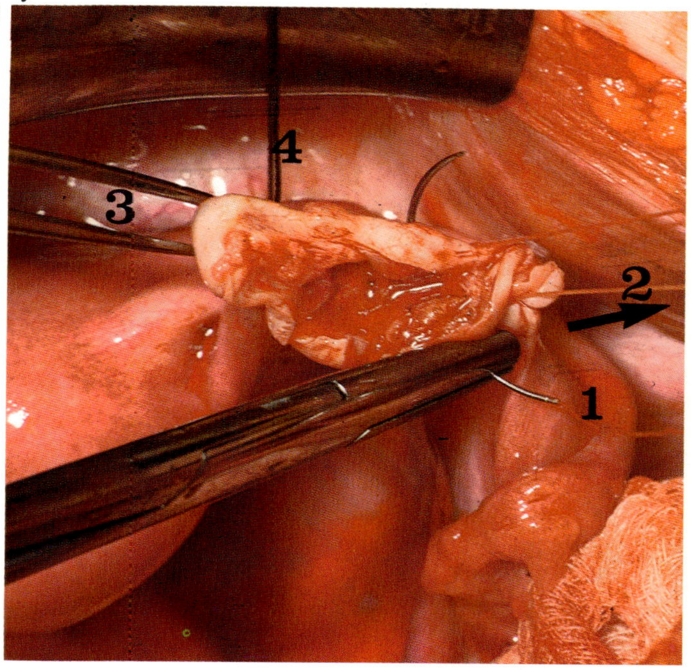

9

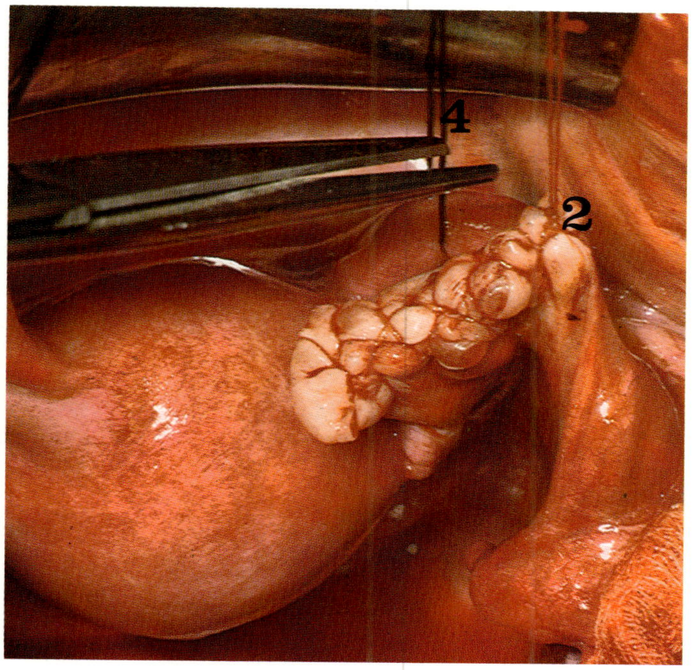

8 and 9 Reconstruction of ovary
About one-half of the ovary remains and the open surface presents as a V-shaped narrow trench. This is closed in the long axis of the ovary by an over-and-over No. 00 PGA suture (1) with the stitches at 0.5 cm intervals to approximate the edges and control bleeding. The end of the anchor stitch (2) is held in the direction of the arrow and dissecting forceps (3) supports the other pole of the ovary. Suture (1) returns by the same route and picks up more superficial bites of the corresponding ovarian edges between each deep stitch to complete haemostasis by an X-effect. It is tied to the initial anchor stitch at (2) and is about to be cut short.

10

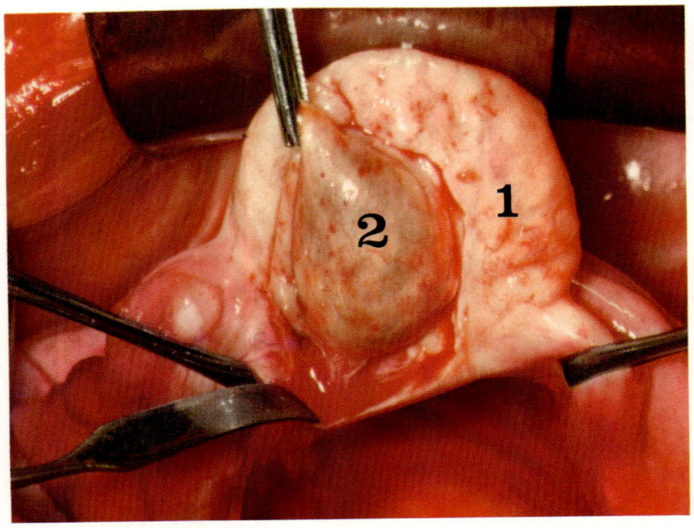

11

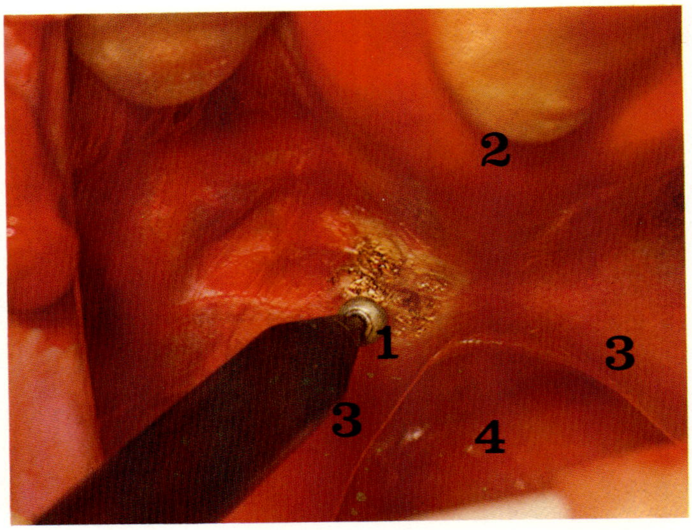

10 Enucleation of endometriomatous cyst
The endometriomatous cyst (2) on the left ovary (1) is sufficiently small to be shelled out in routine fashion and the ovary will be reconstituted as already described.

11 Diathermy treatment of endometriomatous plaque
The commonest site of endometrioma in the pouch of Douglas is at the attachment of the utero-sacral ligament. If there is distortion and evidence of blood collection it is better to excise the affected area. In lesser cases treatment is to fulgurate the area with diathermy. A ball electrode (1) is suitable and is being used in the photograph. The uterus is numbered (2) the utero-sacral ligaments (3) and the pouch of Douglas (4).

Ventrosuspension

In treating endometriosis by conservative surgery it is generally agreed that ventrosuspension should be added to the procedure. There are two main reasons for doing so:

1 In spite of treatment endometriosis tends to continue developing in the region of the utero-sacral ligament attachments and in the pouch of Douglas. It is clearly correct to anticipate such a development by lessening the opportunity for ovary and tube to become adherent to the pelvic floor.

2 Dyspareunia is a severe and disabling symptom which may independently contribute to infertility by discouraging coitus. Conservative ovarian surgery alone seldom completely relieves the patient of either dyspareunia or backache but the pain of both can be considerably ameliorated by elevation of the adherent and congested ovaries from the posterior pouch. Ventrosuspension gives a real prospect of relief in such cases. The main steps of the operation are illustrated on pages 77–78.

12

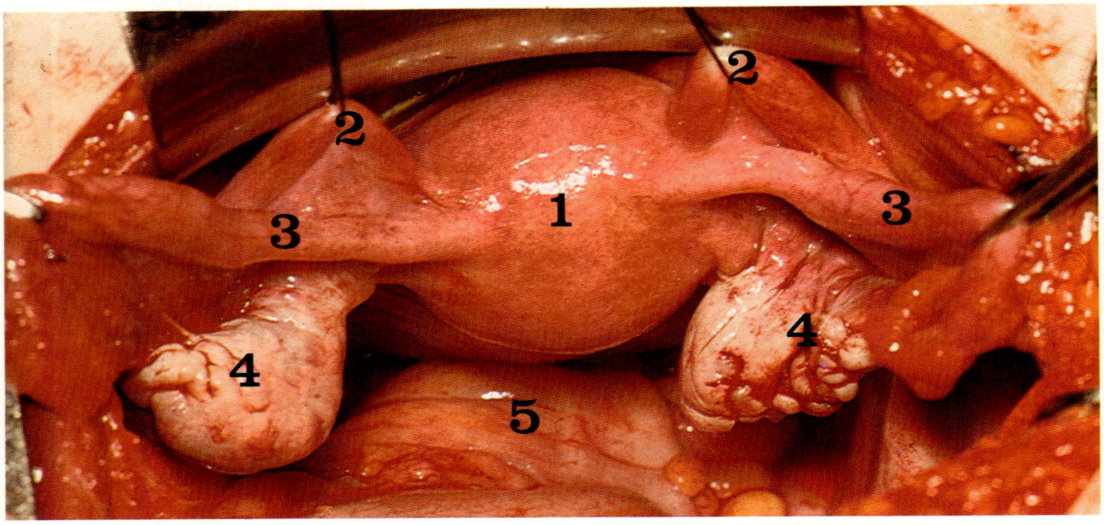

12 General appearance before ventrosuspension
The appearances are those at the end of the operations just described. The uterus is numbered (1), the round ligaments (2), the fallopian tubes (3), the ovaries (4) and the rectum (5). The uterus tends towards retroversion and the stay sutures encircling the round ligaments will draw them extra-peritoneally to be fixed to the rectus sheath as shown in subsequent photographs.

13

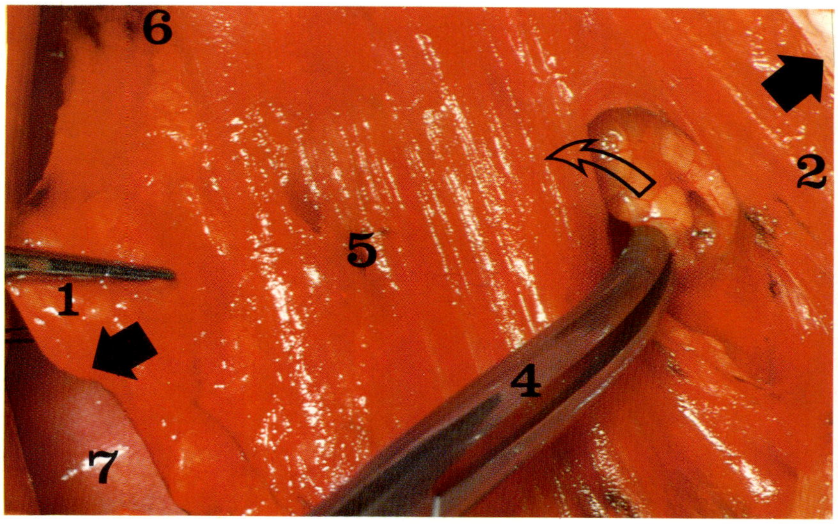

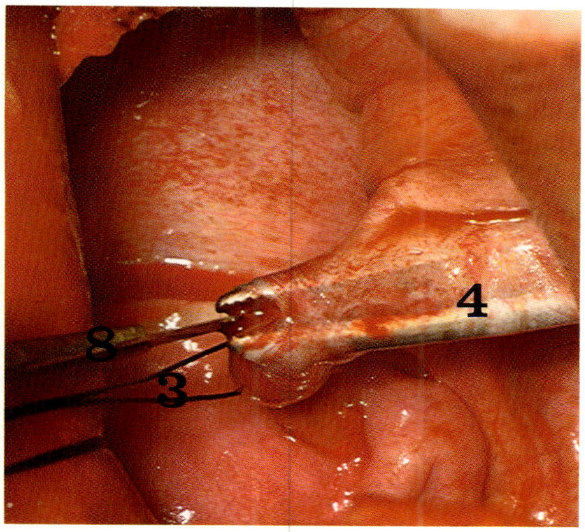

14

13 to 16 Extraperitoneal approach towards and retrieval of right round ligament

In **Figure 13** the peritoneal edge (1) and the edge of the rectus sheath (2) are drawn apart by forceps in the direction of the broad arrows to expose the rectus muscle (5). A round ligament (or Phillips') forceps (4) is introduced lateral to the muscle and travels extraperitoneally towards the traction suture on the right round ligament in the direction of the open arrow. The symphysis pubis is in the general direction (6) and the small intestine seen in the wound is numbered (7). The points of the forceps which are first aimed towards the inguinal ring and then follow the round ligament medially and cephalad are kept under direct vision through the peritoneum. They are immediately beneath it and clear of the inferior epigastric vessels. In **Figure 14** the round ligament traction suture has been reached and the jaws are opened and the stretched peritoneum incised by the scalpel (8) where arrowed so that

15

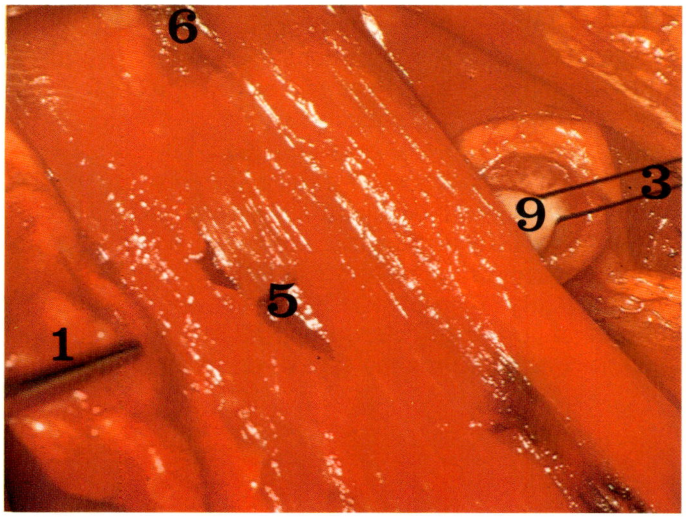

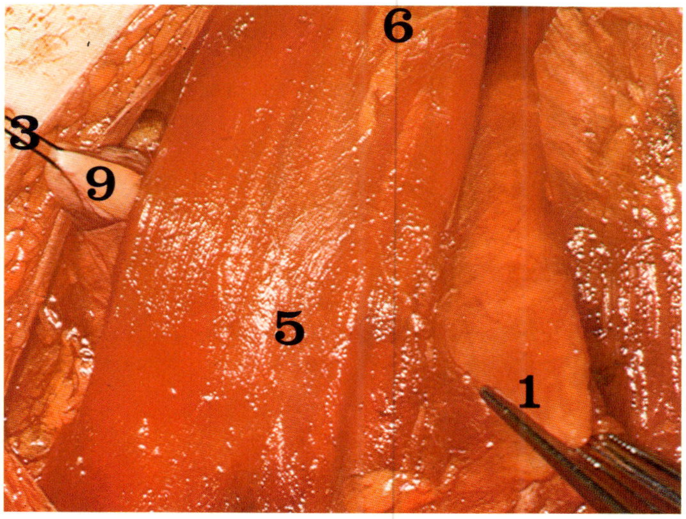

16

the traction suture (3) can be fed on to the forceps (4) and drawn back along the path of the forceps. In **Figure 15** the forceps has been withdrawn and still holds the suture (3) which brings the apex of the round ligament loop (9) into the rectus sheath lateral to the muscle (5). The same procedure is carried out on the left side and the apex of the retrieved left round ligament loop is numbered (9) in **Figure 16.**

17

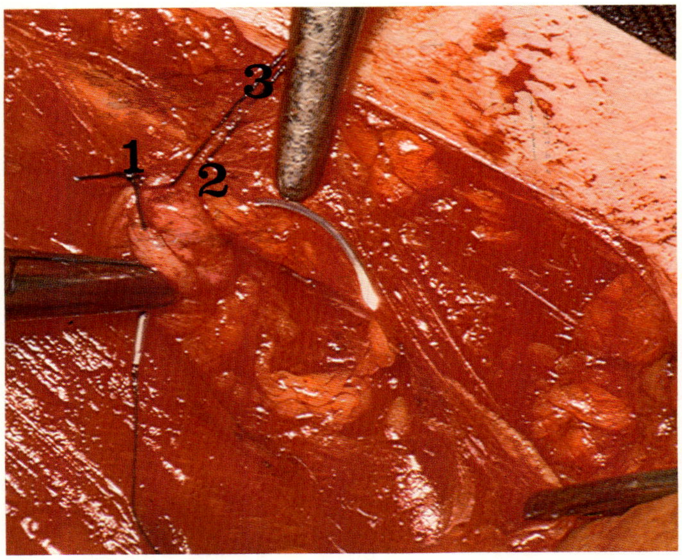

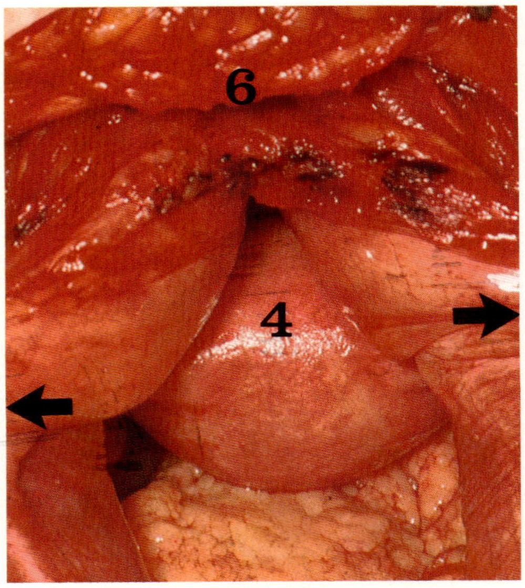

18

17 and 18 Attachment of right round ligament to rectus sheath and appearance at completion of operation
The loop of the round ligament is sutured to the inner aspect of the lower leaf of the rectus sheath. **Figure 17** shows the first stitch in position and cut short (1) while the needle indicates the placement of the second (2). **Figure 18** shows how the uterus (4) has been drawn forward to the symphysis pubis (6) by the repositioned round ligaments.

Increase in fertility following treatment of endometriosis by endocrine and by surgical methods

In early cases a choice exists between the oral contraceptive steroids and the antigonadotrophic drug, Danazol. An overall pregnancy rate of 43 per cent was obtained by Greenblatt et al (1974) when using the latter and 50.8 per cent was reported by Kistner and Patton (1975), with pseudopregnancy only. When such treatment fails or when the stage of the disease indicates the need for surgery it is helpful to know what success rate might be expected.

Jones and Rock (1980) studied figures from 10 recent series with a total of 795 cases and a pregnancy rate of 59 per cent. This pregnancy rate was of course inversely related to the extent of the disease. They concluded that 50–60 per cent of patients with infertility due to endometriosis externa will become pregnant following conservative surgery. Any such pregnancy is most likely to occur within 24 months of the operation. Kistner and Patton reported a 76 per cent rate but 96 per cent of the patients were under 32 years of age, they only had surface ovarian involvement and there were no other factors apparently contributing to the infertility. In contrast, 106 patients with the more usually encountered peritoneal involvement and adhesions had a pregnancy rate of only 38 per cent.

Ovarian cystectomy for simple ovarian cysts

In ovarian cystectomy for infertility the prime consideration is that the benefits should outweigh the disadvantages. The laparoscope has provided proof, if that were needed, that peritoneal and peri-ovarian adhesions commonly follow haemorrhage resulting from ovarian surgery and these may cause tubal kinking or occlusion. The first question one must ask is whether cystectomy is really necessary and except where they are sufficiently large to constitute an obstetric hazard or there is doubt about their pathology there are few occasions when these cysts need to be removed.

If and when operation is indicated the procedure should be carried out with the utmost care and precision. The outstanding requirement is optimal haemostasis and this implies careful reconstruction and suturing of the ovarian tissue with fine needles and suture materal. The minimum amount of ovarian cortex should be removed and all raw areas should be covered with visceral or parietal peritoneum.

9: Operations on the fallopian tube

This section is being written at a time of evolution in the practice of tubal surgery and it is not yet clear how it will eventually develop.

It is likely that much of this work will eventually be done as a microsurgical subspecialty and for that reason an acknowledged expert, Mr Robert Winston has been invited to describe and illustrate not only the techniques but the general principles of operating under the microscope (Chapter 10). For the present, neither the facilities nor the necessary specialist training in microsurgery is generally available so that for the forseeable future most tubal operations will be done by predominantly macrosurgical methods. In isolated communities and in developing countries the prospects must be even more long term.

The operations described and illustrated here in Chapter 9 are appropriate to all these latter circumstances and are presented to instruct those with limited facilities and/or those who have not had specialist training.

Pre and postoperative management

It has not been the policy of the Atlas to advise on such matters but there are particular considerations in the general control of tubal surgery. A separate list of basic policy items is set out in Appendix C.

Operative technique and equipment

Macrosurgery can be made more precise and successful by the use of the fine instruments and non-absorbable sutures and by taking advantage of any microtechniques or equipment which may be available. Optimal access with minimal tissue trauma is important and tubal blood supply must always be respected; haemostasis must be meticulous. Handling of tissues should be minimal and angled glass rods are used to support the tubes and ovaries. Peritoneal moisturisation is maintained continuously and a jet of saline is directed at the site of diathermy cutting to lessen the risk of burning the tissues. The form of abdominal wall retraction, the vaginal packing and the modern diathermy equipment seen in Chapter 10 are now used routinely by the authors. Former less satisfactory methods are sometimes seen being used in Chapter 9 but they have been superseded in practice.

Splinting

Polythene rods or tubes are often essential splinting equipment at operation but majority opinion is now against their retention postoperatively – when it is felt that they do more harm than good. They are probably unnecessary since there is evidence that fibrin is quickly laid down at any site of anastomosis and confers stability with an hour of the completion of the operation (Winston 1978). The authors have gradually been discarding postoperative splints while obtaining improved results.

Tubal operations applicable to the treatment of infertility

1 Salpingolysis
2 Salpingostomy
3 Operations to overcome cornual occlusion
4 Operations to restore tubal continuity following sterilisation.

The procedures are dealt with separately although in practice they are often combined. Thus salpingolysis is frequently a necessary preliminary to salpingostomy and may indeed also be required prior to the other two operations. Two salpingolysis operations are illustrated to demonstrate how surgical treatment must be adapted to meet different requirements. In salpingostomy two cases demanded the different managements illustrated; a salpingostomy operation using a Mulligan hood prosthesis is also described. For cornual occlusion the tubes are shown being reimplanted in the uterus by two different methods and the advantages and disadvantages of each are discussed. Utero-salpingostomy may well have advantages over both but it is a frankly microsurgical procedure for a specialist surgeon and the technique is described in Chapter 10, page 153. Provided there has been no gross destruction by diathermy the operation of tubal anastomosis is straightforward (as described here).

Results of tubal surgery

In this chapter a limited number of recently published figures are quoted to set what might be an attainable target for each condition as it is dealt with in the Atlas. The principal criterion in this context is not the percentage of patients who subsequently achieve a pregnancy but the percentage who achieve a live birth. Any such statistics however are still suspect if one accepts the points raised by Cooke (1978). He maintains that the impact of treatment can only properly be measured against the limited data available on the incidence and prognosis of infertility, that there is often wide divergence between operability rates and cases operated on, that follow-up data are collected in widely varying fashion and that conception rates take no account of subsequent abortion and ectopic pregnancy. Israel and March (1976) saw more than 2000 patients over a four year period and performed 155 laparoscopies and 83 conservative operations. Their yield was 9 full term pregnancies and 10 abortions and ectopics.

Salpingolysis

This is the most frequently required infertility operation and its purpose is to separate adhesions which distort the fallopian tubes; it is understood to include the release of periovarian adhesions when these are present. All degrees of severity are encountered and are treated individually on certain established surgical principles. Two representative cases are described here. The first entails simple lysis of the fallopian tube with repair of the traumatised peritoneum of the broad ligament (page 80). The second deals with the familiar and difficult problem of a pelvis which has previously been the site of recurrent or prolonged inflammation and where the tubes are bound down and distorted by multiple fibrous adhesions (pages 83–85).

Salpingolysis: A mild case of tubo-ovarian adhesion

The less severe cases tend to follow recession of ovarian endometriosis or previous non-recurring pelvic infection and the adhesions are generally old, avascular and tenuous. The tube may be sufficiently kinked to prevent the passage of dye or opaque medium when injected through the cervix; sometimes the adhesions involve the lateral mesosalpinx and partially cover the ovary so that there is doubt as to whether there is terminal blockage of the tube. The fimbriae are often found to be intact once freed so that the problem is partly one of temporarily disturbed tubo-ovarian transport of the ovum. The degree of deciliation in such cases is not severe.

The operation is a simple one, effecting lysis of the tube and ovary by defining and displaying the adhesions on angled glass or fine metal rods before dividing and excising them with fine scissors which should be of diathermy type if vascularity demands it. There is likely to be some disturbance of the mesosalpingeal surface which may lead to adhesions and any defect is repaired with fine (6 × 0 prolene) sutures. Control of bleeding is essential for the same reason (Swolin 1975).

1

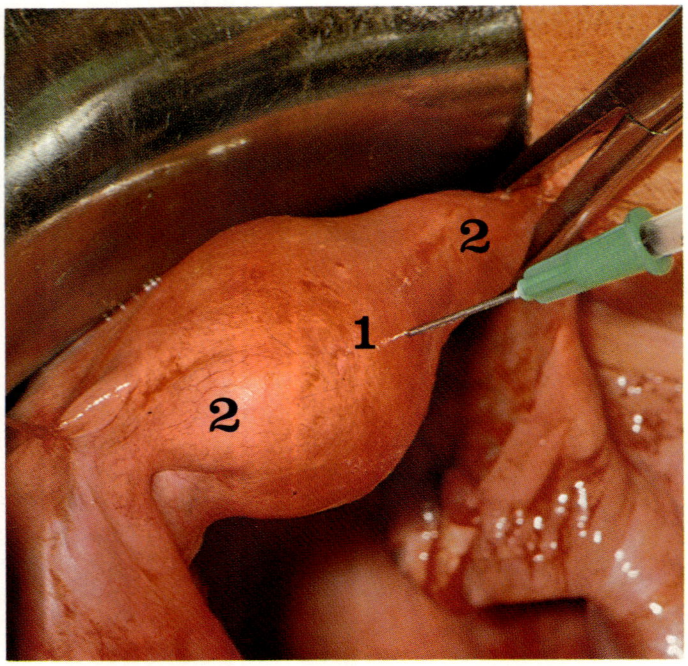

2

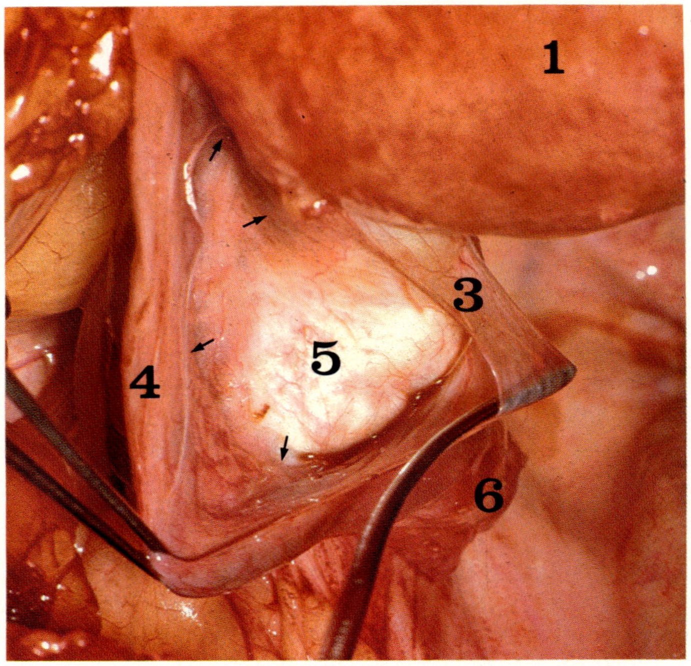

1 and 2 Condition at laparotomy
Both tubes were known to be blocked. The cervix was occluded preoperatively and in **Figure 1** methylene blue is injected into the uterine cavity (1) to outline the tubes as far distally as possible. The uterus is noticeably distended and under pressure from the injection as are the inner ends of both tubes (2). **Figure 2** shows the ampullary-fimbrial junction of the left tube attached to the lower posterior aspect of the uterus by a fibrous band (3) which kinks and effectively blocks the tube. The ampullary portion (4) is drawn around the ovary (5) which is itself bound down by multiple adhesions (arrowed). The fimbrial end of the tube is seen at (6).

3

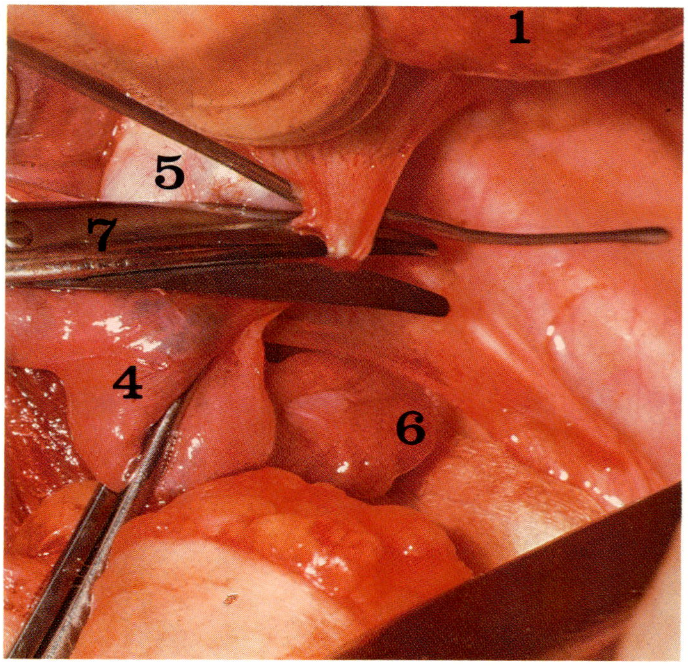

4

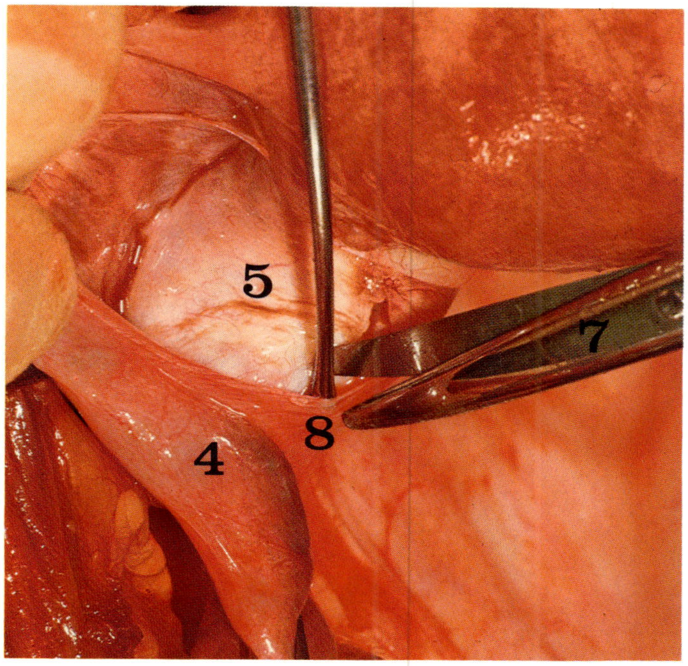

3 and 4 Division of tubal adhesions to uterus and ovary
The broad fibrous adhesion between the left tube and the uterus is displayed on a curved probe in **Figure 3** and is divided with scissors (7) close to the tube to avoid raw protrusions which might cause further adhesions. As the tube falls laterally the fimbrial end is clearly seen. In **Figure 4** the tubal adhesions to the left ovary (8) are divided and the tube is now freed and in normal position. The blue dye is seen through the thin wall of the distally occluded and distended tube in these, and the two following, pictures.

5

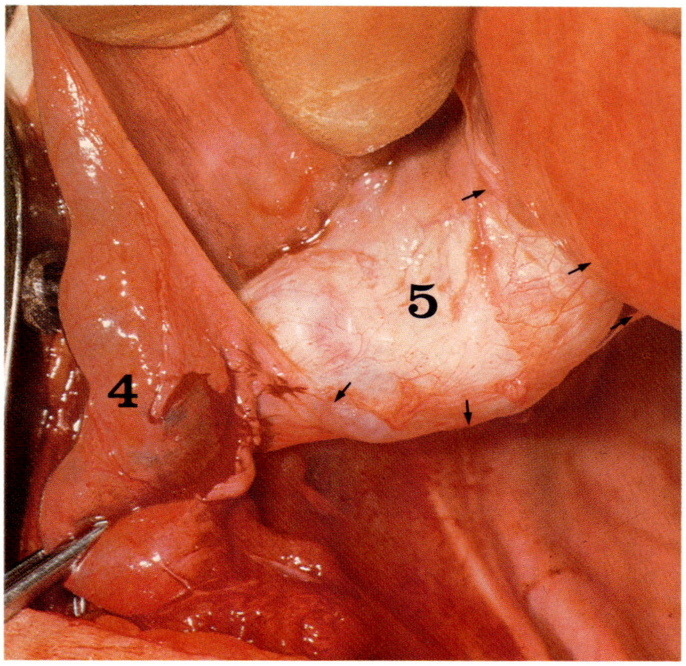

6

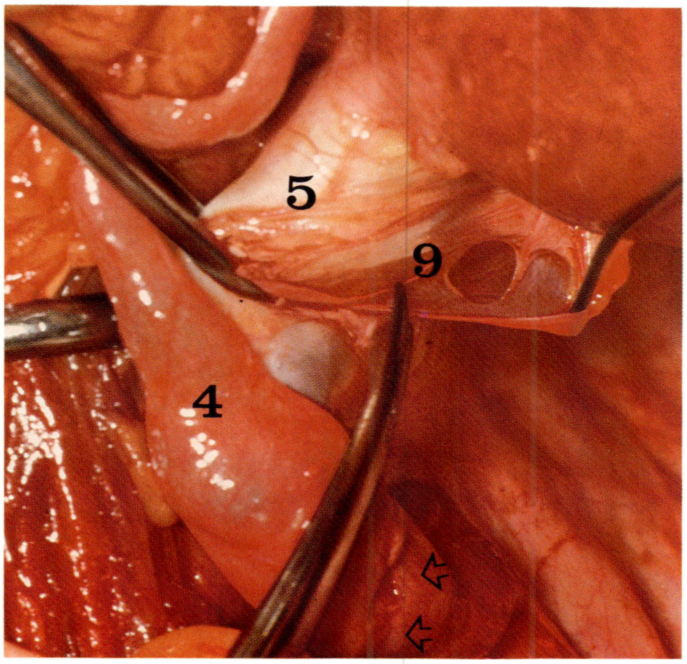

5 and 6 Release of left ovary from its periovarian adhesions
The multiple avascular periovarian adhesions are indicated by fine arrows in **Figure 5**. The ragged edges of those already divided are seen on the left of the photograph and this tissue should be removed preferably with bipolar diathermy scissors since there is some free blood indicating vascularity. In **Figure 6** release of the ovary continues medially at (9) and once freed from the uterus and pelvic pouch it assumes a normal position. The photograph shows a raw area on the tubal surface where it was separated from the uterus (open arrows) and which will have to be repaired.

7

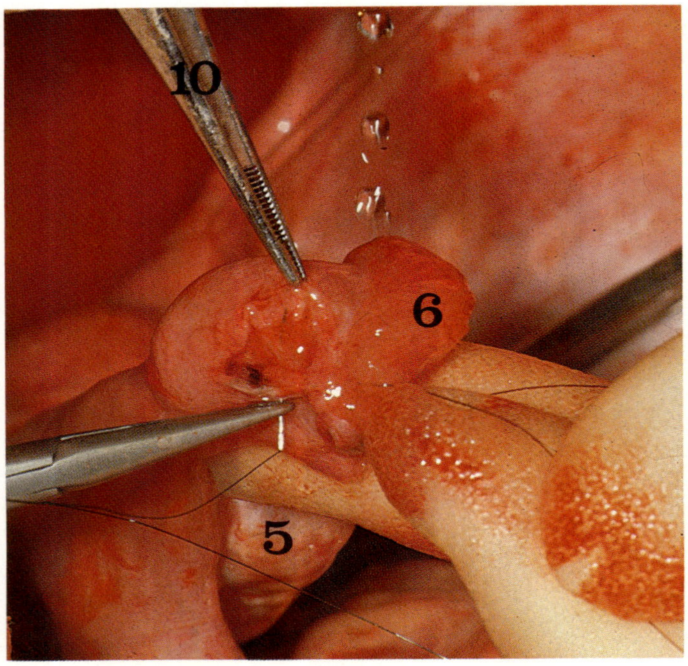

8

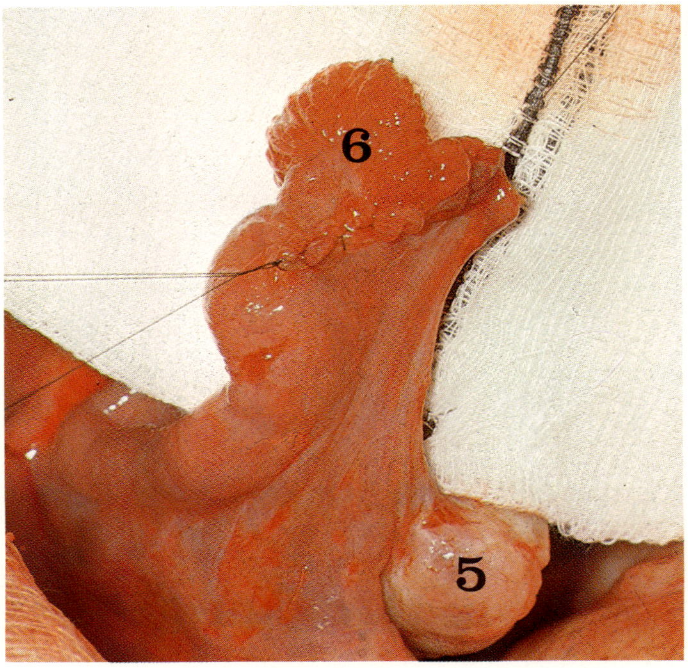

7 and 8 Repair of damage to peritoneal coat of left tube
Figure 7 shows the fimbrial end of the tube (6) with methylene blue dye in the pelvis so that the lumen is now open. The defect on the serosal wall, which would quickly form adhesions with adjacent structures, is being closed by a continuous suture of 6 × 0 prolene. The tube is steadied by the finger and fine dissecting forceps (10) and a stream of saline keeps the field clear of blood and dye. In **Figure 8** the defect has been closed and is displayed between the two ends of the prolene suture.

Results obtainable from salpingolysis operations

The results of salpingolysis in this first group are excellent. Up to 50 per cent of patients conceive and in 35–40 per cent the pregnancy goes to term. Cooke (1978) found that in a total of 286 cases reported in the literature there was an overall 45 per cent pregnancy rate. Only Horne et al (1973) reported their term pregnancy rate: 42 per cent in 33 cases.

It is almost impossible to obtain meaningful results for the second group. The divided adhesions are so rapidly replaced by new ones that only an occasional patient becomes pregnant. The majority require fimbriolysis at least and generally some form of salpingostomy in addition to lysis. They tend to be classified as salpingoplasty or salpingostomy cases and, as in the latter, results are poor.

Salpingolysis: A severe case of (pelvic) adhesion following pelvic infection

Multiple and dense peritubal and periovarian adhesions may follow a severe pelvic endometriosis but are much more likely to result from pyogenic infection. It was seen in Chapter 1 that acute salpingo-oophoritis from an ascending infection may cause surprisingly little residual damage provided it does not become chronic and recur. If it does and there are subsequent recurring exacerbations the severity of the pathology is directly proportionate to the frequency with which these occur (Westrom 1980). Another well recognised cause of fibrosis and tubal blockage is a peritonitis resulting from a ruptured appendix or appendix abscess and particularly if there was wound drainage. The case described here had such a history.

Surgical management is conducted along established lines. First the omentum and then the large and small intestines are mobilised and elevated from the pelvis. The fallopian tubes are meticulously and gently freed from their enveloping adhesions by sharp dissection if necessary and the ovaries are elevated from the pelvic floor in turn.

In some of these cases such lysis frees the fimbrial ends and dye injected into the uterine cavity escapes from the tubal ostia. If it does not and there is a blockage at the outer end of the tube a fimbriolysis or salpingostomy may also be required. In all such operations the surgeon must aim to disturb the tissues as little as possible and leave the pelvis dry with an intact peritoneal coat so that there is minimal basis for further adhesion formation. Even so the prognosis cannot be other than poor.

9

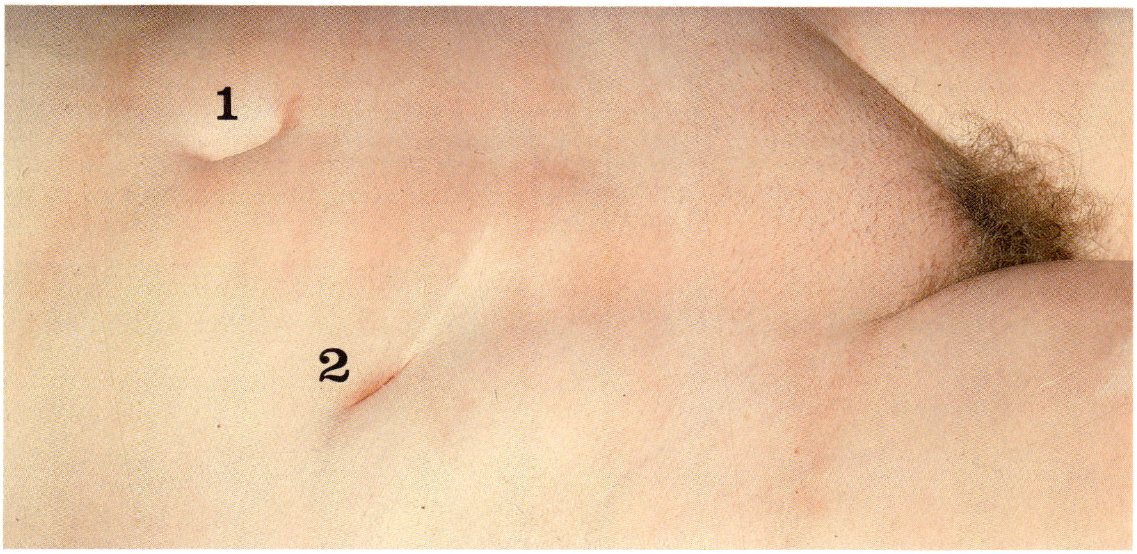

10

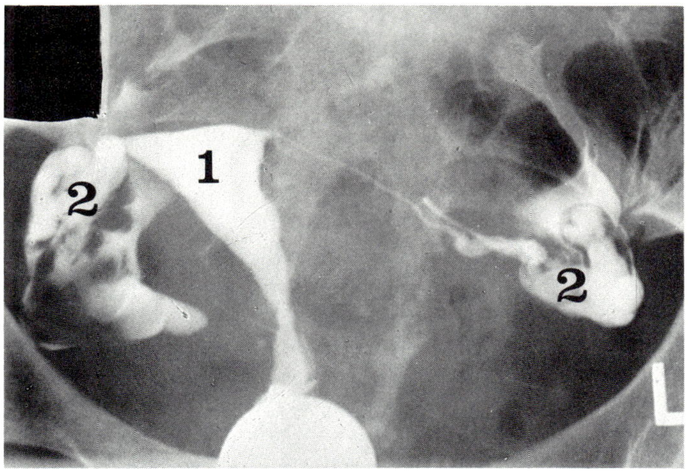

9 Abdominal scars from previous pelvic peritonitis
The patient in this case suffered from rupture of an acutely infected and obstructed appendix with widespread peritonitis when aged 12. The wound broke down and discharged leaving an indrawn distorted scar (1) and the site of a stab drain is seen at (2). Recovery was slow and in such circumstances severe pelvic adhesions frequently result in infertility.

10 Hysterosalpingogram
The ampullary portion of both tubes (2) is distended but there is peritoneal spill which is localised presumably by peritubal adhesions. The asymmetry and lateral elongation of the left tube suggests displacement by such adhesions. The uterus is numbered (1).

11
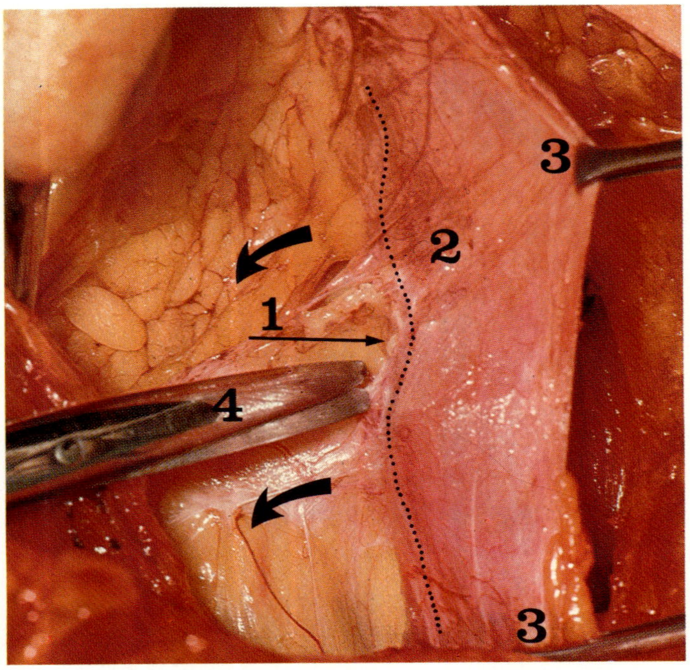

12
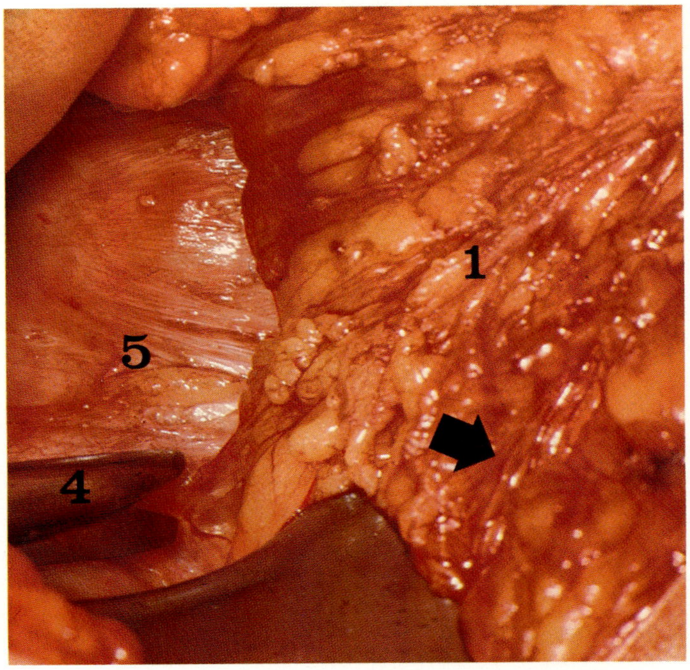

11 and 12 Release and upward displacement of adherent omentum
In **Figure 11** the omentum (1) is firmly adherent to parietal peritoneum (2) on the right side just medial to the dotted line. The peritoneal edge is held taut by tissue forceps (3) and scissors (4) find a plane of separation where arrowed.

The omentum is then rolled medially in the direction of the curved arrows. In **Figure 12** it has been freed well laterally and is now gently detached medially from the surface of the bowel (5). It is tucked under the upper wound edge in the direction of the broad arrow where it is retained by an abdominal pack.

13
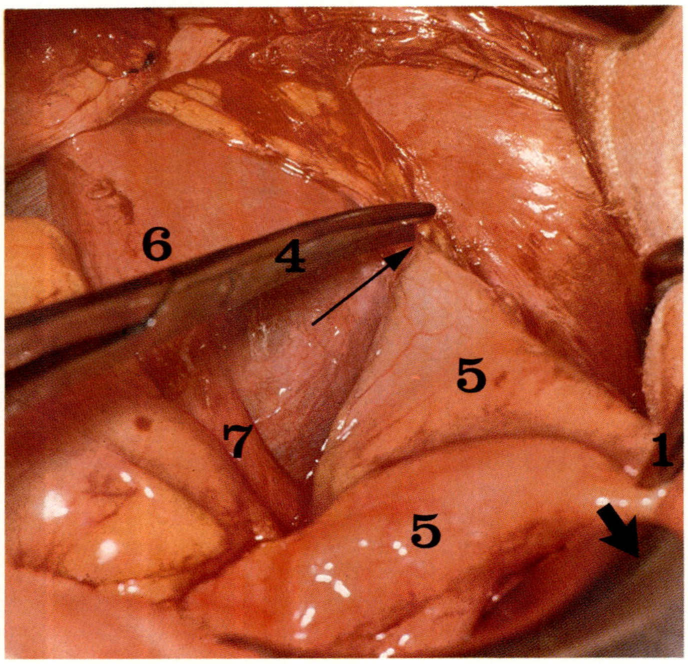

14
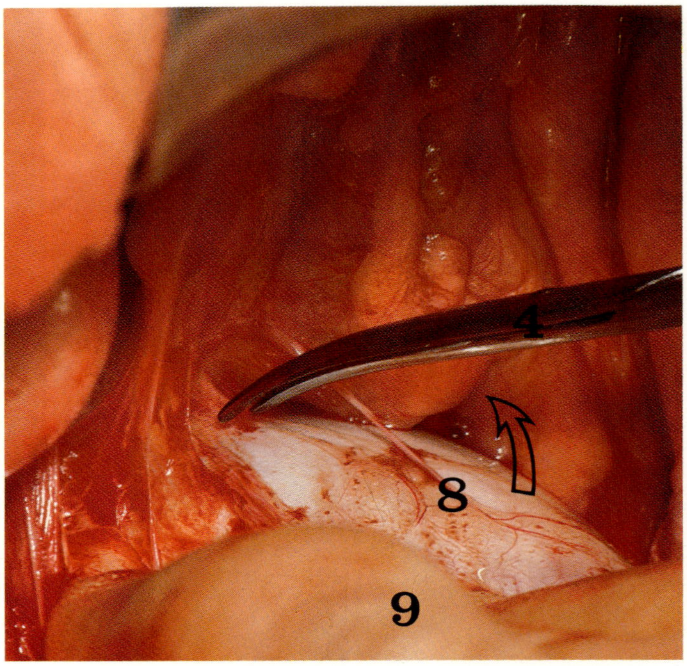

13 Release of small intestine from uterus and right fallopian tube
Coils of small intestine (5) are held laterally by dissecting forceps (1) in the direction of the broad arrow while scissors (4) release an adhesion to the anterior aspect of the uterus where arrowed. The small intestine is then packed off with the omentum. The uterus is numbered (6) and the right tube (7).

14 Right tubo-ovarian cyst defined
Retraction of the uterus reveals a thick-walled tubo-ovarian cyst (8). This is defined by scissors and the surgeon's finger (9) elevates it in the general direction of the curved arrow. Such cysts are of retention type replacing a previous abscess and inevitably rupture when disturbed.

15

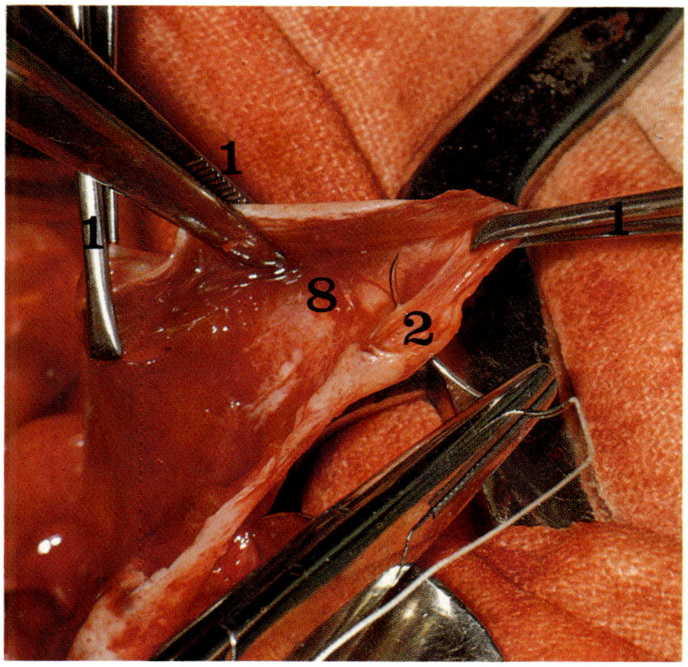

16

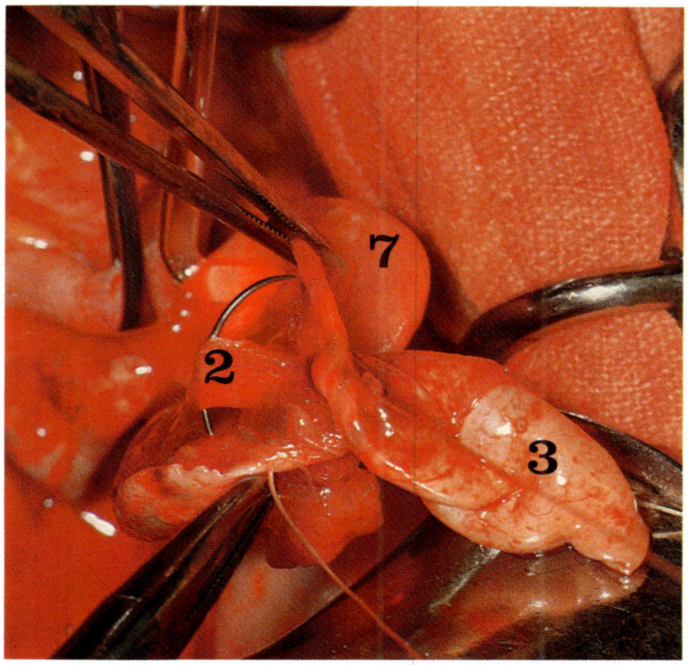

15 and 16 Reconstitution of right ovary
The spread out ovary (8) had largely formed the wall of the cyst and is seen being held open by dissecting and tissue forceps (1) in **Figure 15**. Reconstruction and compaction of the ovary in two layers is commencing with a No. 00 PGA suture on a round needle (2) and in **Figure 16** the process continues. As the ovary is closed and decreases in size it recedes medially to reveal the fallopian tube above (7) curving laterally and with a surprisingly healthy looking fimbrial end (3).

17

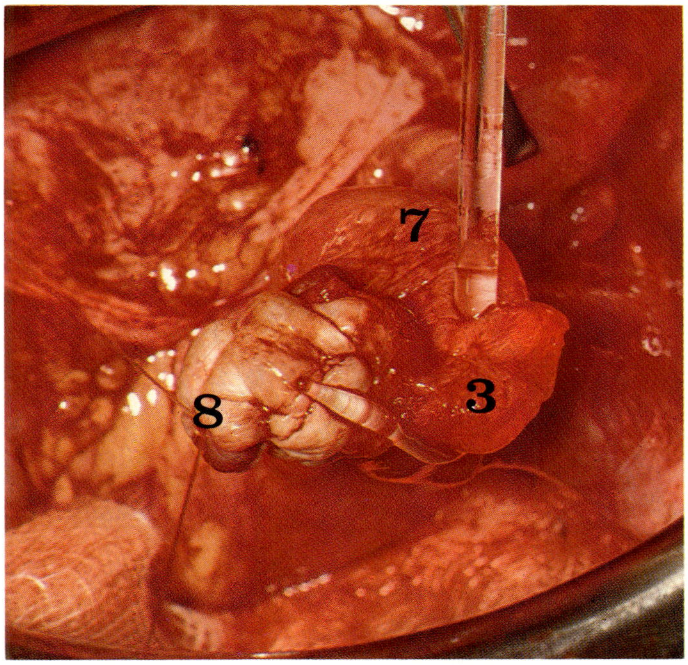

18

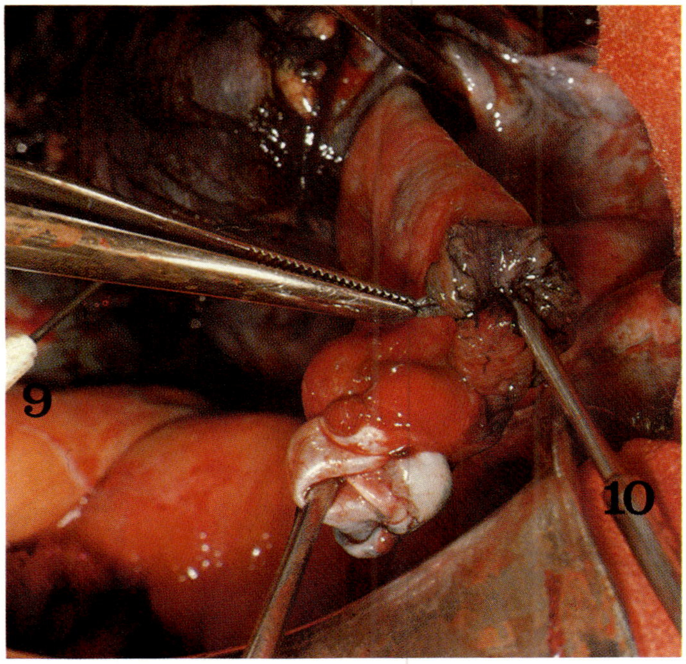

17 and 18 Salpingolysis and ovarian reconstruction complete: tubal patency established
The second layer of sutures in the ovary (8) is being tied off and it is seen that the gonad is now of normal size and approximately normal shape. The tube (7) curves round above it in normal position and the fimbrial end (3) is supported on a curved glass rod for display purposes. The cervix was occluded vaginally before opening the abdomen and methylene blue dye is injected (9) into the uterine cavity in **Figure 18**. It is seen escaping from the end of the tube which is denoted by a probe (10).

Salpingostomy

Various surgical procedures come under this general heading and suggestions for a better nomenclature have been advanced. The 'Miami' classification has much to commend it and is reproduced in Appendix C. The term salpingostomy should always be taken to denote the surgical opening of the distal part of a completely blocked fallopian tube.

Three operations are described in this section and one of these should meet the requirements of most cases. The first is essentially a fimbriolysis in which the freed fimbrial edge is sutured back as a cuff. The second is the classic case of a sealed hydrosalpinx being opened by a plastic procedure and the third deals with the application of a Mulligan hood.

Surgical techniques are influenced by the need to keep the tubes open postoperatively whereas the damage already done to these structures by infection is the major factor in causing infertility. They are fibrotic and immobile with ciliated epithelium replaced by squamous cells and the whole oocyte transport system is compromised.

1: Salpingostomy by fimbriolysis and eversion suture at the ostium

Careful and gentle separation of agglutinated and adherent fimbriae may sometimes result in opening the lateral end of the blocked tube. The fimbriae themselves may appear surprisingly normal and on occasion the surgeon may decide not to interfere further. Such a limited procedure is attractive if the tissues appear very normal; on the other hand it would clearly be over-optimistic to expect the majority of such tubes to remain open on their own and for that reason a series of fine sutures is generally inserted to fold back the fimbriae in the form of a narrow cuff.

19

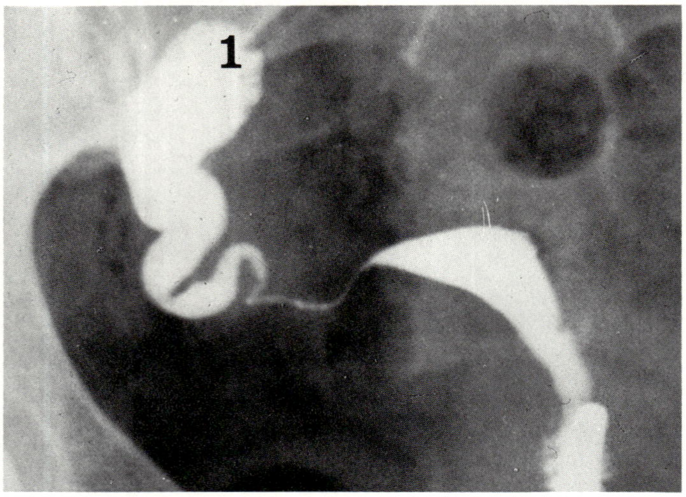

19 Hysterogram
The right tube is distended with no spill and the fimbrial end is occluded. The thin linear pattern at (1) could indicate phimosis. (See page 94.)

20

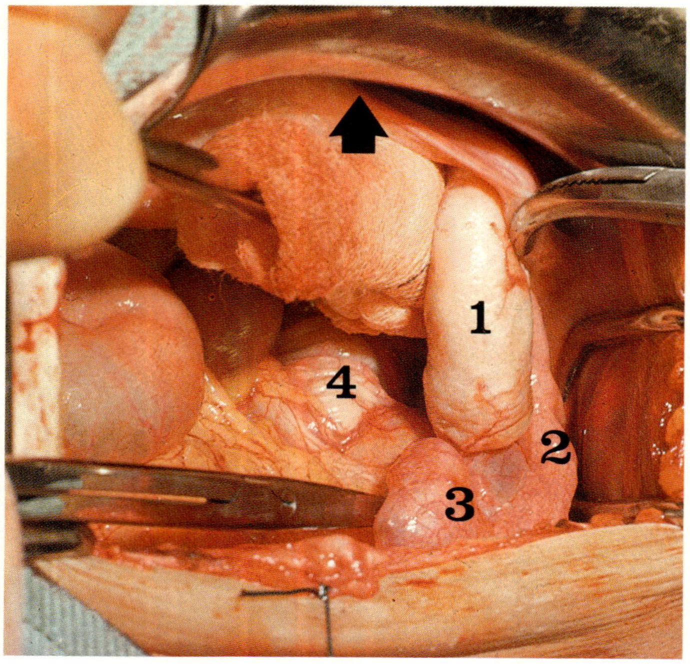

20 Appearance at laparotomy
The uterus is displaced forwards in the direction of the broad arrow to expose the right ovary (1) and the right fallopian tube (2) lateral and posterior to it. The ampullary portion is distended at (3). The rectum is numbered (4).

21

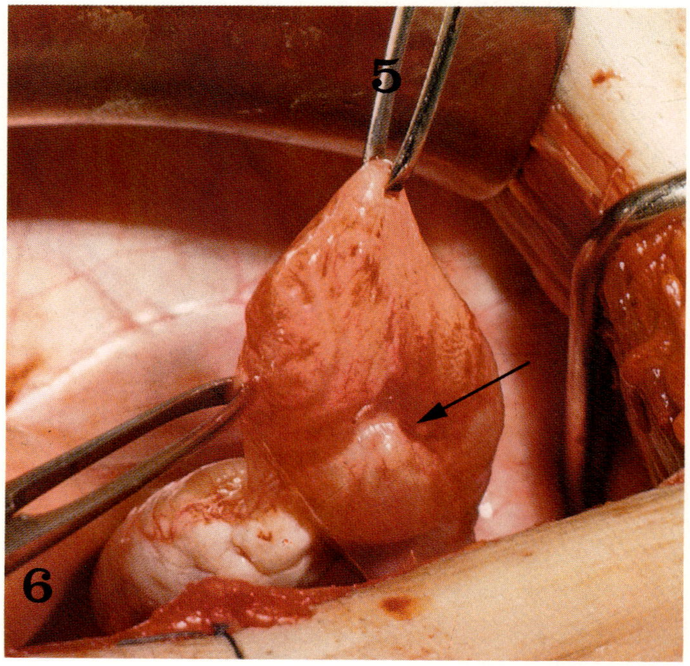

21 Fimbriolysis (i)
The serosal coat of the lateral end of the tube is picked up with very fine tissue forceps (5) and the closed ostium appears to be at the point arrowed. Fine glass probes are gently used to tease the fimbriae apart in an attempt to open the ostium without trauma or bleeding. The uterus is numbered (6).

22

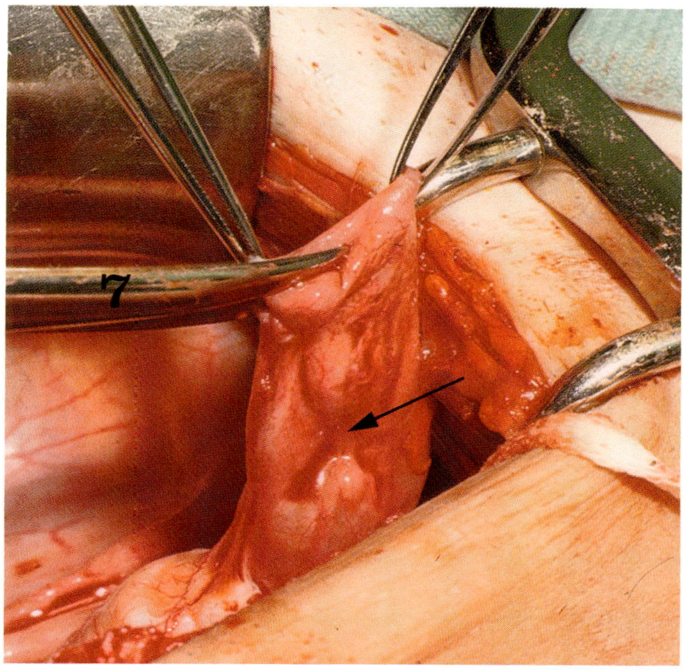

22 Fimbriolysis (ii)
The ostium was open as demonstrated by the commencing escape of dye and its centre is indicated by the arrow. The fimbriae are thick and clubbed together so that the scissors (7) cannot separate them further. Such an ostium cannot be expected to remain open without further surgical attention.

23

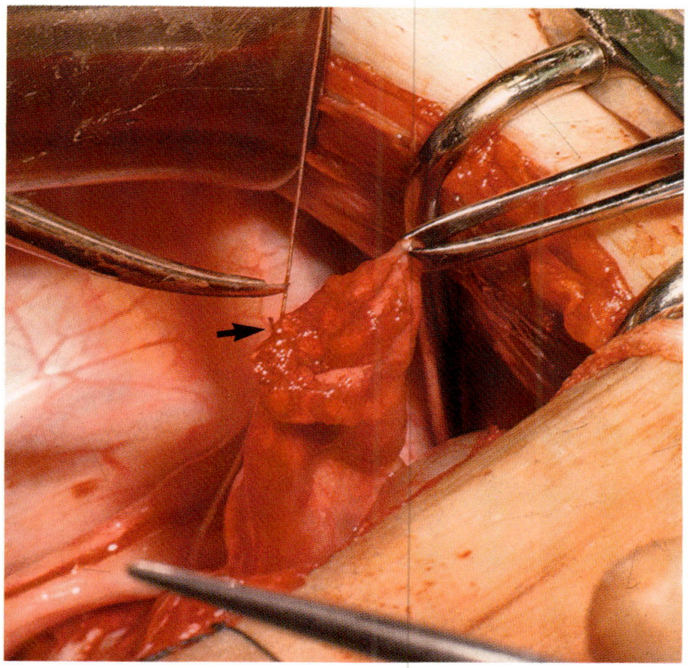

23 to 25 Formation of an eversion cuff at the ostium
The thickened fimbrial rim of the ostium is folded outwards as a cuff by a series of No. 000 PGA sutures in which the needle first picks up the distal edge of the ostium and then the corresponding bite of peritoneum at a distance of 1.5 cm from the edge. As the stitch is tied the edge is

24

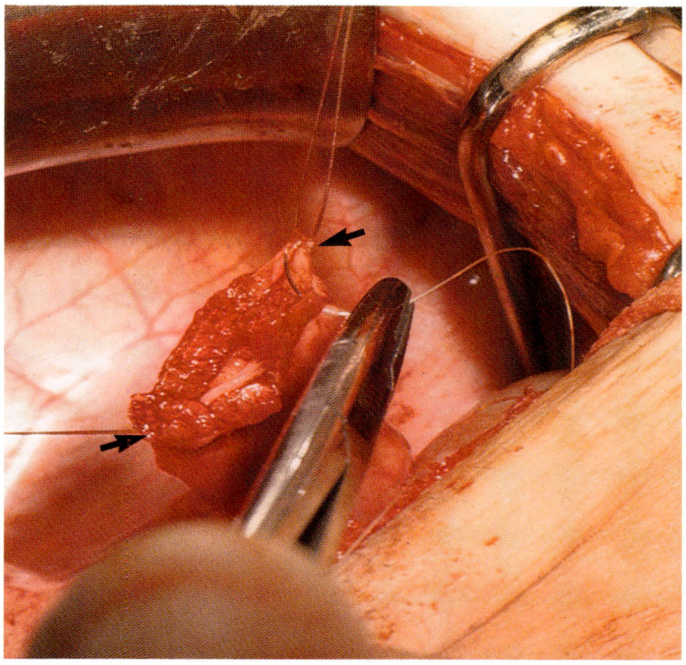

25

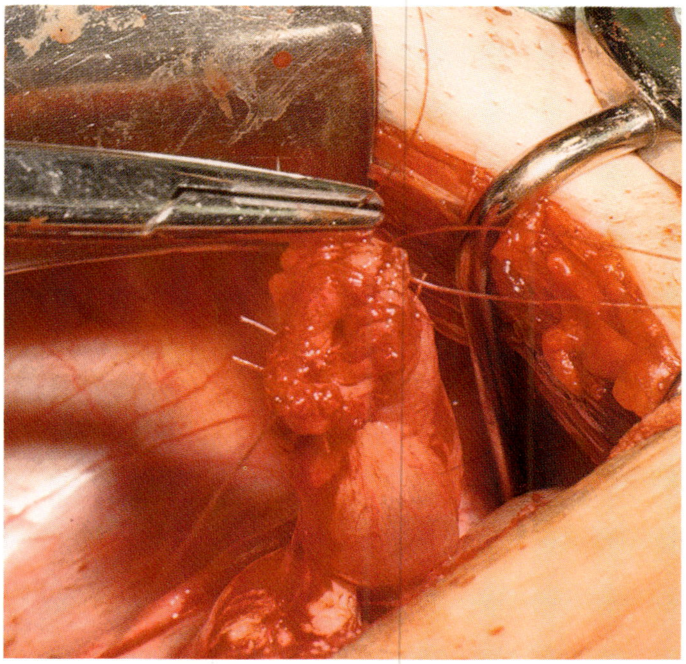

everted and the ostium is opened up. Five or six such stitches are placed at equal distance from each other around the circumference of the opening. **Figure 23** shows the first stitch in place (arrowed) and about to be cut short while the tissue forceps displays the open but stubby fimbrial end of the tube. In **Figure 24** two stitches are in place (arrowed) and a third is being inserted. To suit the surgeon's hand the peritoneum is picked up first before transfixing the fimbrial edge. In **Figure 25** the cuff is complete and the final stitch is being placed. The stitches on the left should be cut shorter; with subsequent knowledge 6 × 0 nylon or prolene sutures would be used in these circumstances.

2: Salpingostomy for hydrosalpinx (stellate cuff operation)

The thickness and fibrosis of the tubal wall varies according to the duration of the pathology; it is assumed here to be of long standing with a thick-walled hydrosalpinx and no discernible ostium. In such circumstances the degree of deciliation will be severe. The prospects of improved fertility are poor but salpingostomy at least provides drainage of the tube and may allow passage of an ovum. The hydrosalpinx is opened and the ends stitched back in a stellate cuff illustrated in the figures. Dye injected into the uterine cavity confirms patency; no attempt is made to intubate the opened tube.

It is advisable to take a biopsy from the apex of one of the opened flaps as a possible aid in prognosis. This is particularly so if one has access to electron microscopy as the ciliated cell count gives some estimate of tubal efficiency (Brosens and Vasquez 1976).

26

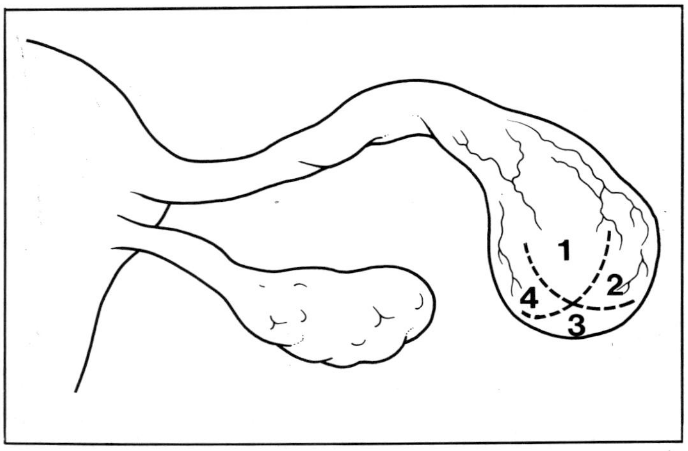

26 Diagram to show site and type of incision*
Each incision is 3 cm long and is at right angles to the other with the intersection over the estimated centre of the ostium. Note the direction of the blood vessels and the placing of the incision between them. Four flaps (1), (2), (3) and (4) with pointed ends are released by the incisions.

Surgical technique

The fallopian tube is mobilised without causing bleeding or creating raw surfaces. Methylene blue dye is injected into the uterus and thence to the hydrosalpinx which it defines and distends prior to its being opened. The supravaginal cervix is occluded by a Shirodkar type clamp and a syringe with an SWG 21 needle injects the dye through the fundus or there are advantages in locking-in a Spackman cannula on the cervix; this avoids extra instruments in the wound, is kinder to the uterus and avoids the leakage of dye into the wound.

The placing of the salpingostomy opening is important in that it should be on the distal end of the tube and yet accessible to the ovarian surface. The aim is to have the intersection of the two incisions as near the centre of the sealed ostium as possible and the surgeon can often be aided in doing so by noting the direction of the blood vessels when the tube is held up to the light. They run distally in this part of the tube wall and the incisions are placed in avascular areas between them as far as that is possible. The incision is made with a fine diathermy needle and unless using microsurgical technique it is probably unwise to use more than the two incisions which result in four flaps of tissue. The apex of each flap is turned outwards and sutured to the serosal coat of the tube with 6 × 0 nylon or prolene sutures as in the diagram.

*More specific instructions on the correct placement of this incision are given on page 142.

Results of treatment in salpingostomy without the use of prostheses

In the type of case described on page 86 moderate success can be anticipated (i.e. 40–50 per cent). Shirodkar (1966) writing of a similar group obtained a 50 per cent pregnancy rate from comparable procedures. (See also results summary, page 132.)

27

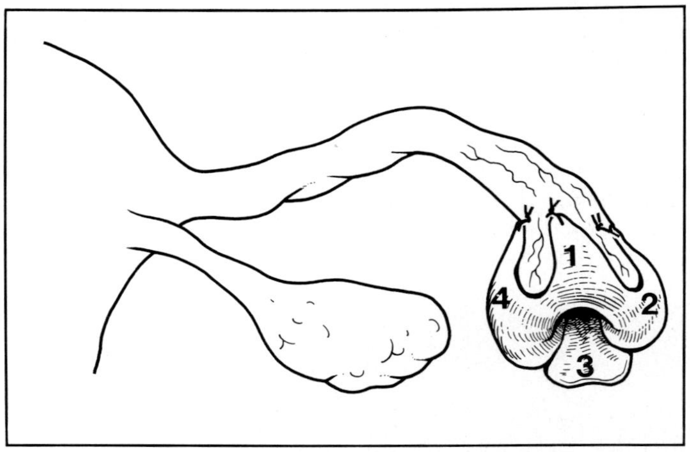

27 Diagram to show stellate cuff salpingostomy completed
The four flaps have all been everted and the apices sutured to the serosal layer of the tube by 6 × 0 nylon sutures. Each is drawn back sufficiently far to give a reasonable imitation of a natural fimbrial end of a tube.

Results from the stellate cuff operation described here are a different matter. They are very poor and carry considerable risk of tubal pregnancy. Shirodkar found that in the absence of fimbriae the pregnancy rate was only 0–5 per cent and Siegler (1969) reported 7 per cent of pregnancies in 119 cases. It may be that microsurgery has something to offer and Winston (1978) considers that with careful selection of cases microsurgery may achieve up to 30 per cent term pregnancies but with a very high risk of ectopic pregnancy. Gomel (1977) had 28 per cent intrauterine pregnancies and Marik (1977) 23 per cent in respective small series.

3: Salpingostomy with the use of prostheses

Investigations subsequent to salpingostomy so often showed the ostia again sealed that methods were developed of artificially keeping them open by inserting inert prostheses. Such operations have been popular over the past two decades and they were encouraged by promising early results. There are several types of prostheses: the authors have tried most of these and prefer the Mulligan hood as the most practical.

It is a great disadvantage that the hoods, having been stitched into place, must be removed by a second operation three months later. The general inclination of the authors is against encouraging the operation but there are circumstances in which it seems to provide the only solution (e.g. where the length of both tubes is mobile and patent, yet the newly released ostia are narrow, raw and without fimbriae and they will clearly seal off again very soon). Because of that and because we understand that many surgeons are using and having some success with prostheses, the technique for inserting Mulligan's hoods is described and illustrated.

Application of Mulligan hood prosthesis

The silastic hood prosthesis* is inert in the presence of body tissue and fluid and is used to maintain patency and cover the raw edge of the fimbrial ostium following salpingostomy.

When the salpingostomy is complete the rim or edge of the opened ostium is picked up by a series of untied and uncut sutures which are equidistant from each other. Four are usually required but on occasion three are adequate. The threads of these sutures are brought through the convex rounded rim of the hood in the same equidistant relationship to each other so that the ostium fits snugly into the concave rim of the hood as the stem enters the tube.

The open mouth of the tube is drawn up towards the inner concave surface of the rim of the hood by pulling on the two threads of each suture and is fixed in position by tying off the sutures in turn. The stem of the prosthesis now extends into the end of the fallopian tube for a distance of approximately 2 cm. Suture of the skirt of the hood to the peritoneum of the tube is essential, otherwise it will become detached.

28

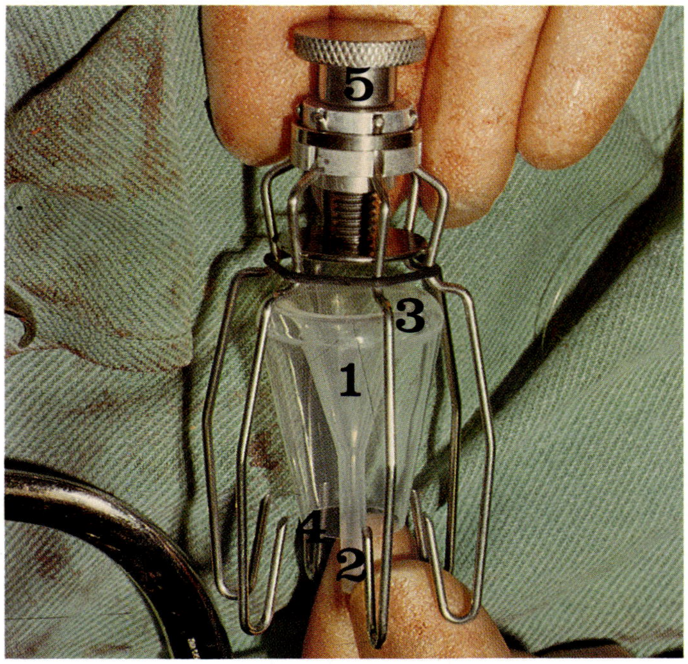

28 Mulligan hood prosthesis with Holter retractor
The plastic hood (1) has a stem (2) which enters the opened terminal lumen of the fallopian tube. The sutures on the end of the tube pierce the rounded rim of the hood (3) to draw the circumference of the new ostium towards the concave inner aspect of the rim in the direction of the fine arrows. The skirt of the hood is numbered (4). A Holter retractor (5) is used to display the hood.

29

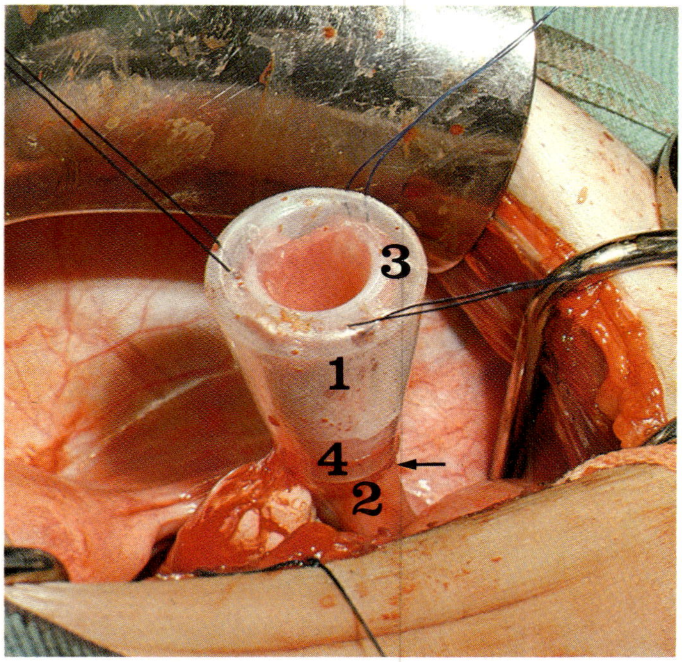

29 Mulligan hood in place on fallopian tube
The hood (1) is in position with the stem within the tube (2). The stitches are ready to be pulled up and tied so that the new ostium lies on the concave inner aspect of the rounded rim (3). There are only three stitches in this case and they are equidistant from each other. The skirt of the hood (4) is sutured to the peritoneal coat of the tube at the level of the fine arrow.

*Marketed by Dow Corning Corporation Medical Products Division, Midland, Michigan, USA.

Stage I: Mobilisation of fallopian tubes and definition of ostium on left side

30

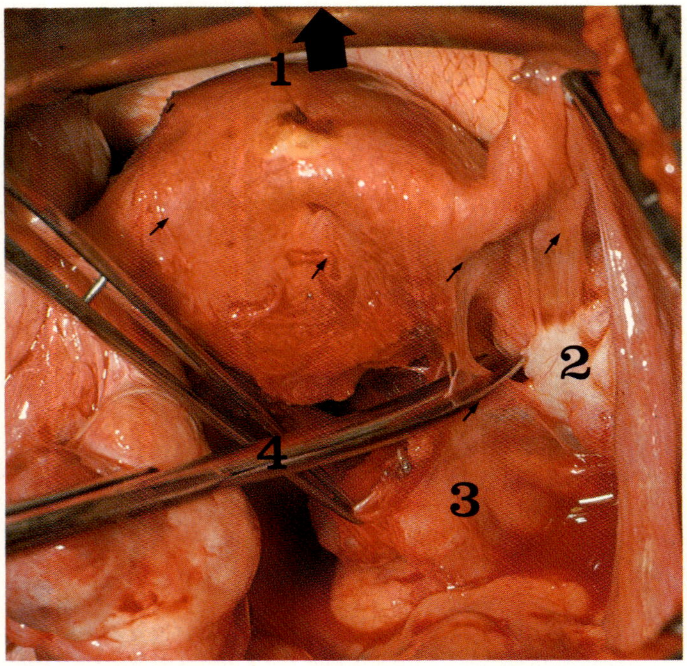

31

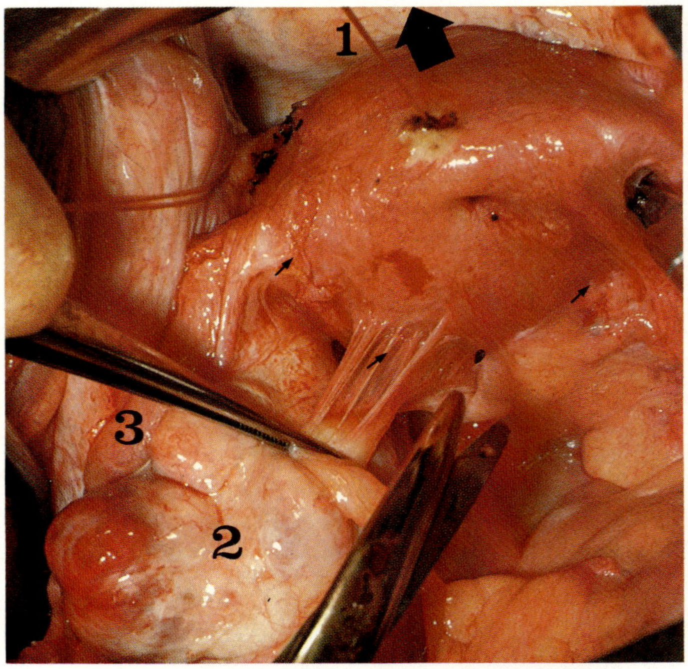

30 to 33
The degree of pelvic adhesions resulting from old chronic pelvic infection is indicated by the fine arrows in **Figure 30**. In that photograph upward traction (broad arrow) on a fundal supporting suture (1) displays the adhesions around the right ovary (2) and also around the right tube (3) which is being freed with the fine scissors (4). In **Figure 31** a similar release of the left appendages is in progress and the same numbers are used. In **Figure 32** the left tube has been freed and elevated from its adhesion to the pelvic floor.

32

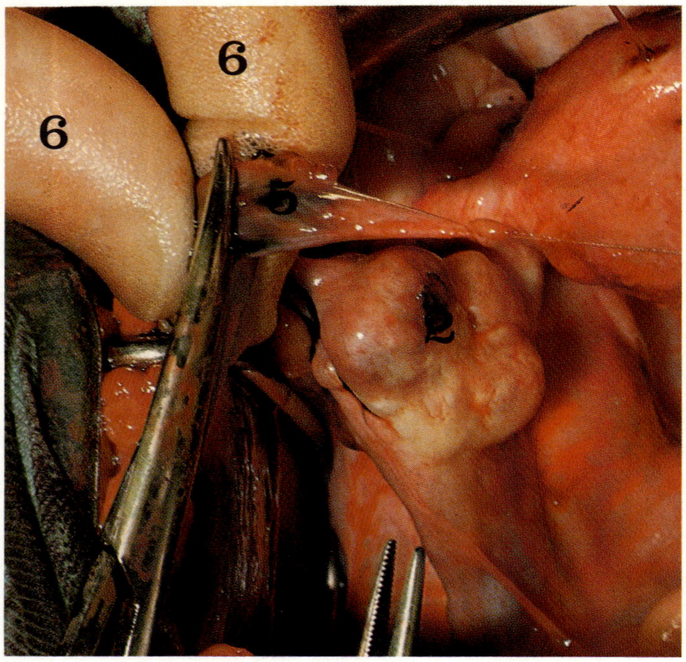

33

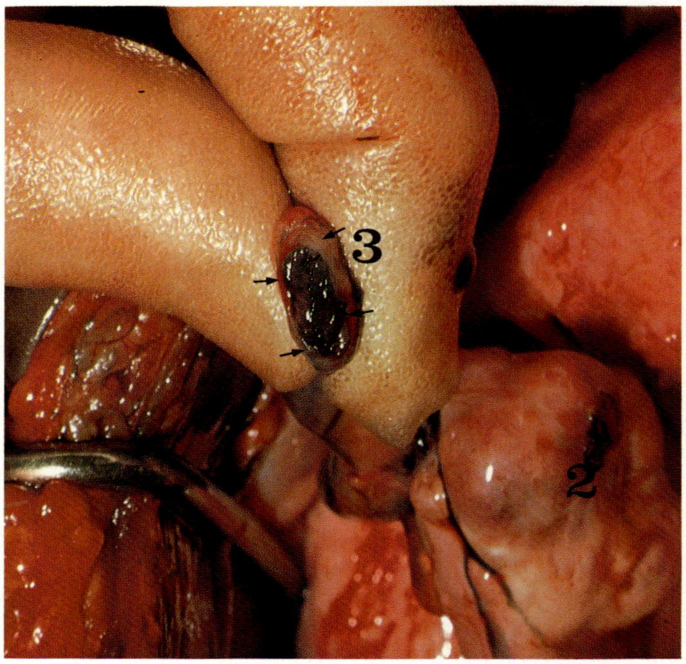

The most lateral portion (5) is held between the surgeon's forefinger and thumb (6) and (6) and shows clearly that there are no recognisable fimbriae. The fimbrial end is replaced by a sheet of fibrous tissue or thick adhesion which is being cut across with scissors in a search for an ostium. The tissue is avascular so that it can be cut without fear of bleeding. **Figure 33** shows the open end of the tube (3) with the circumference of the ostium indicated by fine arrows. Judging by its size it probably represents the lateral ampullary portion of the tube. It is of suitable size for fitting with a Mulligan hood and no further preparation is necessary.

Stage II: Preparing left tubal ostium for application of Mulligan hood

34

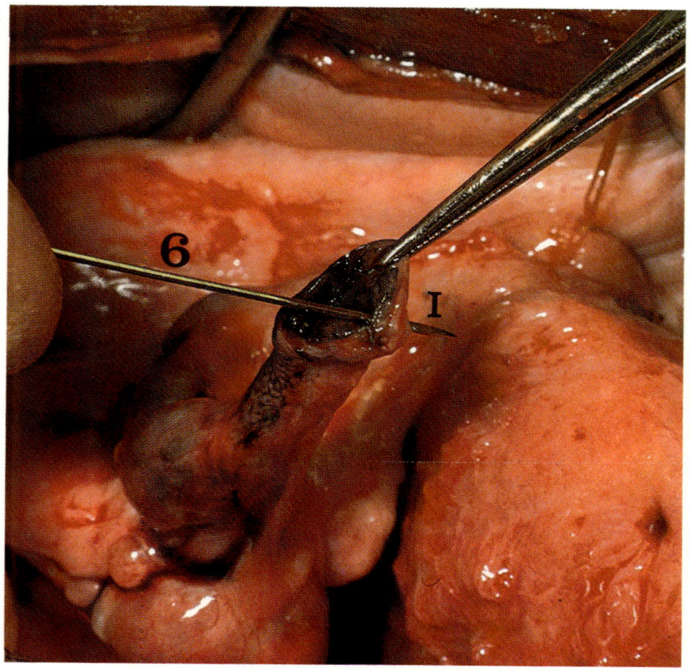

35

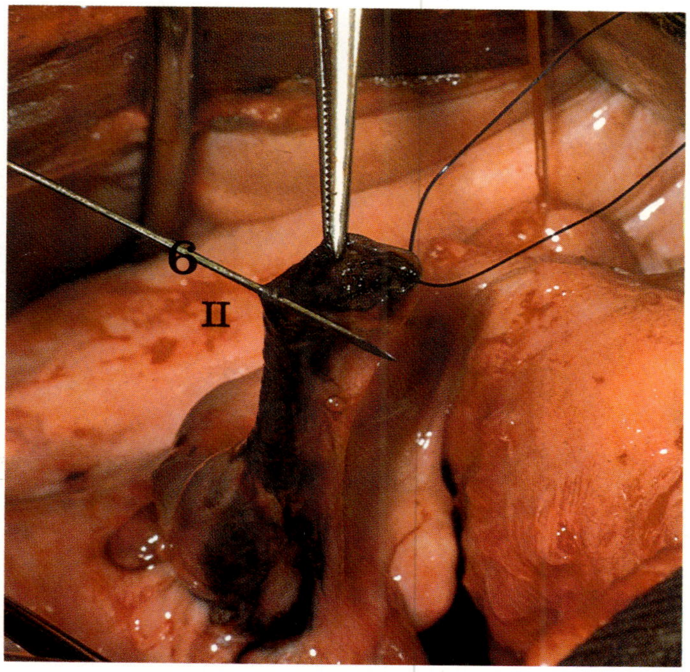

34 to 36
The seromuscular coat of the circumference of the new tubal ostium is transfixed by a series of equidistant sutures (in this case four), the end being left long to subsequently anchor the tube to the prosthesis. In **Figure 34** the first of these (I) is being placed with the ostium steadied by a fine dissecting forceps and the atraumatic needle (6) carrying a No. 3 × 0 nylon suture. In **Figure 35** a second suture (II) is being inserted and in **Figure 36** all four are in place (I, II, III and IV).

36

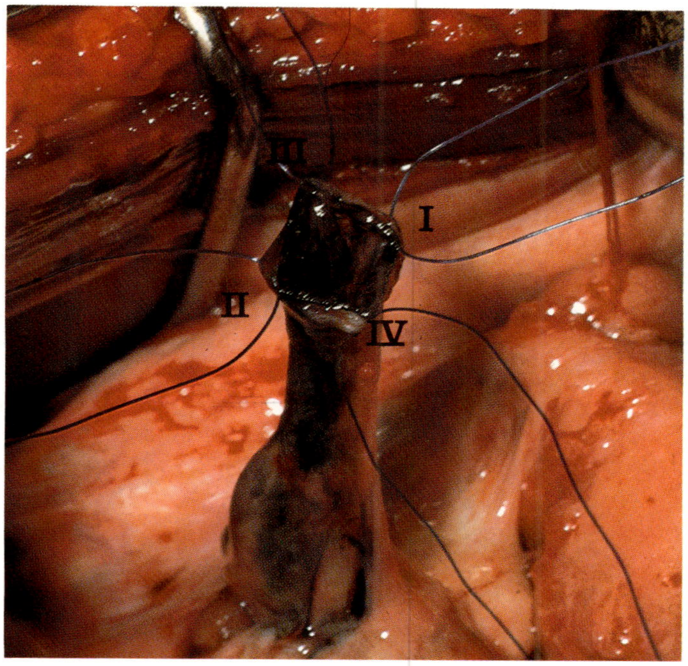

Stage III: Application of Mulligan hood to left tube

37

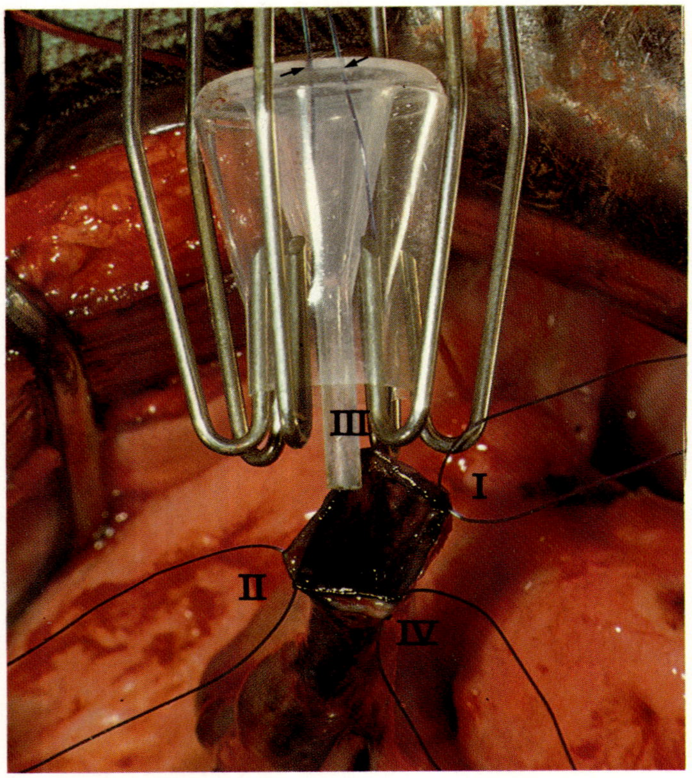

38

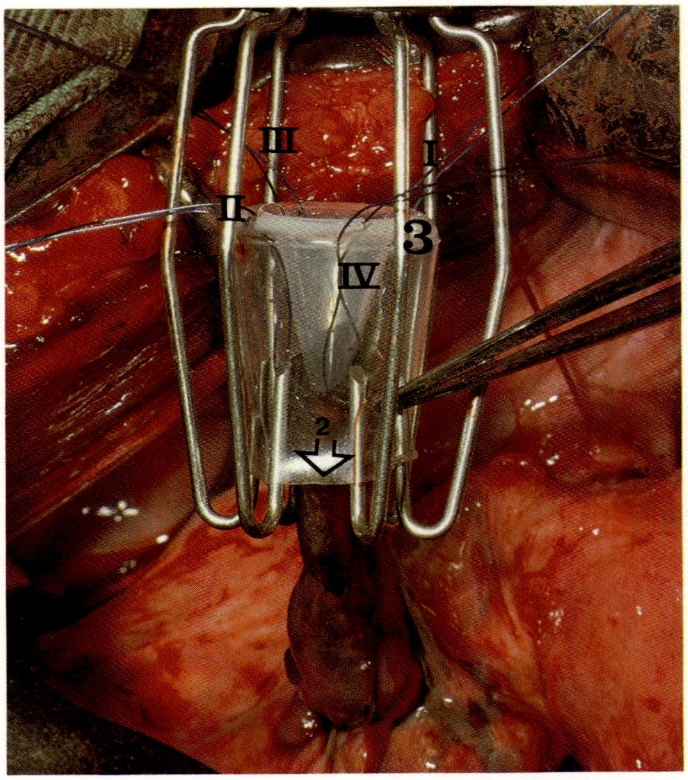

37 and 38

The prosthesis is now fitted on to the end of the fallopian tube in the manner illustrated. The double ends of each of the four uncut sutures (I, II, III and IV) are threaded on needles and after entering the space between the stem and the skirt of the hood they traverse the rounded rim of the hood at a distance of 5 mm from each other. When drawn upwards and tied on the convex side of the rim of the hood each suture fixes the corresponding part of the ostial circumference on the concave side of the rim.

Using the same numerals for the prosthesis as in **Figure 36** the ends of suture III are in place in **Figure 37** and can be followed to where they pierce the rim of the hood (arrowed). If this is taken as the 12 o'clock position then the other sutures will be placed as follows – suture I at 3 o'clock, suture II at 9 o'clock and suture IV at 6 o'clock. The open end of the tube is ready to receive the stem of the hood which will be inserted in the direction of the open arrow. **Figure 38** shows the ostium of the tube being drawn up towards the concave surface of the rim (3) by the sutures I, II, III and IV. Sutures I, II and III have been pulled up more firmly than suture IV which is momentarily left loose for demonstration purposes. The stem (2) (and arrowed) is now within the lumen of the tube.

The Holter hood retractor is not essential equipment and is not normally used by the authors. It may reduce the amount of handling of the fallopian tube and can be of advantage to the surgeon without skilled assistance. In these circumstances it acts as a display scaffolding on which the progressive steps of the operation can be seen as they are completed.

Stage IV: Securing Mulligan hood in left fallopian tube

39

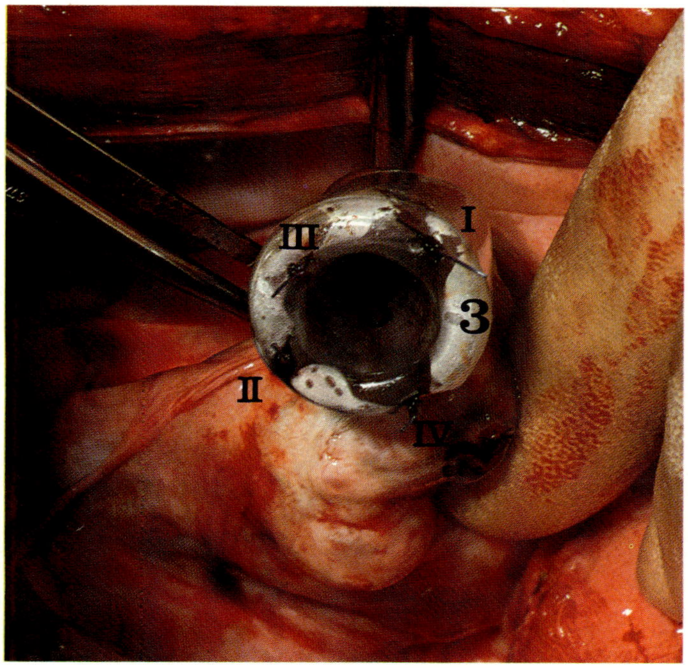

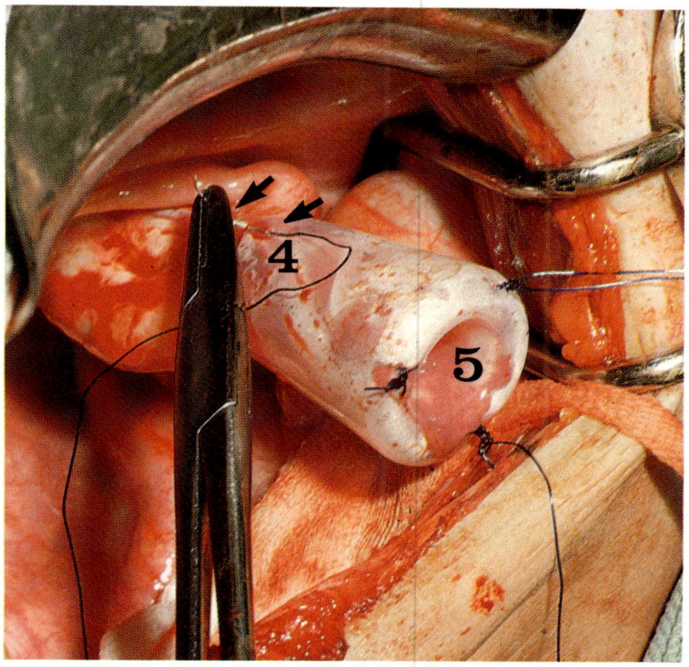

40

39 and 40

The tied off sutures I, II, III and IV in **Figure 39** have drawn the circumference of the ostium to the concave side of the rim of the hood (3) where indicated and it is apparent that they are equidistant from each other. The stem of the hood is now fully inserted into the lumen of the tube. The wide end of the hood (5) lies over and in close proximity to the ovary; it is obviously important to try and retain the features of the normal pick-up mechanism.

The hood would now appear to be firmly anchored to the tube but experience has shown that it will become detached unless the skirt of the hood is also sutured to the peritoneal coat of the tube. **Figure 40** shows the method of suturing. The arrows indicate where the needle has traversed first the skirt (4) of the hood and then the serosal coat of the fallopian tube. Two further similar equidistant stitches on the edge of the skirt would be adequate in this case. This photograph is of the right tube and had three instead of four anchor stitches on the rim of the hood.

Stage V: Completing insertion of Mulligan hood in right tube

41

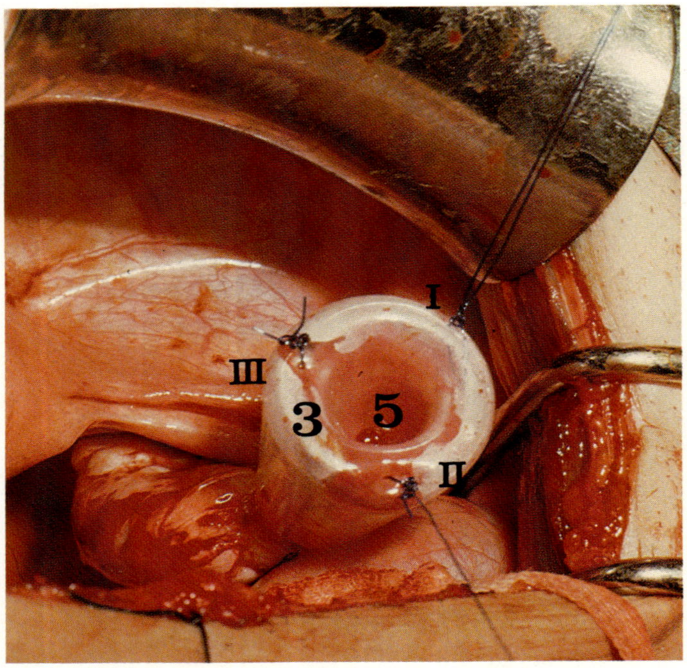

42

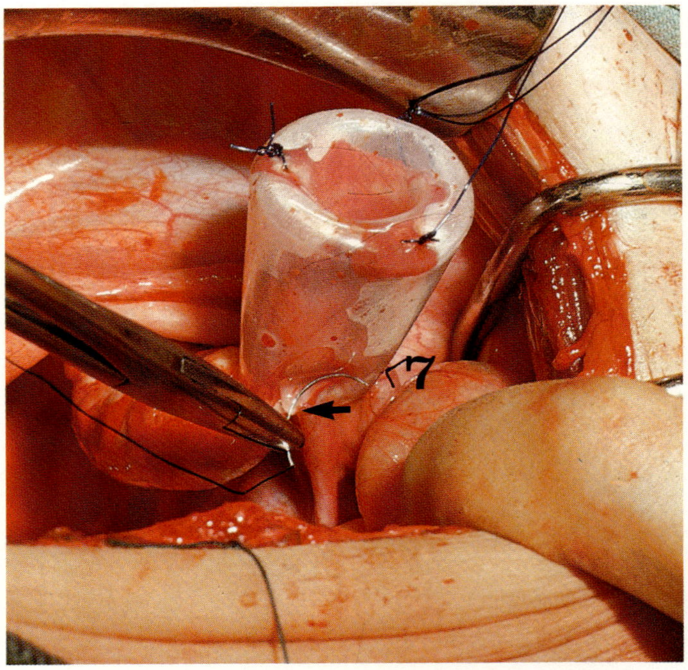

41 and 42
The photographs show a Mulligan hood being applied to the right fallopian tube in the same case. In **Figure 41** the circumference of the tubal ostium has been secured within the rim of the hood by three equidistant sutures in this case – numbered I, II and III, and in the 12, 4 and 8 o'clock positions. Suture III has been cut short, the others are retained as tractors. The rim of the prosthesis is numbered (3) as previously and the open end is (5). **Figure 42** shows the insertion of an anchoring stitch on the skirt of the hood. The needle has traversed the edge of the skirt where arrowed and will then pick up the peritoneum of the tube as in **Figure 40**. One stitch has already been inserted at (7) and a further one will suffice.

Results obtainable from Mulligan hoods

Since study of available figures sometimes aids decision in a particular case it may be helpful to see what has been achieved by the method. Cooke (1978) reviewed all the major series reported and amounting to a total of 284 cases. There was a mean pregnancy rate of 24.6 per cent and a range of 12 to 40 per cent in spite of a tubal pregnancy rate of 57 per cent in 181 cases. The living-child rate calculated from the last six publications was 15 per cent of 215 cases, with a range of 6 to 20 per cent. The ectopic gestation rate was 6 per cent (10 in 159 cases).

Fimbrial phimosis

This condition can be confused with hydrosalpinx but differs from it in that there is a still patent but restricted ostium with a fibrous edge. Some fimbriae are still present and may be mobile. It is frequently difficult to recognise them from hysterosalpingography although a thin linear pattern such as that seen at (1) in **Figure 19** (page 88) should raise suspicions and lead to careful examination at laparoscopy. These cases should not be treated in the same way as hydrosalpinges. The results from gently and very slowly dilating the narrow ostium are much superior to what can be obtained by incision.

Implantation of fallopian tubes into uterus

Tubal blockage involving the isthmal portion has traditionally been treated by implantation of the opened medial end of the tube into the fundus of the uterus. The results of such operations (see page 110) have always been better than the overall figures for ampullary salpingostomy and this is no doubt explained by the fact that tubal peristalsis and ciliary action are intact and the tubo-ovarian pick-up mechanism can still function. Winston (1978) considers that cornual obstruction usually follows low grade endosalpingitis and he has observed that the intramural portion of the tube is rarely blocked. He adds that coexisting hydrosalpinx should be regarded as a contraindication to operation.

The disadvantages of tubal implantation are very obvious. It leads to a shortening of the tube, the new uterotubal junction is an unphysiological one, haemostasis is a problem and the tubal blood supply itself is endangered by compression within the uterine wall.

Winston (1977) using the method of cornual anastomosis reports that nearly 45 per cent of patients with inflamed tubes and 60 per cent who had Pomeroy or diathermy sterilisation subsequently achieved intrauterine pregnancies. The operation however is a frankly microsurgical one which can be technically difficult to do. Winston takes the view that both procedures have a place and that implantation should probably be reserved for those cases where the intramural portion is damaged or cannot be identified or as a second operation where uterotubal anastomosis has failed to produce a pregnancy.

Type of implantation operation

There are three accepted methods of implanting the tubes. In the first the detached and blocked medial end of the tube is removed in continuity with a cone or wedge of uterine muscle at each cornu. The medial open ends of the tubes are introduced into the uterus through wedge- or cone-shaped openings and their split ends stitched to the anterior and posterior endometrial surfaces (**Figure 45**). The second method (**Figure 46**) is similar except that a 7 or 9 mm diameter reamer or cork-borer is used in preference to the knife. A more uniform and smooth-walled tunnel results but access and haemostasis present difficulties and the authors believe that the reamer complicates rather than simplifies the procedure. In the third method (**Figure 47**) the fundus of the uterus is laid open by a transverse incision into the cavity. The open medial ends of the tubes are fish-mouthed as before and inserted and fixed within the uterus under direct

43

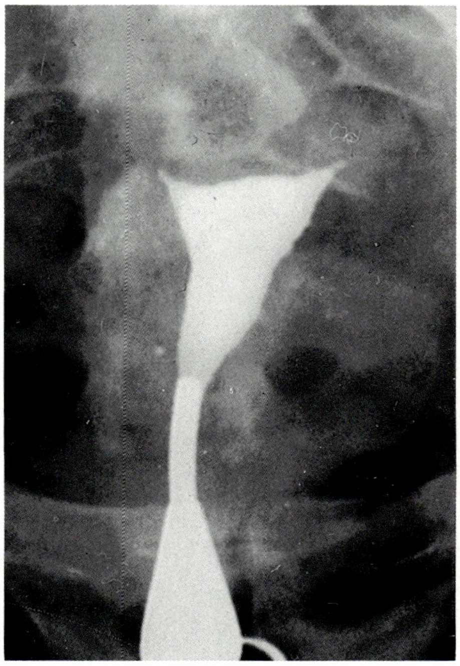

44

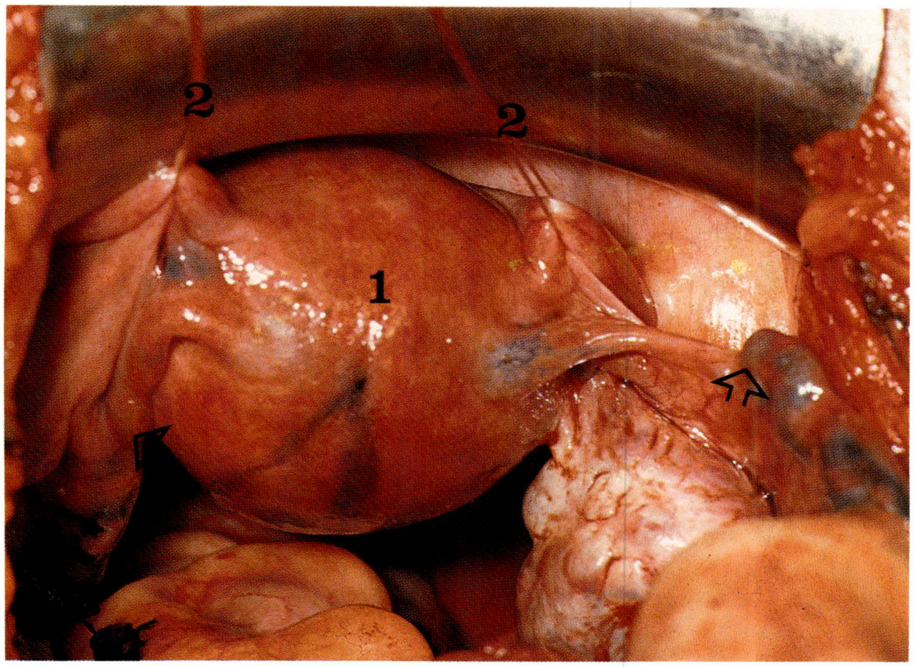

43 Hysterosalpingogram
The radiograph shows complete blockage of both tubes at their medial ends, yet the outline of the uterine cavity suggests that the interstitial part of the tube is patent; present day opinion is that the intramural lumen is seldom occluded.

44 Naked eye appearance of occluded medial ends of fallopian tubes
The uterus (1) is supported forwards by the tractor sutures (2) and (2) on the round ligaments. The medial portion of both fallopian tubes i.e. the whole isthmal portion with the medial end of the ampullary portion is hard and fibrous to the feel. Probes passed into the tubes from the fimbrial ends reach only as far as the open arrows so that the whole of the tube medial to this is useless and will have to be excised.

45

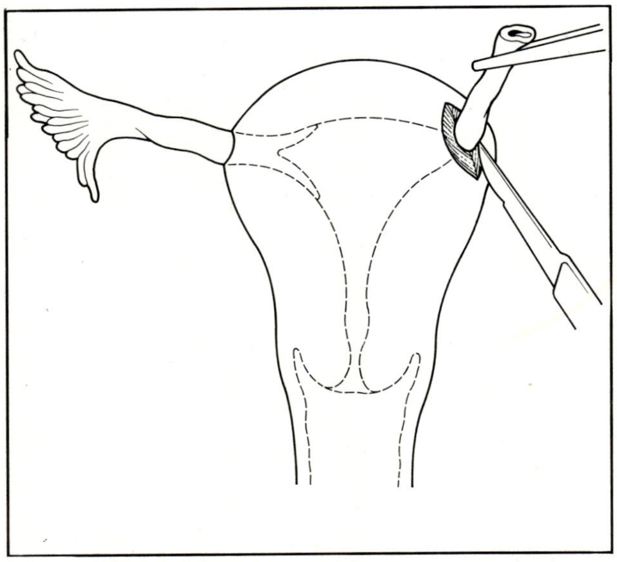

46

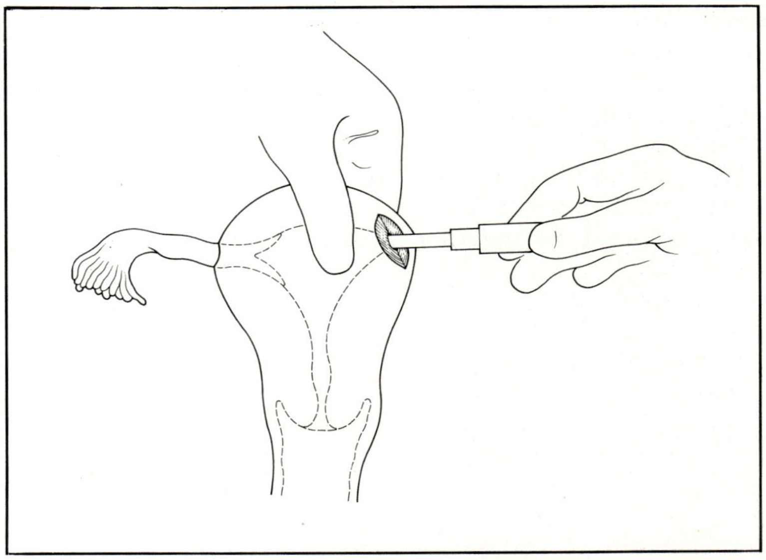

vision. The fundus is then carefully closed. One is working under direct vision and can place the tubes snugly in the uterine wall but the large incision is a likely source of postoperative bleeding and the uterine wall is inevitably weakened.

Whatever method is used and however localised the tubal blockage the surgeon will be dismayed by the ultimate shortness of the implanted tubes. Winston (1978) has no doubt that a shortened oviduct leads to reduced fertility but animal experiments indicate that the effect is greater from ampullary than from isthmal deficiency. In tubal implantation cases the ampulla is not usually implicated and pregnancy certainly occurs in some cases where the tubes appear very short.

47

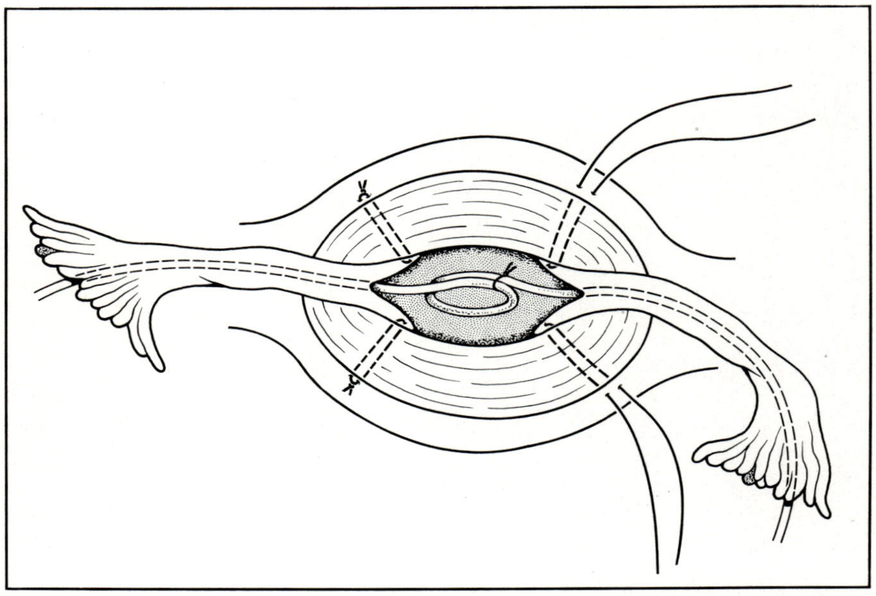

Cone (wedge) method of tubal implantation

The term 'cone' is used in preference to 'wedge' as it represents more accurately what is done in the operation to be described. The lateral extent of the proximal tubal obstruction is defined by passing a fine probe into the fimbrial end of the tube. The tube is transected at that point and the proximal obstructed portion is excised with a cone of uterine cornual muscle to give access to the uterine cavity. Each tube is then implanted as described below. The operation is done under general anaesthesia and it is customary to seek a bloodless field by the use of a uterine tourniquet and bull-dog clamps on the infundibulo-pelvic ligaments. Oozing from the uterine wall when the circulation is restored can be persistent and difficult to eliminate and this recognised problem may account for reported uterine weaknesses at the cornu. In the case described here the uterine and ovarian vessels were not occluded and it will be seen that while the field is certainly not bloodless there is no undue bleeding or clouding of the operative field. If operating under these conditions it is advisable to use a fine diathermy needle when 'coning out' the cornu but not otherwise. This limited use of diathermy is debatably less than ideal, but seems a small price to pay for having immediate control of bleeding throughout the operation. Most surgeons are fully aware that effective clamping of the ovarian artery is more traumatic than they would wish; haematomata are liable to develop at the point of application and can hardly fail to adversely affect the tubal blood supply.

The technique of cone implantation

Stage I: Excision of occluded medial portion of fallopian tube – right side

48

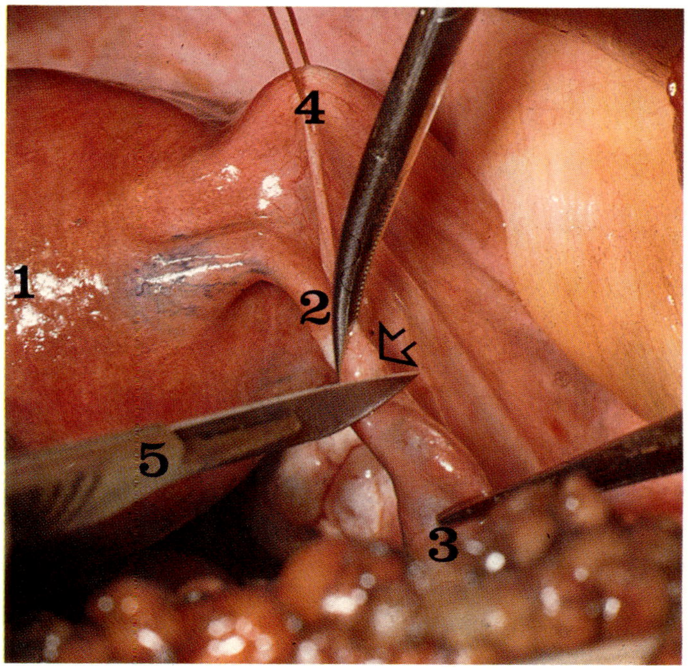

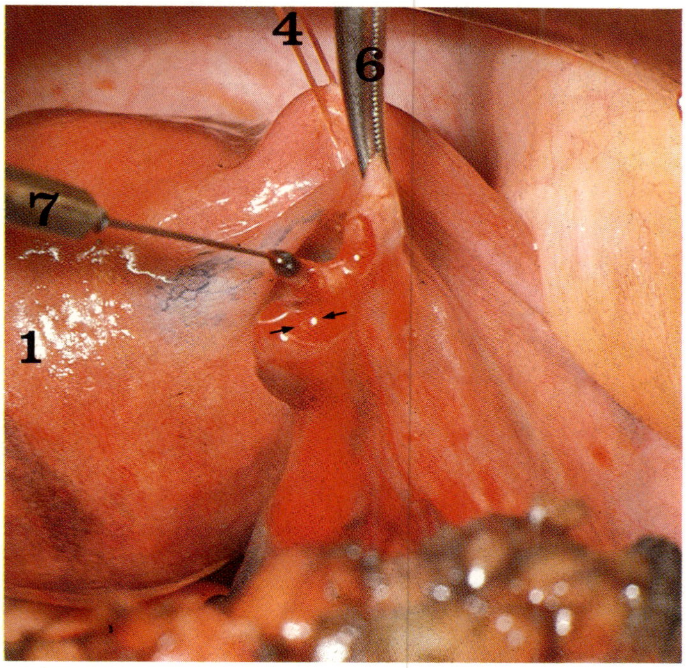

49

48 to 50
In the photographs the uterus is numbered (1), the blocked isthmal part of the tube (2), the patent ampullary portion (3) and the round ligament (4). In **Figure 48** the fallopian tube is blocked as far laterally as the open arrow and it is transected distal to that by the scalpel (5) where there is known to be an open lumen. The open end of the lateral part of the tube is denoted by fine arrows in **Figure 49** and the obliterated medial part of the tube is elevated by fine forceps (6) while the fine diathermy needle (7) seals off a bleeding point. In **Figure 50** the forceps (8) retracts the closed segment of tube and the cotton swab (9) displaces the appendages in the direction of the arrow. A fine diathermy needle is used to 'cone out' the interstitial portion of the tube towards the uterine cavity.

It is most important at this stage to avoid damage to the blood supply in the mesosalpinx. This entails working very close to the mesenteric border of the portion of tube being excised and the aim is to remove the fibrous blocked segment without obtruding on the mesosalpinx at all. The small vessels running parallel to the tube can be seen when the mesosalpinx is lifted up and looked at against the light so that their position is known and they can be avoided.

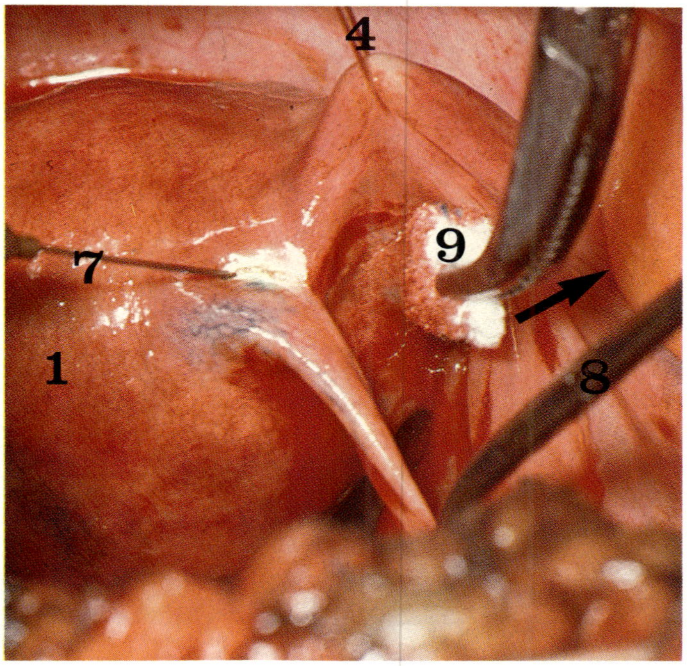

50

Stage II: Preparing uterus and fallopian tube for implantation – right side

51

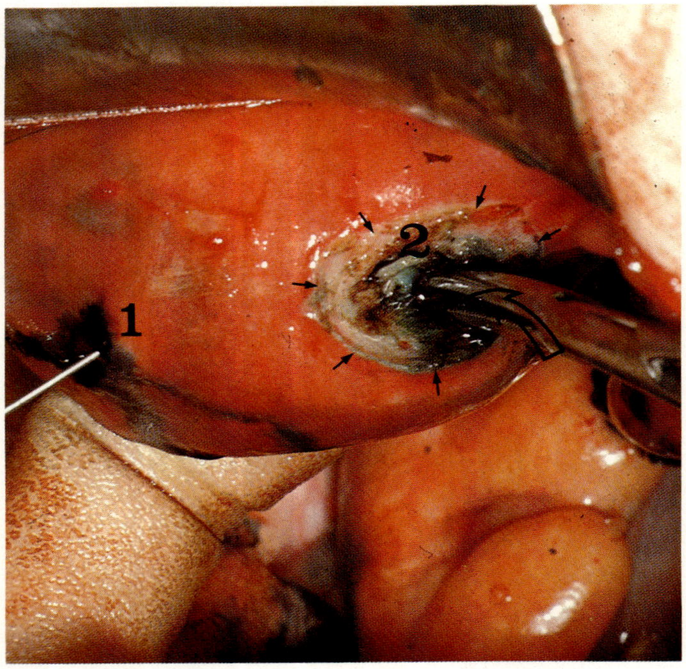

52

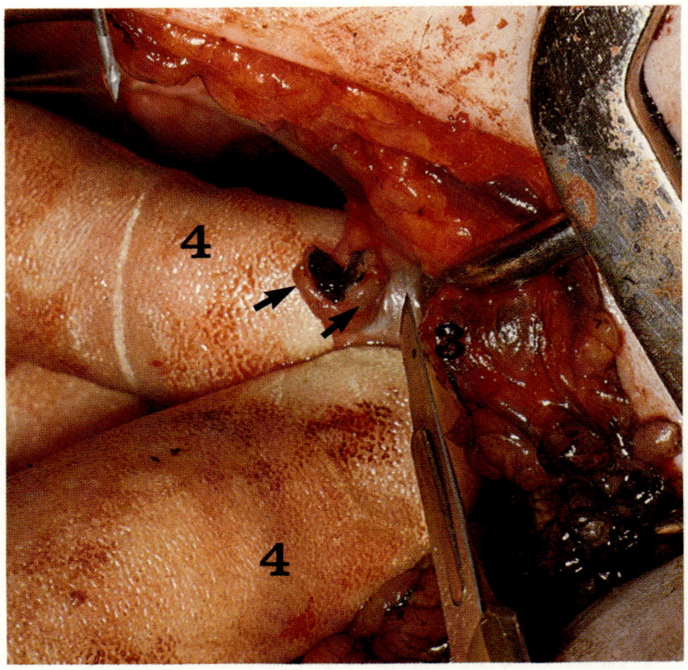

53

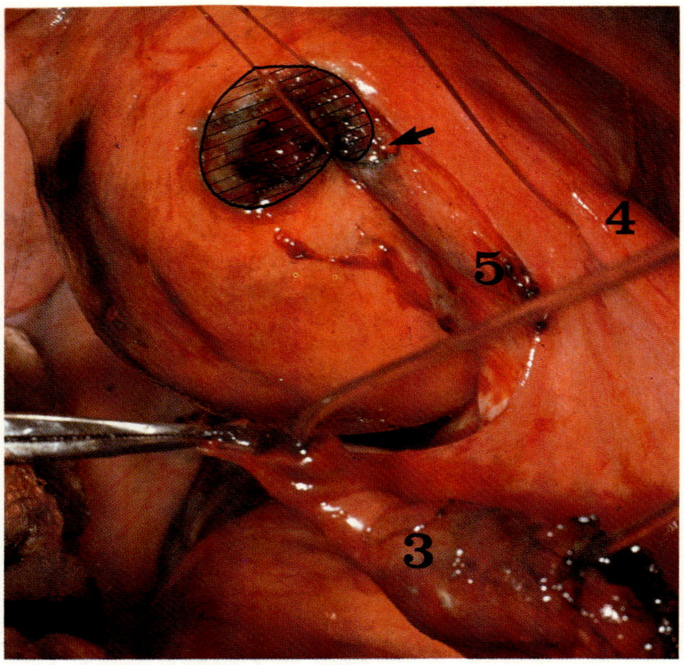

51 to 53
The cervix is occluded by a cannula and methylene blue dye is injected into the uterine cavity through the fundus uteri (1) on **Figure 51**. The 'coned out' cornu (2) gives access to the endometrial cavity and this is confirmed by the escape of dye as the probing forceps is inserted (arrowed). The base of the cone is indicated by fine arrows. In **Figure 52** the medial part of the ampullary tube (3) is held between the surgeon's finger and thumb (4) and (4) and the end is split (where arrowed) to give a 'fishmouth' effect. In **Figure 53** the area of tubal excision merges into the uterine conical opening (2) and is 'toned-in' where it lies above the mesosalpinx (5). It is important to accurately define the point or angle where the conical uterine opening meets the open mesosalpinx because it is from this starting point that the uterine opening is closed around the implanted tube prior to closing the defect in the mesosalpinx. A fine suture of No. 000 PGA material is inserted into the uterine muscle at this point by a round-bodied needle and is left uncut as a guide and retractor. From its position on the side of the uterus the stitch embraces the ascending branch of the uterine artery and it therefore has haemostatic value both when held firmly and when eventually tied off. The ampullary part of the tube (3) is displayed on a plastic tube which occupies its lumen. The fishmouthed medial end is clearly seen. The round ligament is again numbered (4). The level of the angle suture is indicated by an arrow.

Stage III: Preparation of tube for implantation – left side

54

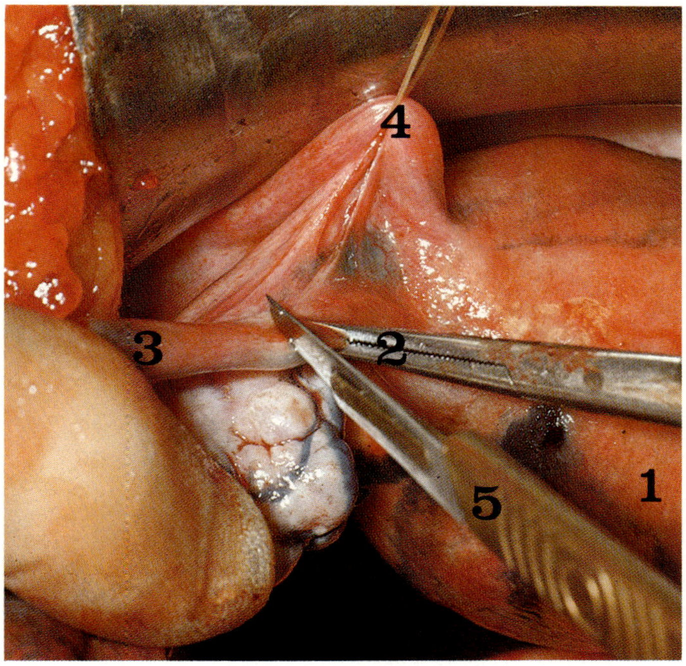

55

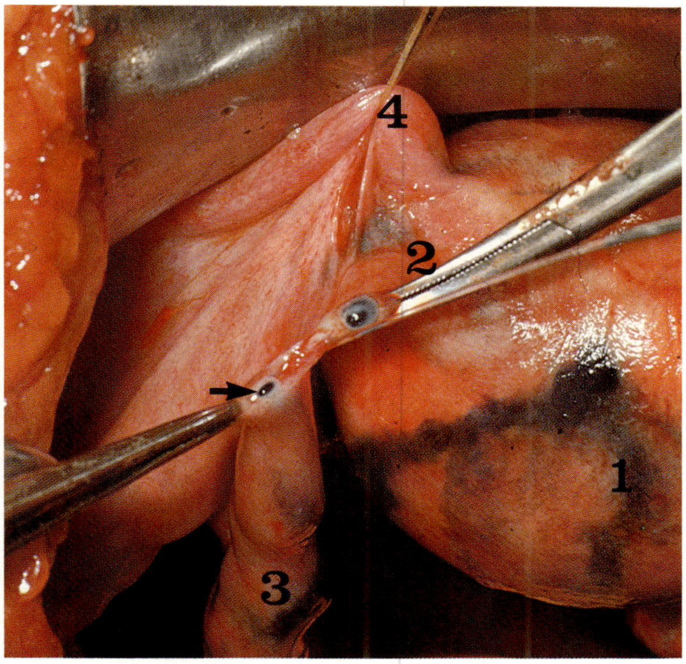

54 to 56
The same numerals are used and similar preparation of the tube is made. The open ampullary end is arrowed in **Figure 55** and where that has been split in **Figure 56**. A stream of saline is directed on the end of the tube as the latter procedure is completed and ensures a clear view.

56

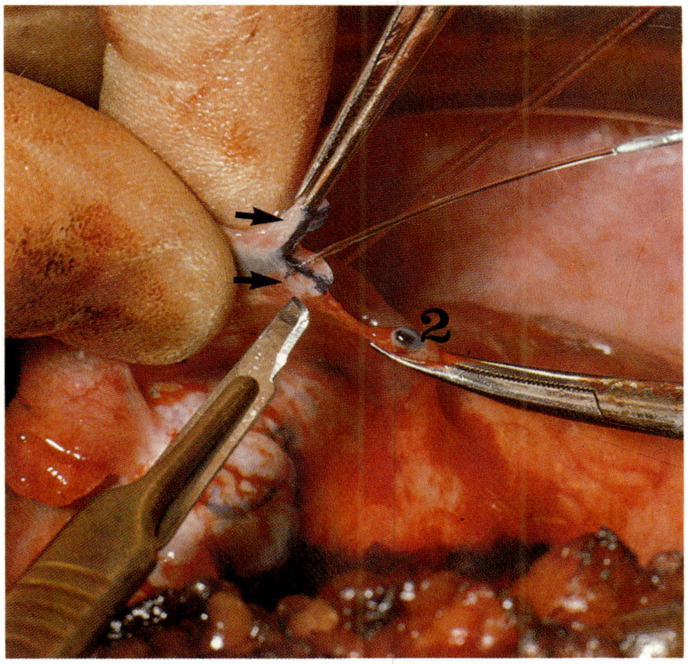

Stage IV: Excision of isthmal portion of tube and uterine cone in continuity – left side

57

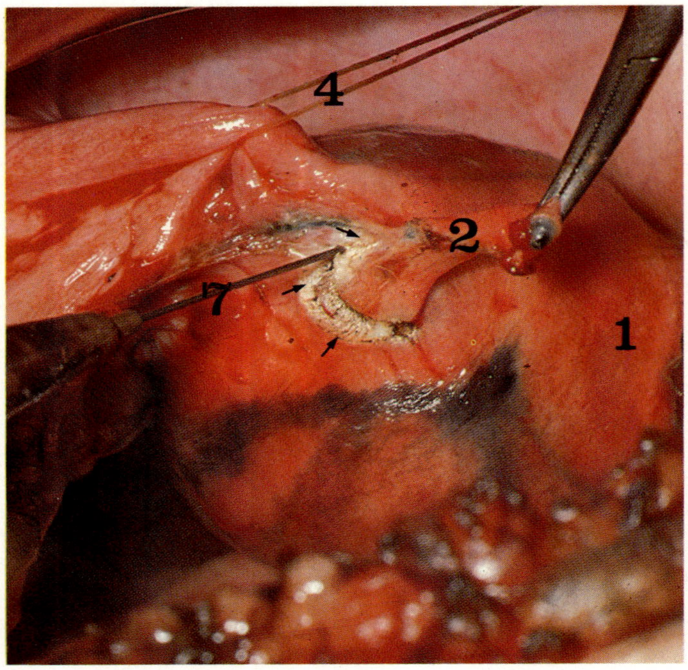

58

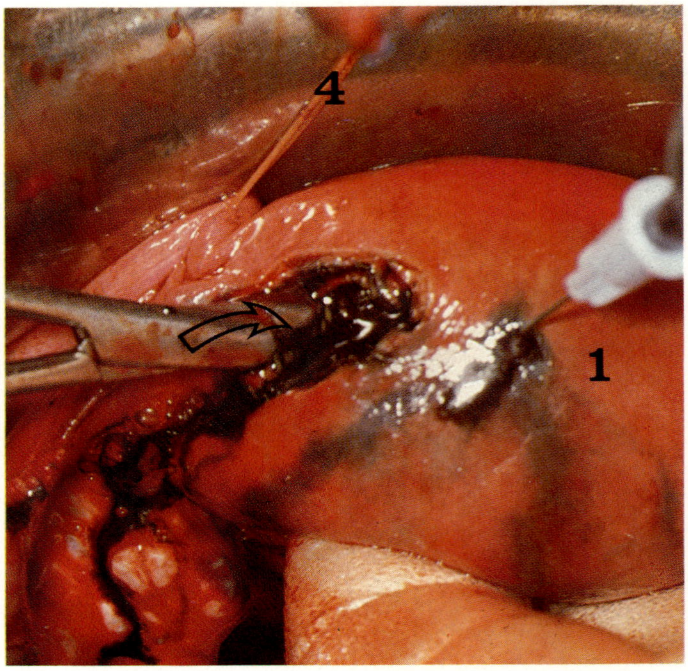

57 and 58
The procedure shown in **Figures 48** to **50** is repeated and the opening into the endometrial cavity confirmed. The same numerals are used.

59

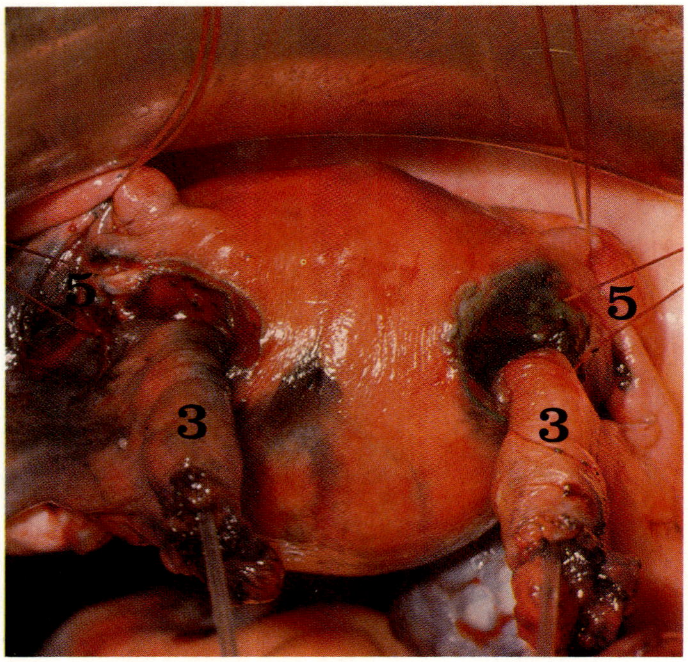

59 Prepared tubes in place for implantation
This photograph shows the prepared tubes (3) and (3) in the position in which they will be when their medial ends are attached to the uterine endometrial wall and the 'coned-out' uterine wall closed around their medial ampullary length. The tractor/guide stitches at the junction of mesosalpinx with uterus are numbered (5).

Stage V: Securing split end of right fallopian tube within uterus

60

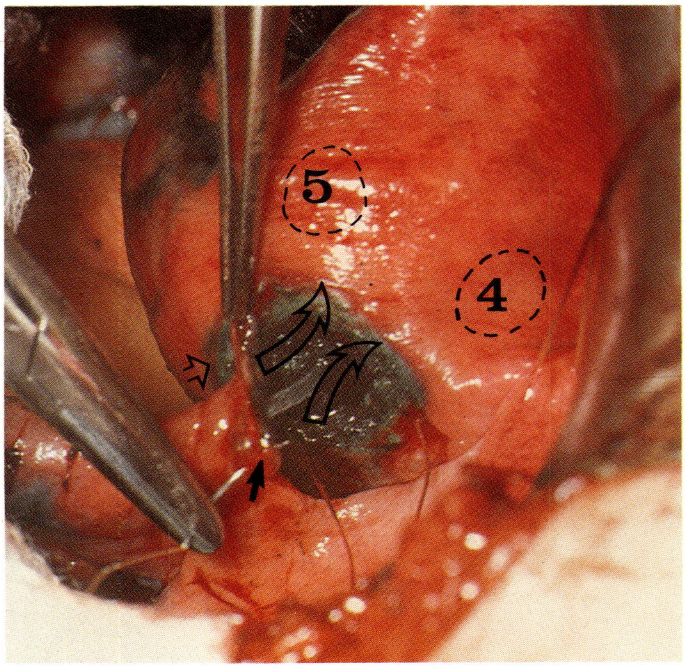

61

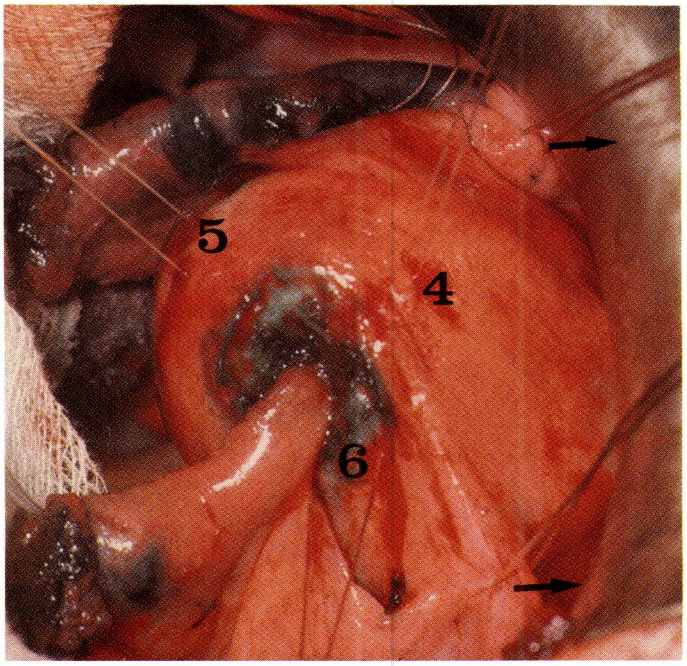

60 and 61
Each of the two flaps of the split opening is transfixed by a No. 000 PGA suture; one will fix its flap to the anterior endometrial surface of the uterine wall, the other to the posterior wall. The two ends of each suture are threaded on to a round-bodied needle in turn and this needle negotiates the conical opening into the uterus before piercing the full thickness of the wall just medial to the cornual opening into the cavity. The two ends of the stitch traverse the uterine muscle and serosa at a distance of 5 mm from each other and when drawn up and tied together on the peritoneal surface they secure the flap to the endometrial surface.

The needle is seen picking up the anterior flap (arrowed) in **Figure 60**. Each end of the stitch will be threaded on to a needle in turn and taken into the uterus along the line of the white plastic tube and out through the muscle thickness of the uterine wall in the area indicated by the dotted lines at (4). The needle will subsequently transfix the other flap (open arrow) and the two ends will emerge on the corresponding part of the posterior uterine wall as shown diagrammatically by the dotted lines at (5). In **Figure 61** the tube is shown drawn into position by traction on the two untied sutures (4) and (5). The angle suture is seen at (6) and mild traction is exerted on the round ligaments where arrowed.

Stage VI: Securing split ends of left fallopian tube within uterus

62
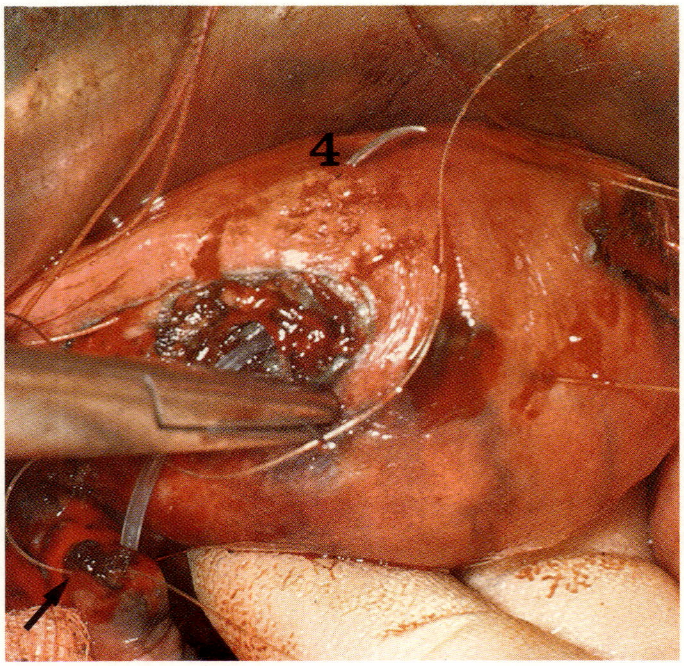

63
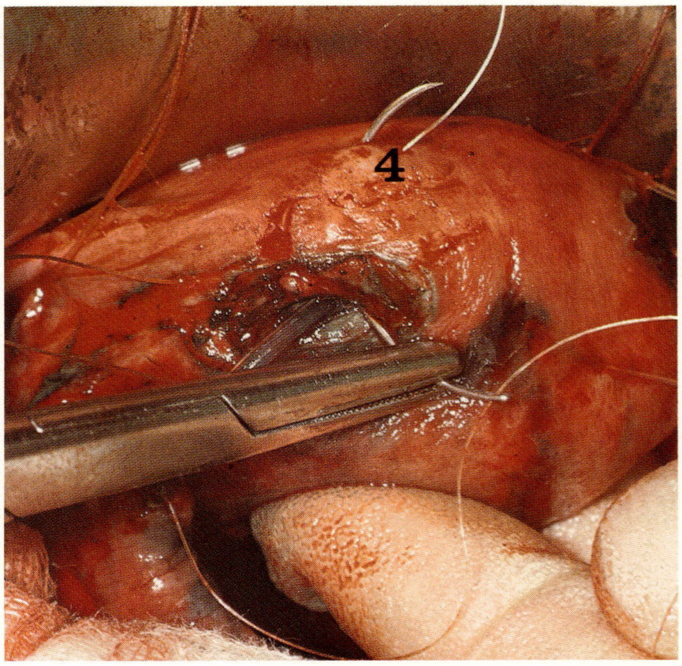

64
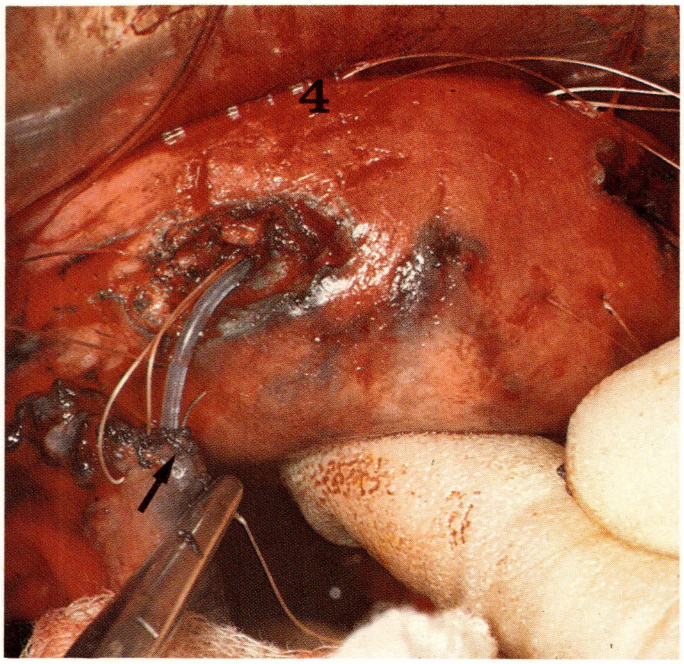

62 to 64
The important step of securing the tubal ends to the uterine wall is shown in more detail in these photographs and the same numerals are used. In **Figure 62** the needle carrying the first end of the stitch on the anterior flap (arrowed) is emerging through the uterine wall at (4), in **Figure 63** the second end follows and in **Figure 64** the stitch is ready to be tied. Meantime a fine needle picks up the other flap (arrowed) in readiness for the procedure to be repeated on the posterior wall.

65

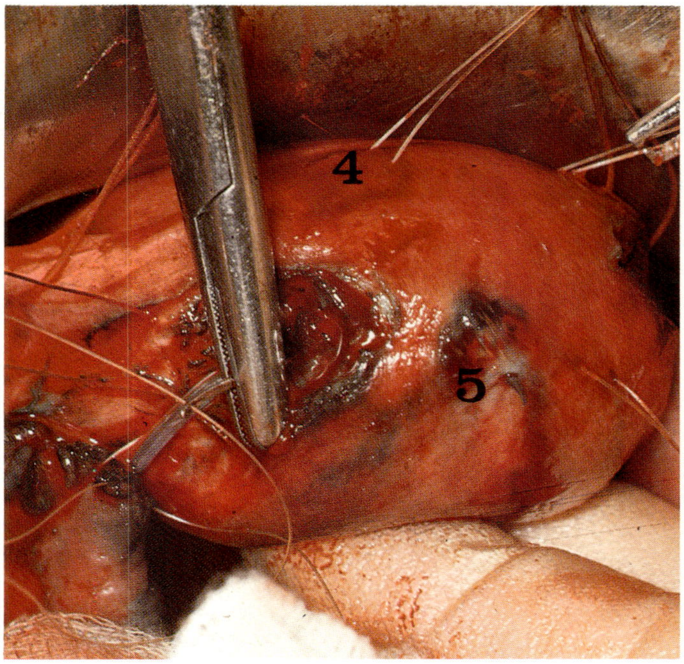

66

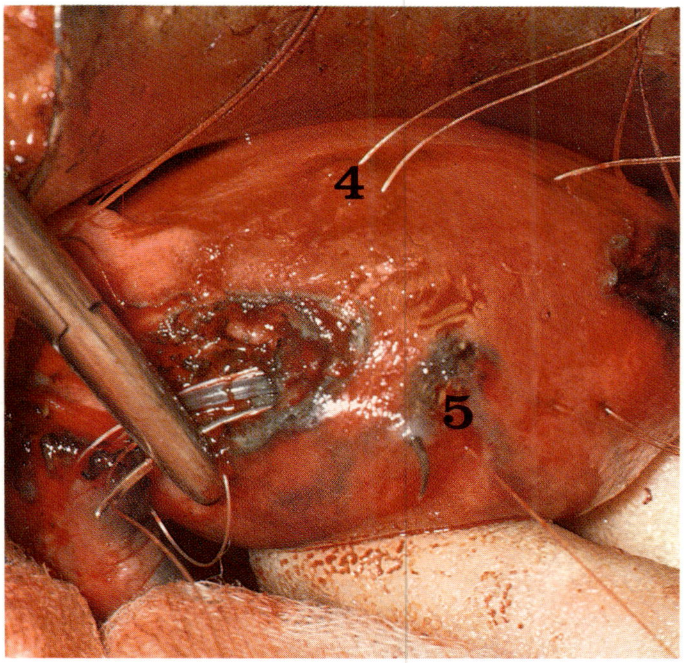

65 to 67
The same procedure is carried out on the posterior flap. The needle carrying the first suture end emerges at (5) in **Figure 65** and the second in **Figure 66**. In **Figure 67** the suture 4 is being tied and suture 5 is in place and ready to be tied. These photographs of the procedure being carried out on the left side show similar stitches already in place on the right side.

67

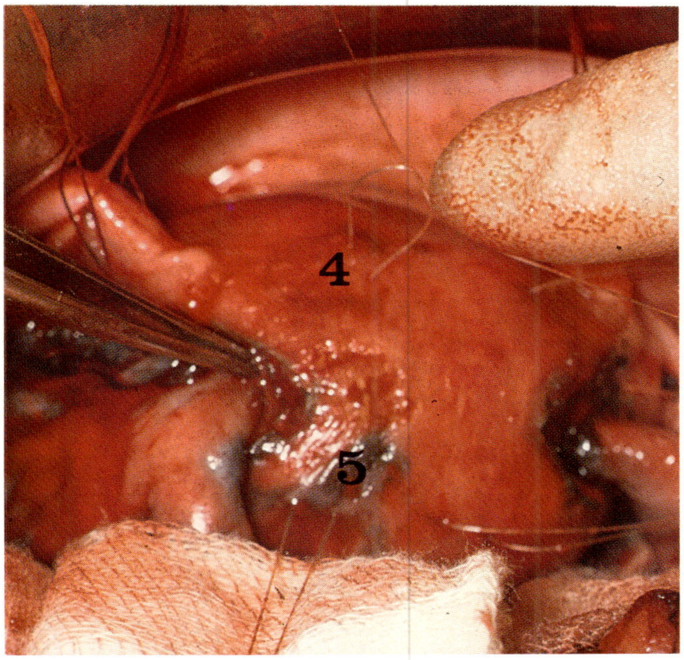

Stage VII: Adjusting cornual opening to fit tubal implant: final appearance

68

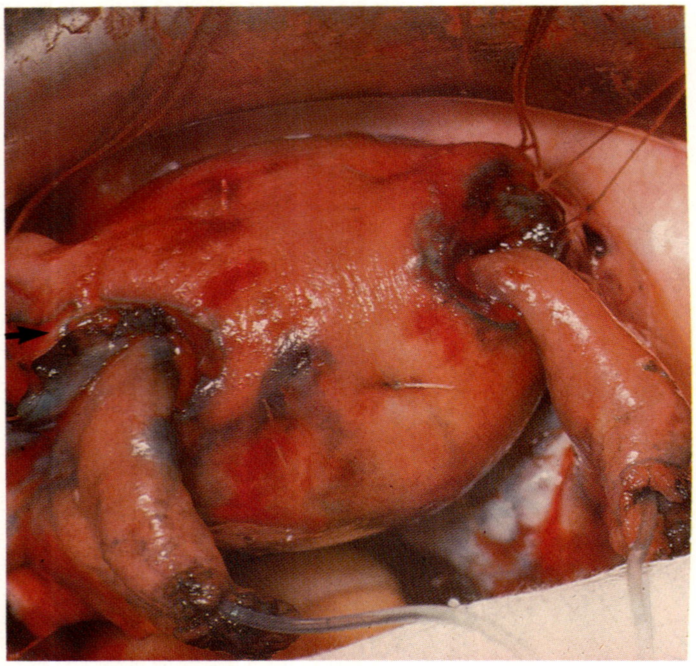

69

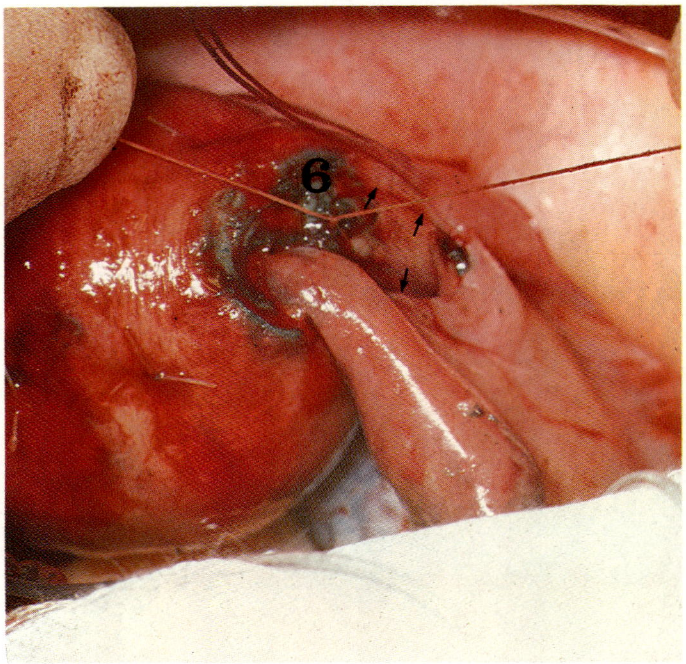

68 and 69
The uterine wall should closely envelop the implanted tube without compressing it and the conical uterine cavity should be closed by fine sutures so that there is minimal or absent raw surface to be seen. In **Figure 68** the first step has been taken by tying off the left angle suture (where arrowed) and the uterine tunnel or cavity is already reduced in size. In **Figure 69** the right-sided angle suture 6 is being tied and is already drawing the uterine muscle close to the tube. The open mesosalpinx is indicated by fine arrows and is subsequently closed by a fine continuous suture.

70

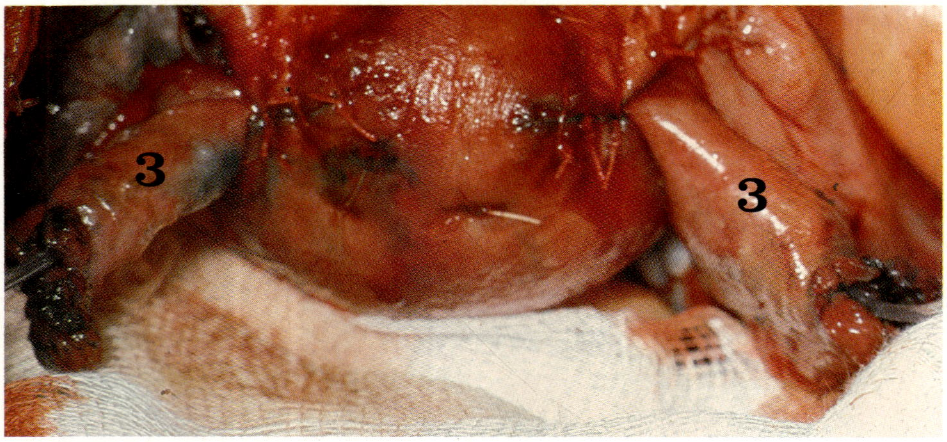

70
Figure 70 shows the tubes finally stitched in position and gives a general idea of the appearances at the end of such an operation. There is some distortion around the tube but no tension and the operative field is dry. The main criticism is that the tubal lengths (3) and (3) do not really seem adequate and this recurring problem has already been discussed. Even so this patient went on to have at least one baby so that an aesthetically pleasing appearance is obviously not essential.

The authors have given up using plastic tubes or rod supports postoperatively in tubal surgery and the tubes seen here were removed at the end of the operation. On the evidence of published reports they seem to confer no advantage and represent an infectious, if not an actual traumatic hazard.

Open method of tubal implantation

The real attraction of this method is that the surgeon is at no time working blind and the medial ends of the implanted tubes can be placed much more accurately within the uterus. The tubes are prepared in the same way as for 'cone' reimplantation and then the uterus is opened across the fundus from cornu to cornu. The tubes are sutured in place and the uterine wall is split so that it can be closed in three layers. The operation is inevitably more formidable, opens up more blood vessels and probably weakens the uterine wall.

The operation is done under general anaesthesia and it is quite necessary to control the uterine and ovarian arteries to ensure a clear operative field. A Bonney's myomectomy clamp is seen being used in the photographs in preference to a rubber tourniquet. This clamp can be very useful as a firm support or scaffold for the uterus in the operation and keeps the fundus of the uterus in the centre of the wound where it is easily accessible to the surgeon's hand.

In the description below many of the manoeuvres illustrated have already been described on pages 97–104 and are not repeated. The steps which are integral to the open method of implantation are of course explained.

71 Assessing extent of tubal occlusion
Methylene blue dye injected into the uterus through the fundus (1) confirms tubal blockage and probes inserted into the fimbrial ends show that this extends as far as the open arrow on each side. The isthmal tube is numbered (2) and the ampullary (3). The Bonney's clamp is seen in the depth of the wound.

72 Preparation of left tube for implantation
The left tube (3) is free and its patency displayed on a plastic tube. The isthmal portion (2) awaits excision. The ovary is numbered (0).

71

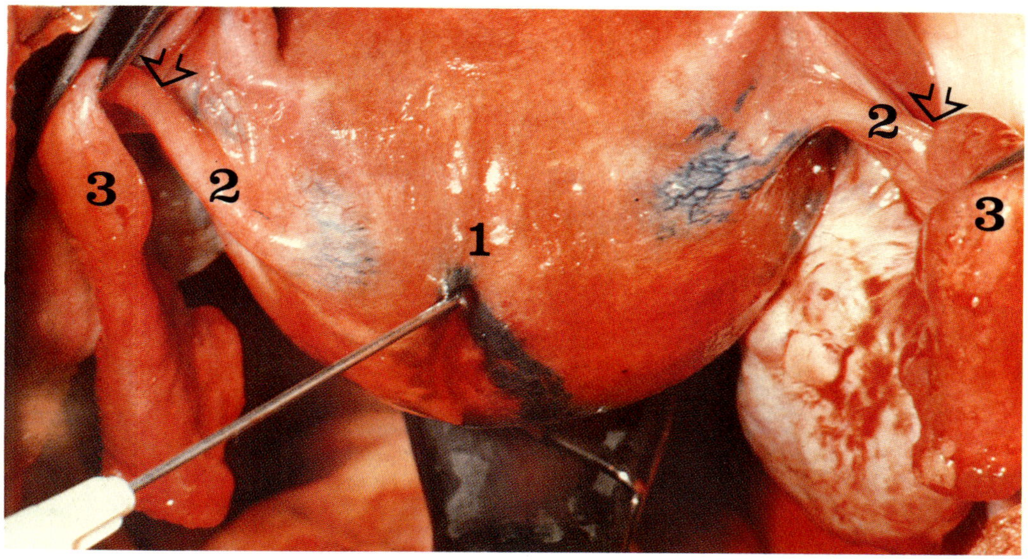

72

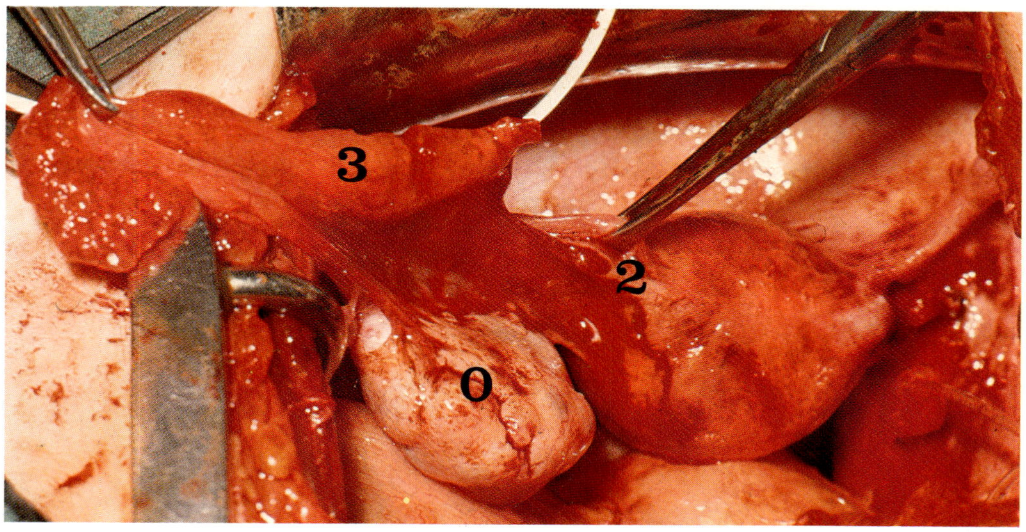

73

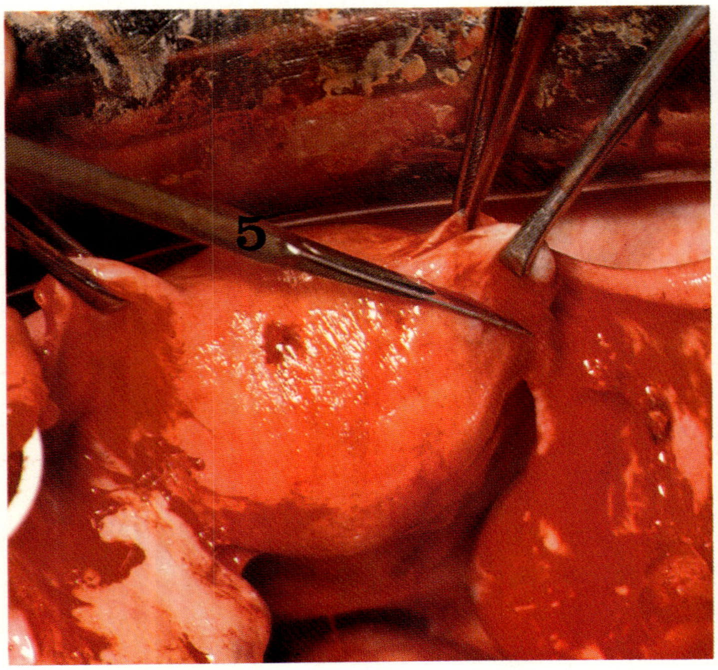

74

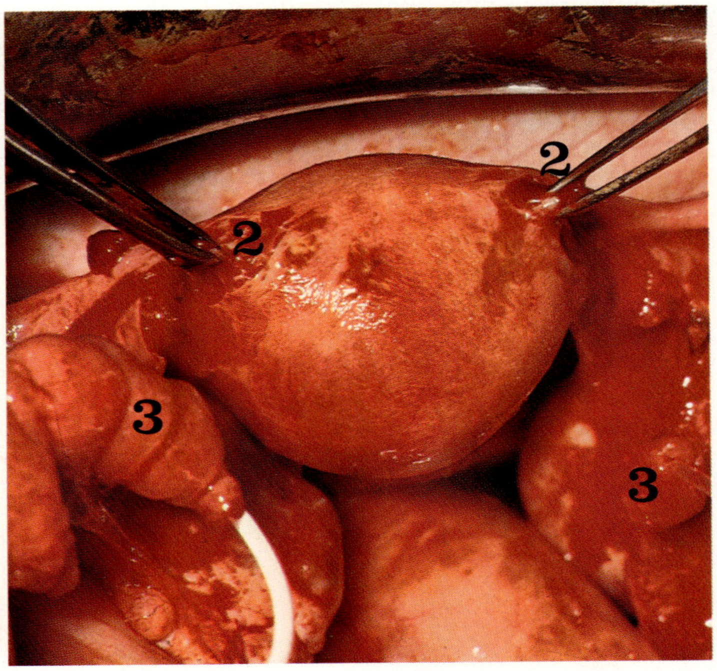

75

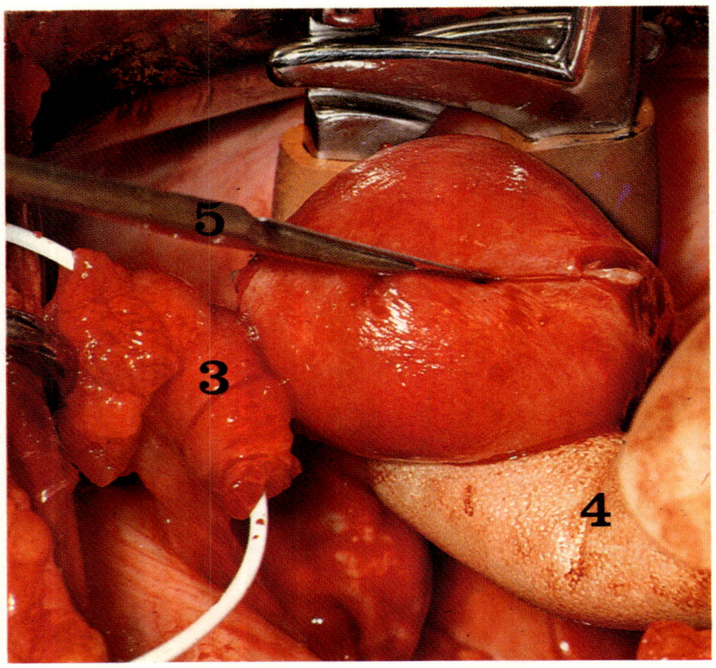

73 and 74 Excision of blocked isthmal tubes
In **Figure 73** the scalpel (5) excises the isthmal portion of the right tube by an elliptical incision with one end towards the fundus and the other towards the angle where the lateral uterine wall meets the mesosalpinx. In **Figure 74** excision of the blocked isthmal tube on the left side has also been completed and there are two elliptical raw areas (2) and (2) at the cornua. Both tubes are free (3) and (3) and have been intubated.

75 Transverse incision into fundus uteri
The uterus is steadied by the surgeon's left hand (4) while the scalpel incises transversely across the fundus from one cornual opening to the other. The incision is made deeply to reach the endometrial cavity.

76

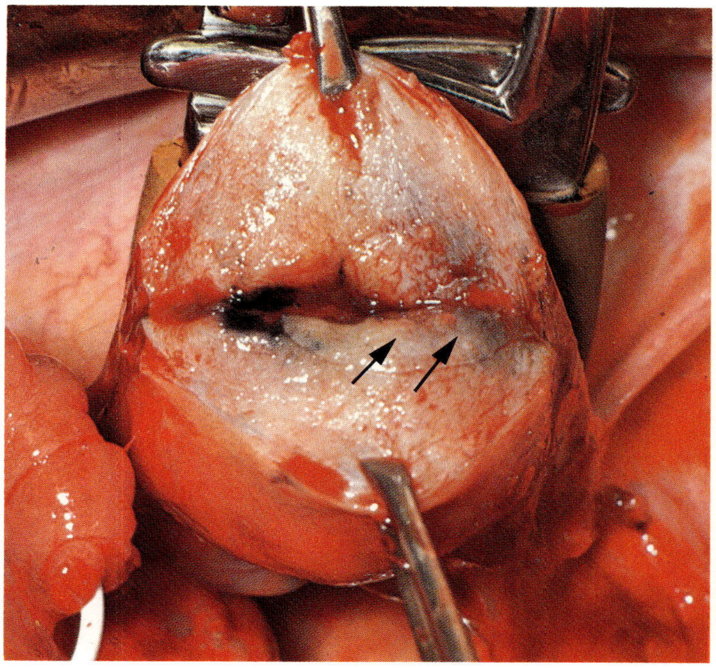

77

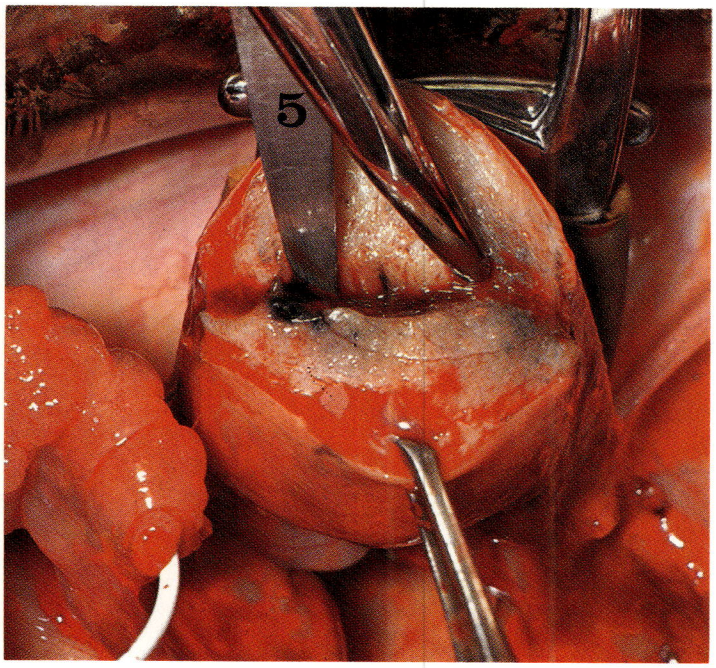

76 to 78 Opening fundus uteri transversely in preparation for tubal implantation

In **Figure 76** the incision is complete and the endometrium can be seen prolapsing into the wound where arrowed. In **Figure 77** the blades of curved scissors (5) are opened to give full access for the tubes and in **Figure 78** the plastic support for the right tube is being introduced into the uterus towards the cervix. Meantime it will be noted that the end of the fallopian tube has been incised to form two flaps as previously (arrowed). It appears to be disproportionate in size because it is near the camera.

78

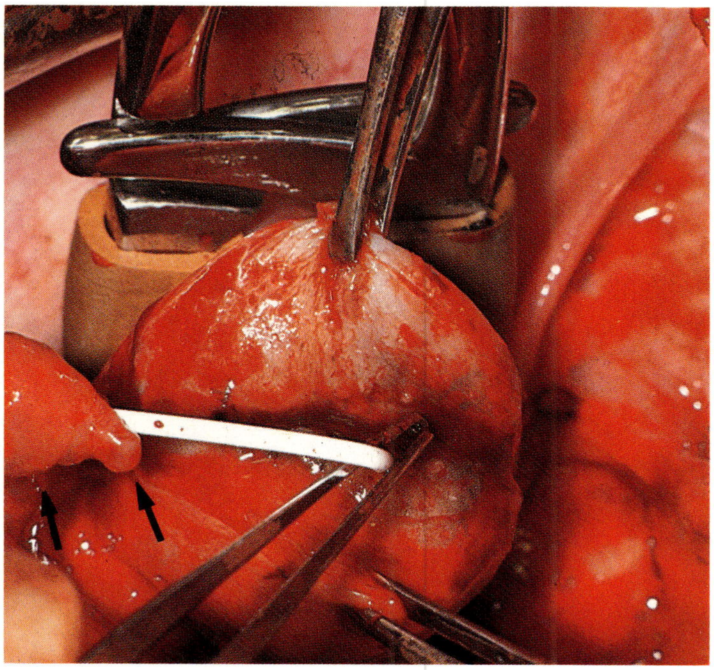

79

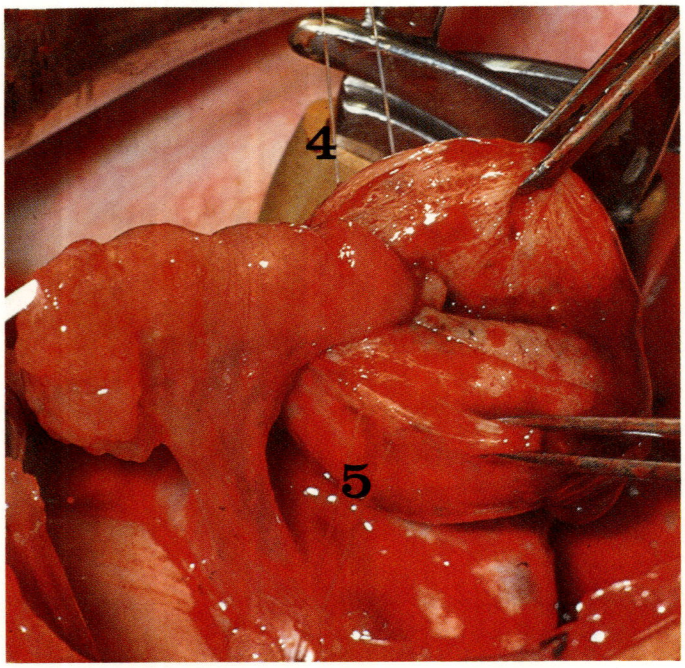

79 Anchoring tube to endometrial surface of uterine wall on left side
The two sutures 4 and 5, each supporting a flap of the fishmouthed tube emerge through the uterine wall, have been drawn taut and are ready to be tied.

80

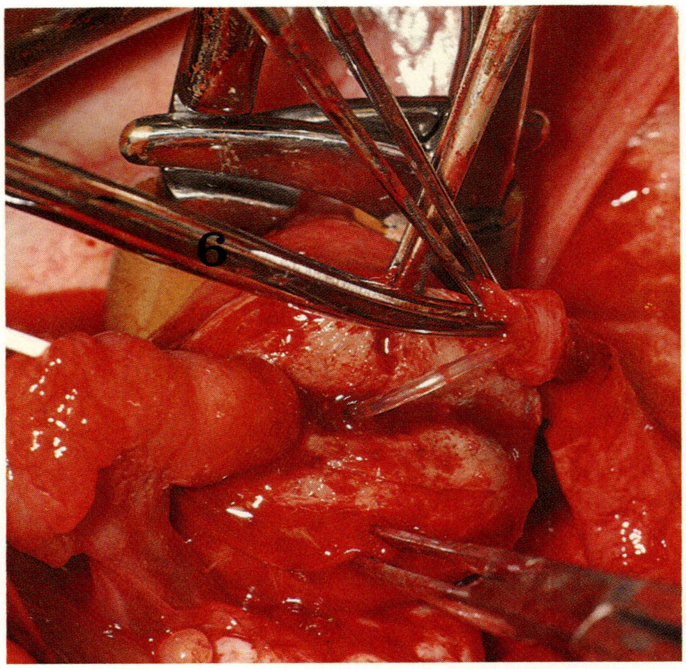

80 Splitting end of right tube prior to implantation
The scissors (6) are incising the end of the tube to open it in fishmouth fashion before implantation into the uterus.

81

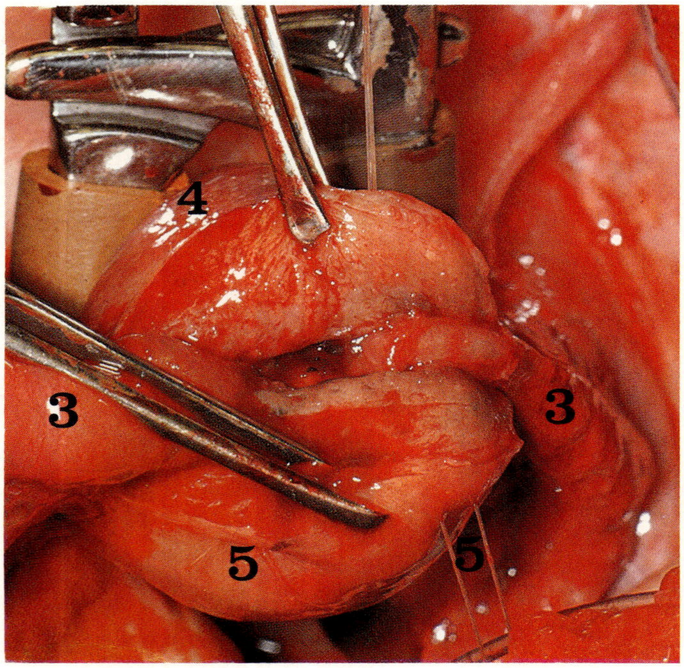

82

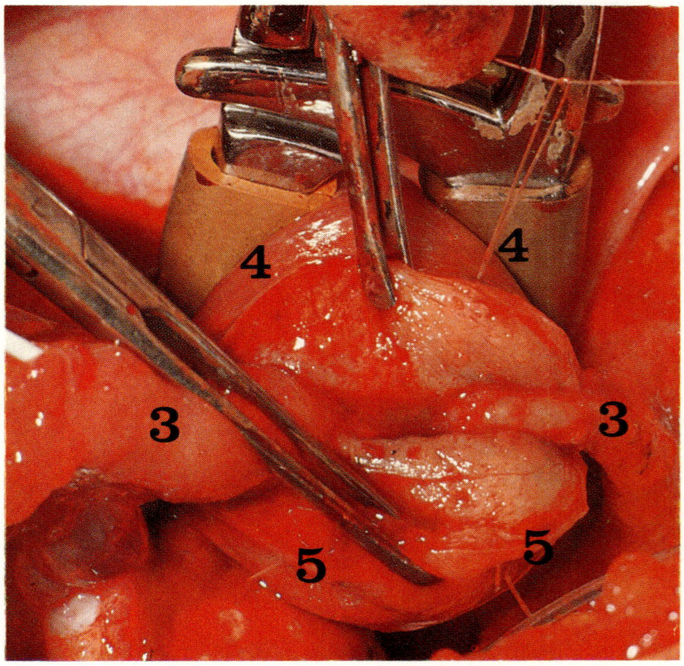

81 and 82 Anchoring tube to endometrial surface of uterine wall on right side
Both tubes (3) and (3) are now in position. In **Figure 81** the anterior and posterior anchor stitches on the left side have been tied off at (4) and (5) while the right posterior stitch 5 is about to be completed. In **Figure 82** the anterior stitch 4 is being secured and both tubes are now tied in place by the sutures 4, 4, 5, 5.

83

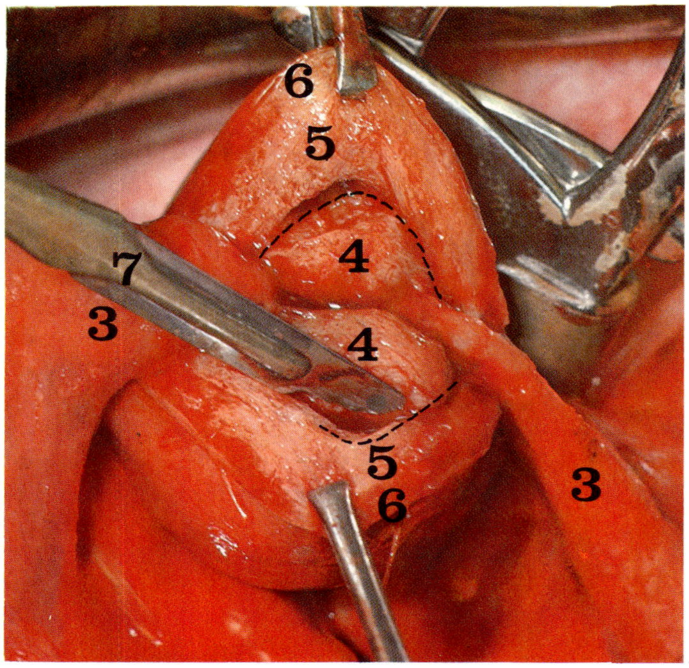

84

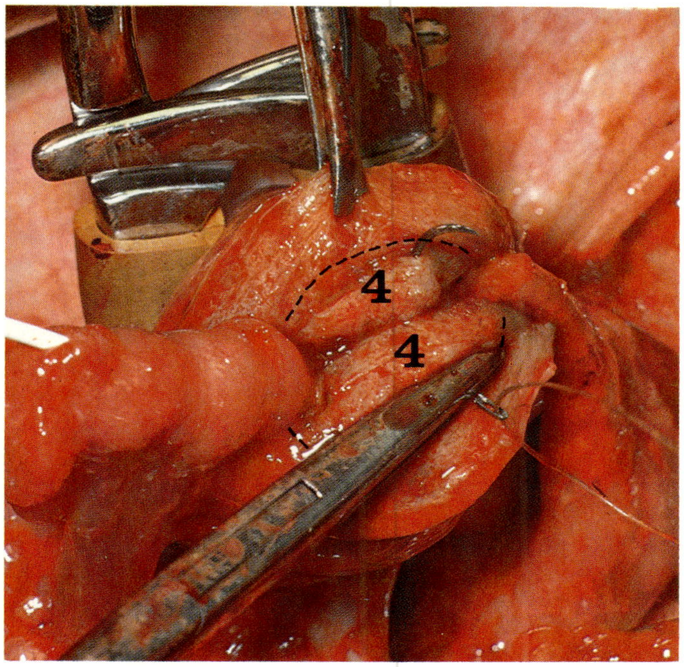

83 to 86 Splitting uterine muscle wall for subsequent three-layer closure

In **Figure 83** the scalpel (7) bisects the thick muscle wall of the uterine fundus anteriorly and posteriorly where indicated by the broken lines so that closure can be completed in three layers: musculo-endometrial (4), muscular (5) and sero-muscular (6). In **Figure 84** the inner muscle layer is being closed by a series of No. 00 PGA sutures which omit the endometrial lining and do not therefore enter or obtrude on the uterine cavity. In **Figure 85** the main muscle layer is being similarly closed by a series of No. 00 PGA sutures. The stitches in this particular case include the

85

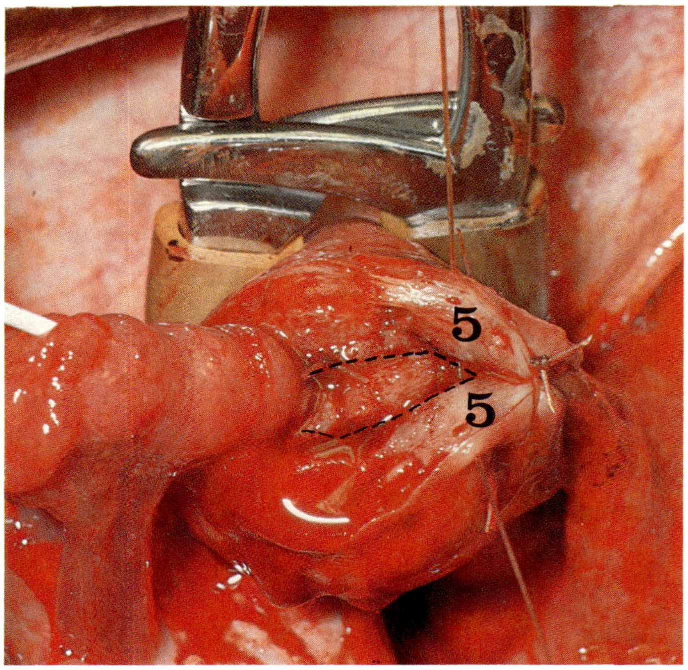

86

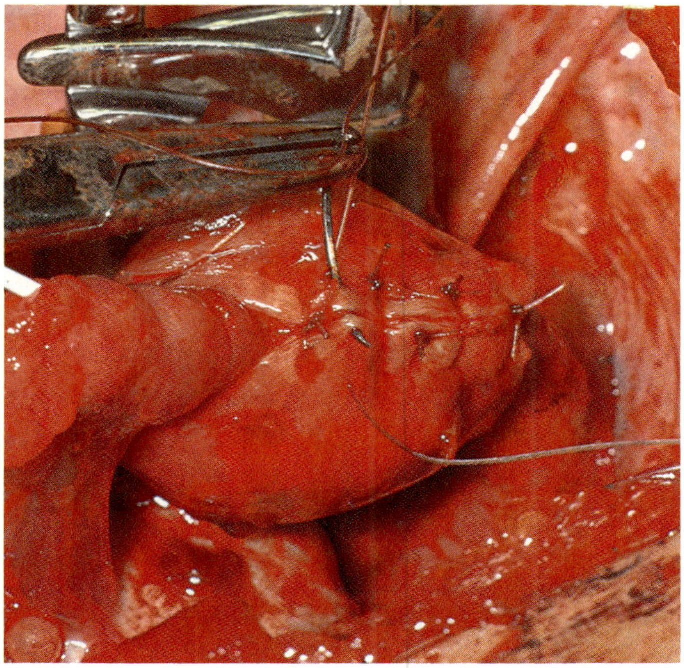

serosal layer so that the subsequent third layer entails only a precise approximation of the sero-muscular edges between the stitches as shown in **Figure 86**. It is preferable to omit the serosal edge when suturing the main muscle layer thus leaving a shallow sero-muscular layer which can be neatly closed by an infolding suture such as described on page 65 of this volume.

87

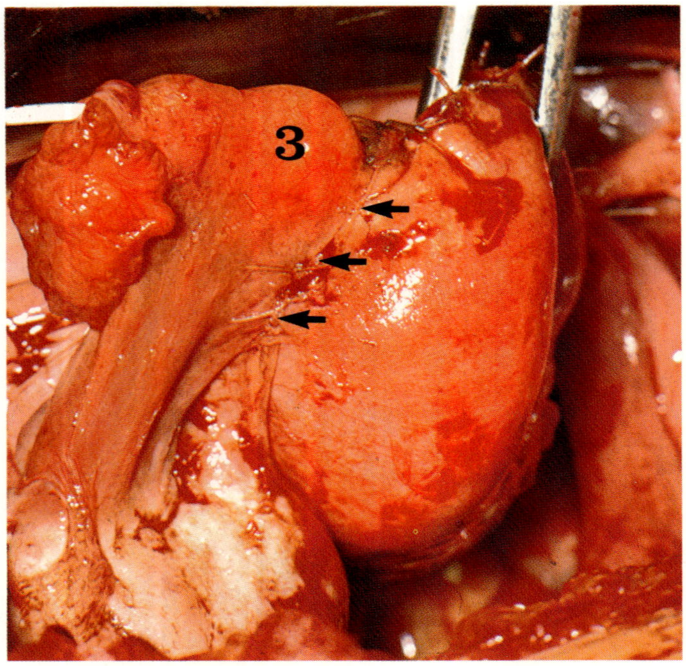

88

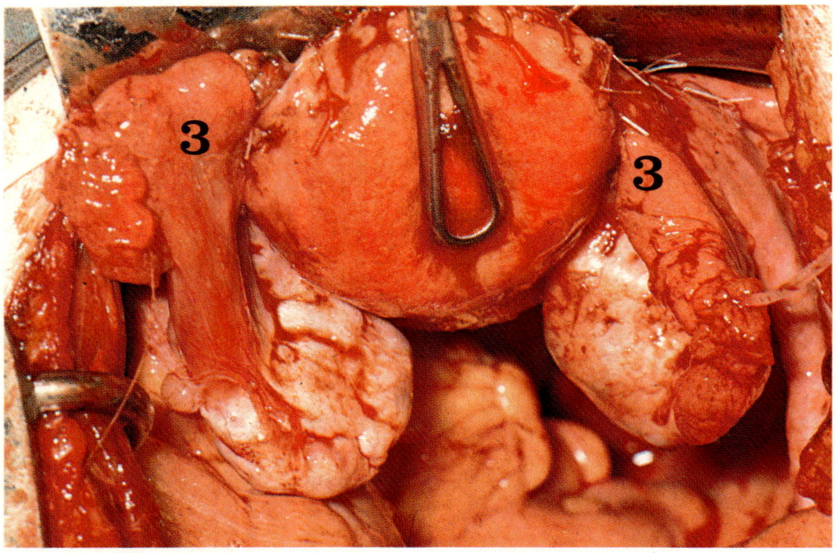

87 and 88 Appearance of uterus and implanted tubes at completion of operation
Figure 87 is a lateral view and shows a healthy looking, if short, tube snugly implanted into the uterus. The clamps controlling the blood vessels have been removed in these photographs and the wound is seen to be dry. The illustration emphasises the importance of closing any gap in the mesosalpinx in the area arrowed. This is effected by inserting a few very fine sutures between the mesosalpinx and the peritoneum on the lateral border of the uterus. **Figure 88** is a general posterior view which shows the tubes of about equal length and in normal position. The tubal splints are seen in situ but were removed before closing the abdomen. The stitches were also subsequently cut shorter; they are left recognisably long to indicate the suture lines in the photograph.

Results of implantation of fallopian tubes into the uterus

Once again there is great difficulty in finding a meaningful average success rate. Mattingly (1977) has studied the published results and gives general guidance in stating that, although the pregnancy rate in some series approximates to 30 to 50 per cent, the number of live births in many reported series rarely exceeds 20 per cent. He adds that there is a high rate of spontaneous abortion and tubal pregnancy in the group.

Results from some of the more recent series with reasonable numbers of patients do not give the live birth rate which is the only true criterion of success. Thus Shirodkar (1960) with much the widest experience of the operation states only that his pregnancy rate was 35 per cent. Hanton et al (1964) had 48 per cent live births in 22 cases, Grant (1971) 26 per cent in 73 cases and Umezaki et al (1974) report 38 per cent success. More recently Douglas (1978) had 9 successful pregnancies out of 19 operations (a success rate of 50 per cent).

If one seeks information on technique from success rates it is worthy of note that Hanton did not use splints and it may be of significance that in some of the older series reported the best results were also obtained without the use of splints. There is no evidence that either wedge excision of the cornu or a reamer technique is superior to the other. Hanton and Grant both used a reamer but Shirodkar discarded the reamer in favour of open implantation after 140 cases. Douglas found poorer wound healing with reamed cases than in those with excision. As Kistner and Patton (1975) remark, perhaps the technique of the surgeon is more important than the type of procedure.

Anastomosis of the fallopian tube

Reversal of previous elective tubal sterilisation is increasingly being requested by patients; the many factors influencing these developments are well known and need not be considered here. Patients unfortunately do not understand the difficulty and sometimes the impossibility of effecting such a reversal, although they accepted the operation as irreversible in the first place and in many cases sought firm assurance that it would indeed be so. Surgeons have felt that they could not afford mistakes about the finality of the operation and this is manifest in the use of unduly radical and traumatic procedures. In laparotomy sterilisation the whole mid-segment of the tube and sometimes the whole tube is excised; in the Irving procedure the medial end of the tube is deeply buried in the uterine wall. Laparoscopic sterilisation has been taught to be incomplete unless the tubes are destroyed by electro-coagulation diathermy for a distance of approximately 1 cm at two different points on their length. Nothing less it was felt could remove the fear of failure and possible subsequent litigation. There is of course no prospect of tubal reconstruction where such measures had been taken.

Yet there has been a gradual change in attitude during the past decade. Some surgeons in anticipation of unlikely but possible reversal requests have made a point of ligating the tube close to the uterus and maintaining the rest of the structure intact because they believed that reimplantation into the uterus was the most successful method of doing so. The intention was more important than the actual technique for the end result of such surgery generally allows of reversal either by reimplantation or end-to-end anastomosis.

When it is possible to do the latter operation there are many advantages over tubal implantation. Microsurgeons in fact have shown that it is an easy and relatively successful operation if there is adequate remaining tubal length.

The practice of laparoscopic sterilisation has been influenced by similar anticipation and there is increasing appreciation of the fact that it is not necessary to completely destroy the tubes to effect sterilisation. Clips or rubber bands applied locally to the tubes have disadvantages but if properly placed are probably only marginally less effective than destructive procedures and still allow the patient to change her mind in a world of increasing complexity and uncertainty. The gynaecologist, meantime, remains in a situation where it seems that he cannot win. It may be that the public will have to accept slightly less than perfection in sterilisation if they are to retain the facility of occasionally having it reversed.

When approached with a request for reversal the clinician must respond with the utmost caution. The history of the case and the record of the sterilisation operation may be available and give some indication of the possibilities; in nearly all instances laparoscopy must be undertaken to assess the situation and proper discussion of its possibilities will have to await the findings at examination. Even if after full investigation the surgeon agrees that an attempt be made to reconstitute the tubes the patient must fully understand that further obstacles may be revealed at laparotomy, that only a percentage of such operations succeed and that there is an increased risk of tubal pregnancy. The psychological and emotional climate in these cases is such that patients are apt to close their minds to these prudent reservations and brook no further delay in treatment.

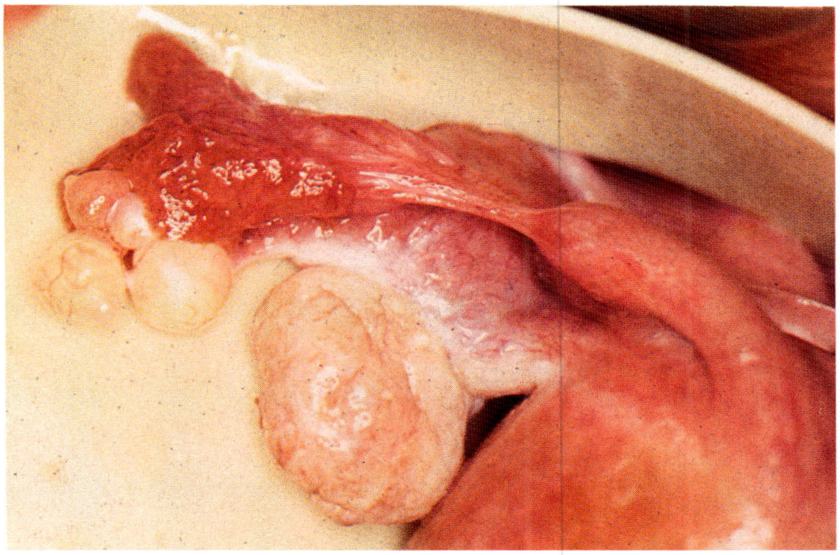

89

89 Destructive effect of diathermy coagulation on left fallopian tube
Laparotomy appearance where the whole lateral part of the fallopian tube has been destroyed by diathermy coagulation. The frequently employed method of fulguration at two points on the isthmo-ampullary portion of the tube is likely to result in such an appearance and there is of course no prospect of surgical reconstruction in the circumstances.

Anastomosis of fallopian tube – technique

Provided the two remaining portions of tube are of sufficient length and the calibre of the two ends approximately the same the operation is comparatively straightforward. The first essential is to dissect out and prepare two ends for anastomosis. Dye is injected along the tube from the uterine end and a fine probe passed from the fimbrial ostium so that the site and extent of the blockage can be defined. The affected sector is invariably atrophic and embedded in a mass of fibrous tissue. This fibrous bloc must be completely excised and the fine diathermy point is used for that purpose. Any blackened coagulated tissue is removed with fine scissors and the aim is to prepare the two ends for approximation with the circular muscle identifiable and the serosal coat intact. When the fallopian tube has been intubated or splinted on a plastic tube or rod the lumen projects from the muscle in nipple-like fashion.

Stay sutures are then inserted into the adjacent edges of the mesosalpinx thus ensuring that the tubal ends are brought together and 'set up' for suture to each other (see **Figures 96** and **97** on page 115).

Suture of the tubal ends must obviously be done with great precision and **Diagram 98** on page 115 reinforces the illustrations which follow. Microsurgeons advise the use of 8 × 0 nylon sutures on a round-bodied needle for this step but for the circumstances envisaged here 4 × 0 nylon on a considerably larger needle is much easier to work with and is recommended.

When the muscle has been approximated, the serosal layer is closed by a series of 4 × 0 or even 6 × 0 interrupted prolene stitches. This closure is carried on to the mesosalpinx anteriorly and posteriorly so that the area of anastomosis is completely smooth.

90

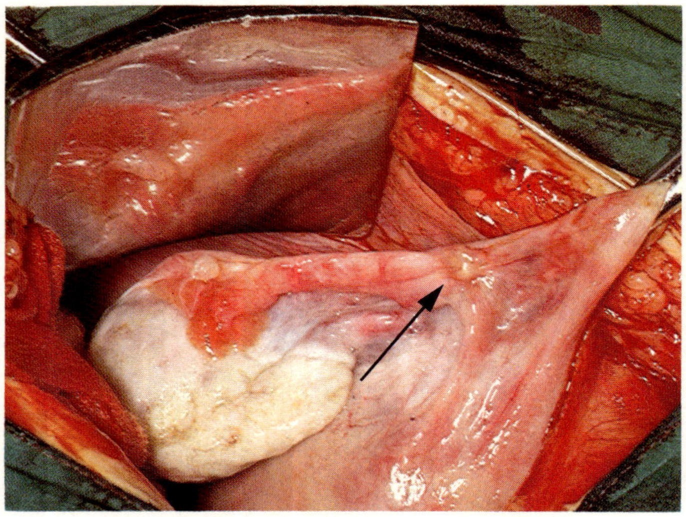

90 Appearance of left fallopian tube following tubal ligation sterilisation by the Oxford method
A small loop of tube has been tied off where arrowed. There is adequate remaining length of healthy tube and anastomosis has every prospect of success.

91

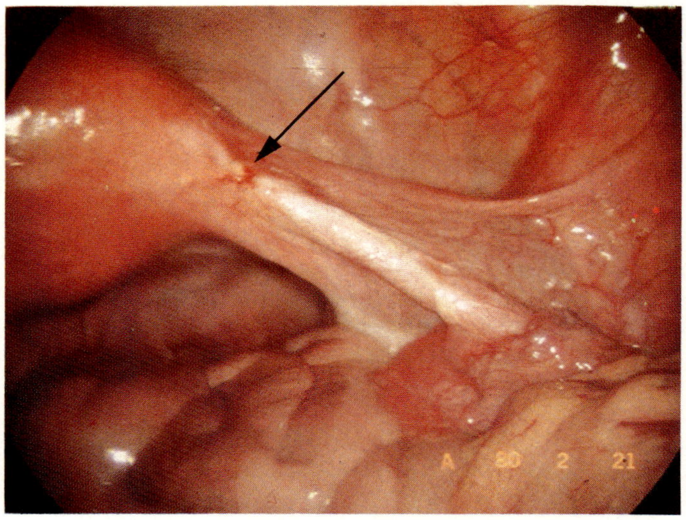

91 Laparoscopy appearance of right fallopian tube following localised diathermy coagulation.
The tube has been sealed by diathermy coagulation in one localised area. Damage is limited and successful anastomosis should be possible.

Stage I: Excision of occluded segment and preparation of tube for anastomosis

92

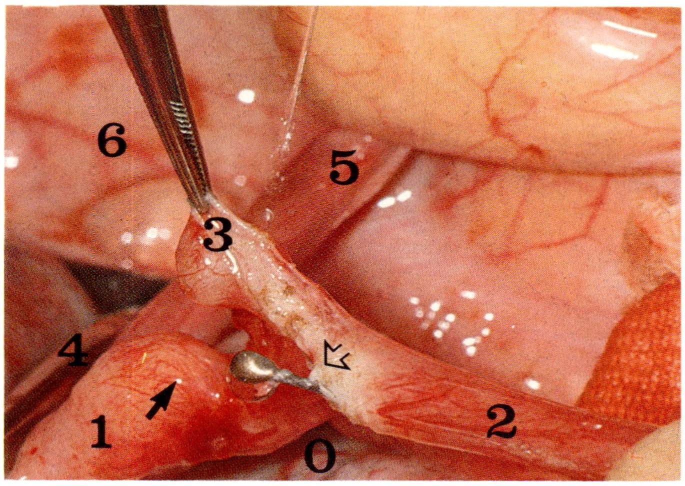

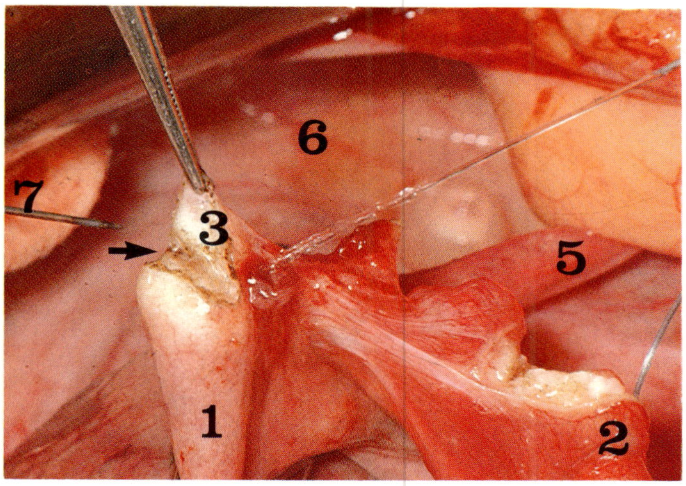

93

92 Exploration and definition of occluded area of right fallopian tube
The medial (1) and the lateral (2) portions of the tube overlie the ovary (0). Fine forceps pick up part of the intervening mesosalpinx (3) to show the area of separation and the divided ends of the tube. A wire probe introduced into the lateral portion of the tube protrudes to indicate the open lumen (open arrow) and the lumen of the medial portion is within the rounded area of fibrous tissue in the region of the solid arrow. The uterus is numbered (4), the round ligament (5) and the bladder (6). A jet of saline is directed at the area being dissected and has the dual function of cooling the tissues being divided by diathermy and keeping the operative field clear of blood to aid visualisation as the tubal lumen is sought.

93 Diathermy excision of blocked ends of fallopian tube
In this photograph the lateral end of the tube (2) has been identified and splinted. The main part of the fibrous mass (3) is held in the forceps and the diathermy needle (7) is seeking the lumen of the medial end of the tube (1) where arrowed. The tubal blood supply in the upper mesosalpinx will probably have been interrupted by the sterilisation operation but every care should be taken to ensure that the existing vascular supply to the two freed ends is preserved. Intrusion into the mesosalpinx is not necessary and should be avoided. The numbers are as previously and the jet of saline is again visible.

This photograph introduces an important cautionary point. The diathermy needle is excising fibrous tissue, but it is also defining the medial end of the tube and the current used should be no stronger than is absolutely necessary. There is an area of tissue blanching where the medial tubal stump is being defined and this will have to be excised with the cold knife before anastomosis is commenced. In this instance the diathermy current is seen to have been too strong.

Stage I: Excision of occluded segment and preparation of tube for anastomosis *continued*

94

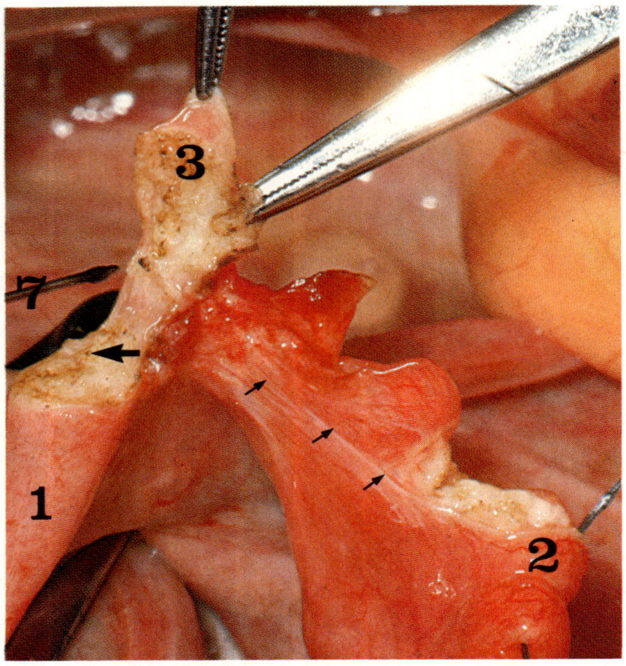

94 Continuing excision of fibrous tissue and identification of tubal ends
The diathermy needle (7) has now encountered the tubal lumen (where arrowed) and the blue dye can just be seen. The dissection leaves the two reopened ends very far from each other and emphasises how much of the tube has been sacrificed in the sterilisation operation. The upper posterior edge of the mesosalpinx is indicated by fine arrows. The blanching seen on the medial end of the tube has largely cleared but removal of a thin annular sector is necessary because of possible damage to its blood supply and also because there is visible tissue charring on the cut surface.

95

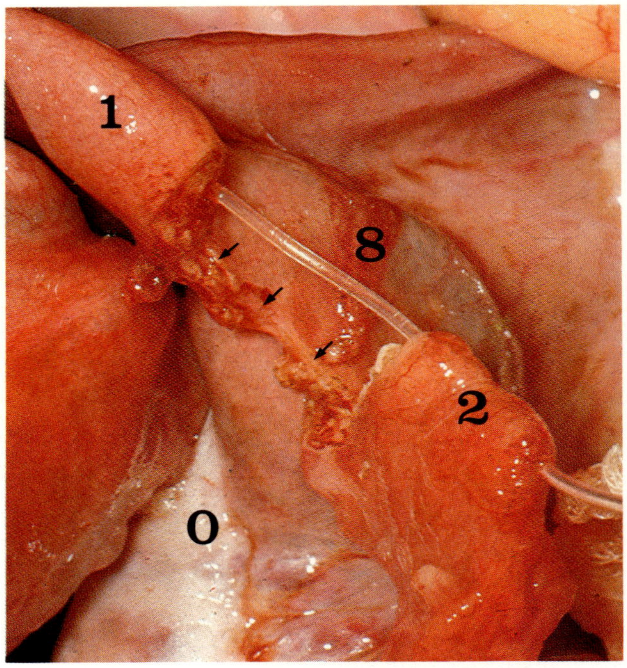

95 Adjacent ends of right fallopian tube prepared and splinted
The distance separating the two ends of tube is again very obvious. The plastic tube which acts as a splint has been advanced into the medial end towards the uterine cavity. The area is clear of fibrous tissue but there are some adhesions (8) which will have to be removed. In this view the upper anterior edge of the mesosalpinx is seen and identified by fine arrows. The medial end of the tube has been trimmed of all tissue damaged by the diathermy current.

Diagrams for anastomosis of fallopian tube

Figures 94 and **95** show the considerable distance between the ends to be joined and the reasons for this have been explained. In anastomosis the first step is to approximate the upper border of the mesosalpinx in such a fashion as to bring the open tubal ends into close proximity and this is shown in **Figures 96** and **97**. The two ends of the tube are designated 'M' for medial and 'L' for lateral and the mid-point of the open mesosalpinx is numbered (3) and is represented as the apex of a 'V'. The gap is closed by a vertical line of sutures seen in **Figure 97** and arrowed. The last of the stitches not only draws the mesenteric borders of the tubal segments close together but leaves them tilted outwards at the antimesenteric border to facilitate further anastomosis. The mesosalpinx suture line is of course double because there are two layers of peritoneum and in practice matching stitches are inserted anteriorly and posteriorly in turn as the 'V' gap is closed from below upwards.

Suture of the muscle layer of the tube is best done to a strict and simple pattern. Surgeons are agreed that 4 stitches approximately equidistant from each other around the tube and which pick up a firm bite of muscle on each side while omitting both serosal and ciliary layers give a satisfactory junction. The serosa is closed separately and gives the opportunity of ensuring a watertight junction; the tubal lining is avoided for obvious reasons. The authors believe that it helps to think of the 4 sutures as being in the 2, 4, 8 and 10 o'clock positions when looking medially towards the uterus. Such placements are not of course truly equidistant but are sufficiently accurate for demonstration purposes.

In **Figure 98** the medial end of the splinted tube is designated 'M', the lateral 'L' and the points of entry and exit of the needle carrying the nylon suture in each of the four stitches are shown by small entry and exit circles. The dotted blue lines indicate the intramuscular course of the needle. In all four the serosa and the lumen are omitted from the stitch. Sutures are in black and are shown loosely placed in the 4 and 8 o'clock positions; when these are drawn up and tied the whole mesenteric halves of the tubal circumference will be drawn together. It is important to observe a strict progression and insert the stitches on the mesenteric aspect of the muscle layer first, since the tubal ends are not only already in close approximation there but if one or both of the antimesenteric stitches is tied off before the others access becomes almost impossible.

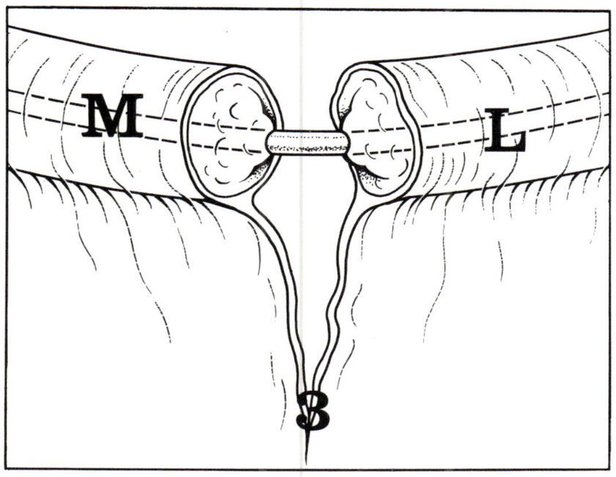

96

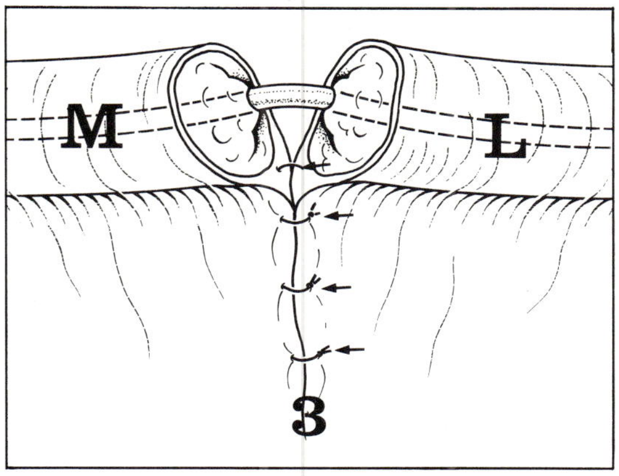

97

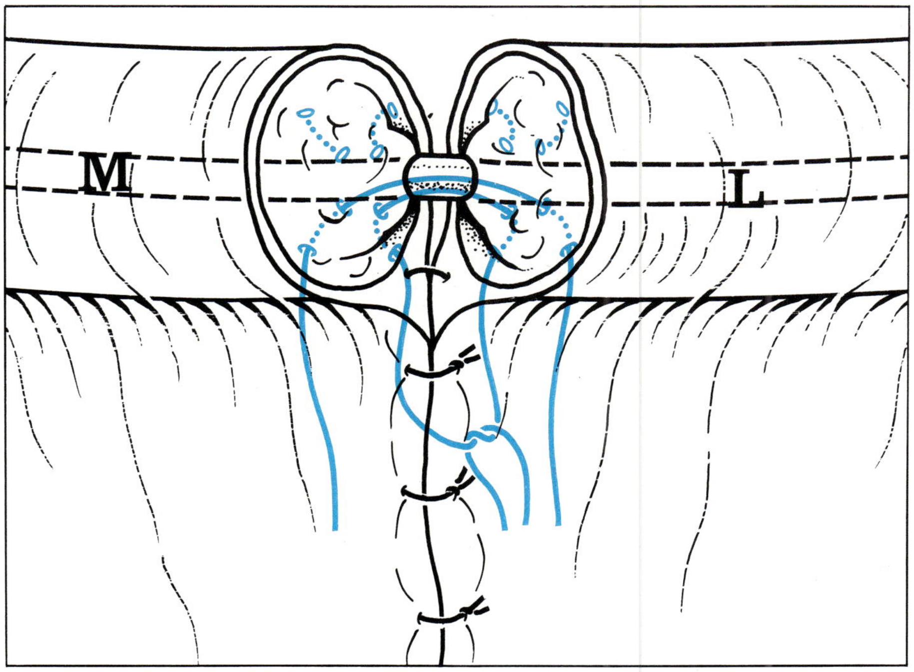

98

Stage II: Suture of mesosalpinx : right fallopian tube

99

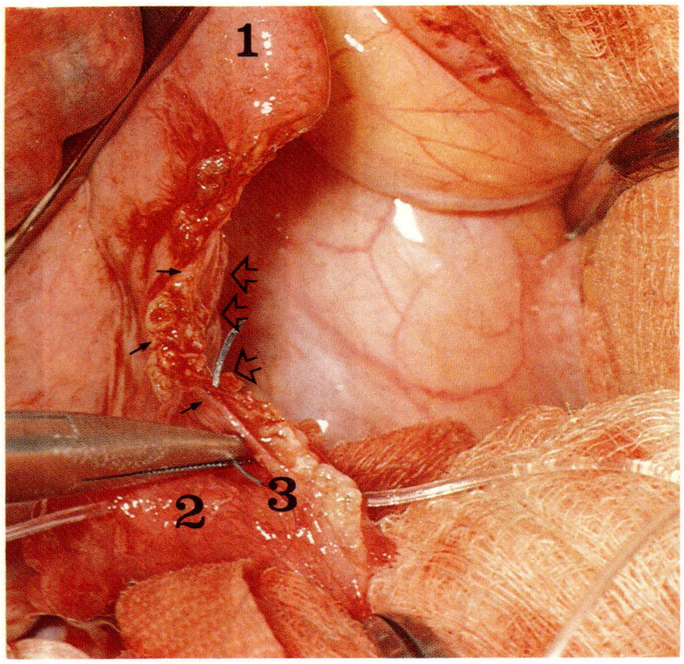

100

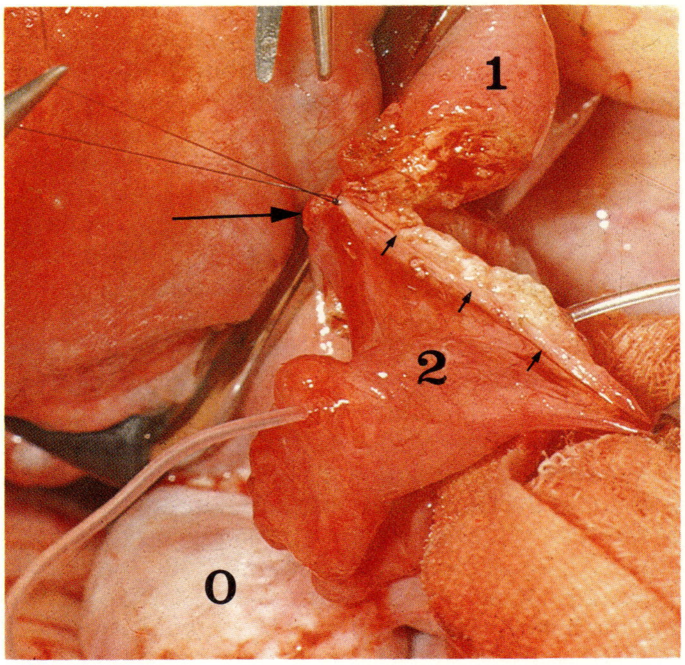

101

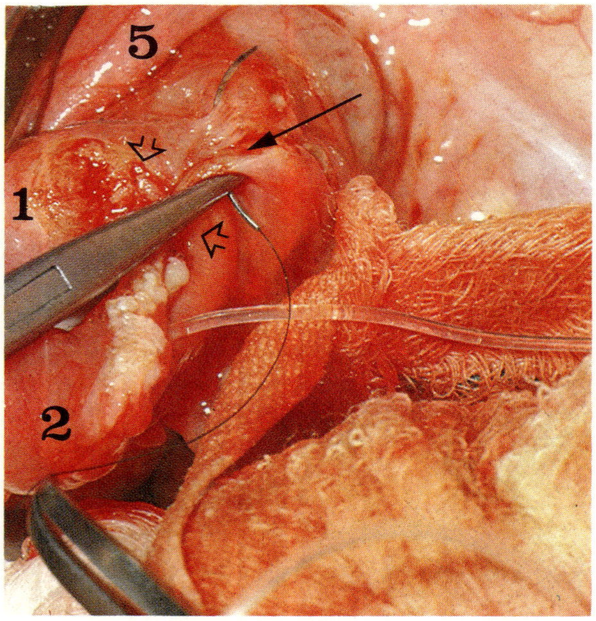

99 to 101
The medial end of the tube is numbered (1), the lateral (2) and the needle holder carrying a 4 × 0 nylon suture on a round-bodied needle (3). The posterior mesenteric edge is denoted by fine closed arrows and the anterior edge by fine open arrows. In **Figure 99** the needle is shown picking up the lateral edge of the posterior layer of the mesosalpinx near the apex of the 'V'. The medial edge is transfixed in turn and this first stitch is being tied off (large arrow) in **Figure 100**. In **Figure 101** the structures have been displaced backwards to allow insertion of the first stitch on the anterior layer of the mesosalpinx (arrowed). The edges of this layer are again denoted by the fine open arrows and the right round ligament (5) helps in orientation of the photograph.

Stage III: Suture of muscle layer of right fallopian tube

102

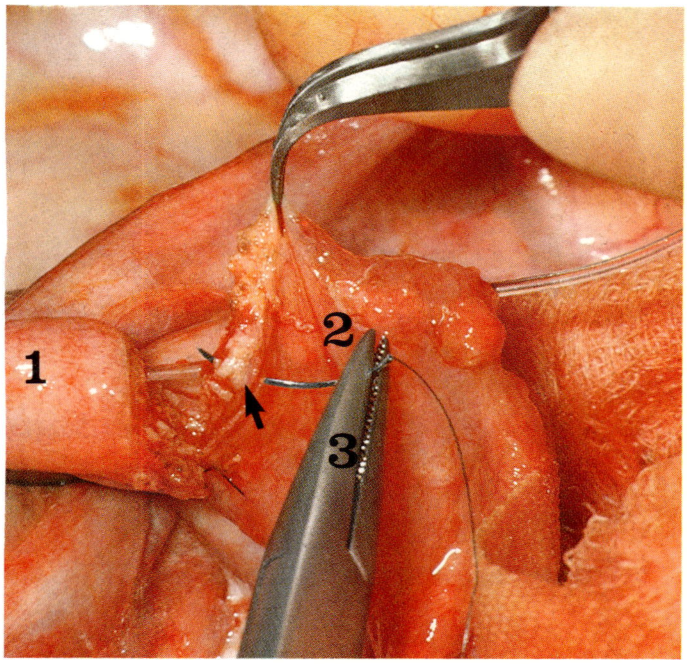

103

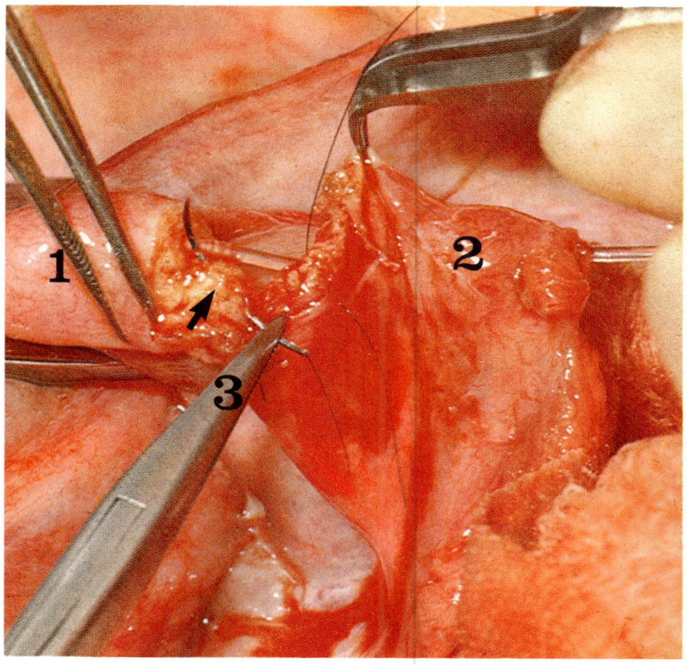

102 to 104 Approximation of ends in 8 o'clock position
In **Figure 102** the needle holder (3) carrying a round-bodied needle on 4 × 0 nylon picks the muscle of the lateral part of the tube (2) (where arrowed) and in the manner shown in **Figure 98**. This corresponds to an 8 o'clock position on the medial part of the tube (1) where the muscle is seen being transfixed by the needle in **Figure 103** (arrowed). The stitch has been drawn up tight and is tied but uncut in **Figure 104** (arrowed). It is clear that the stitch does not include the mucosal or serosal layers of the tube.

104

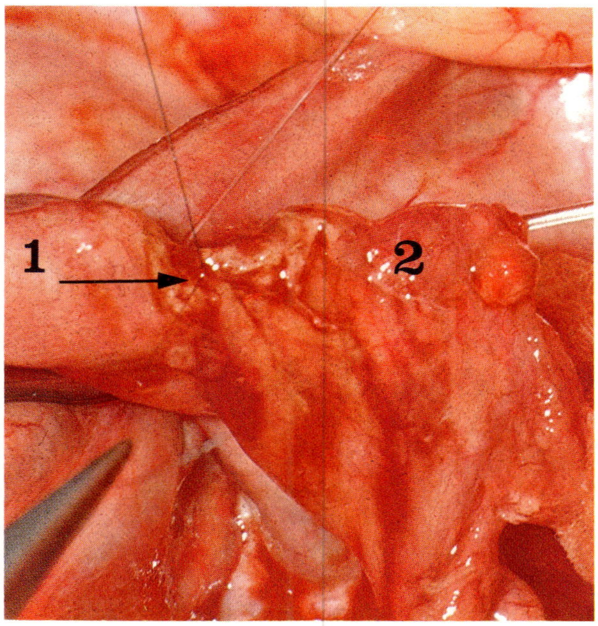

105

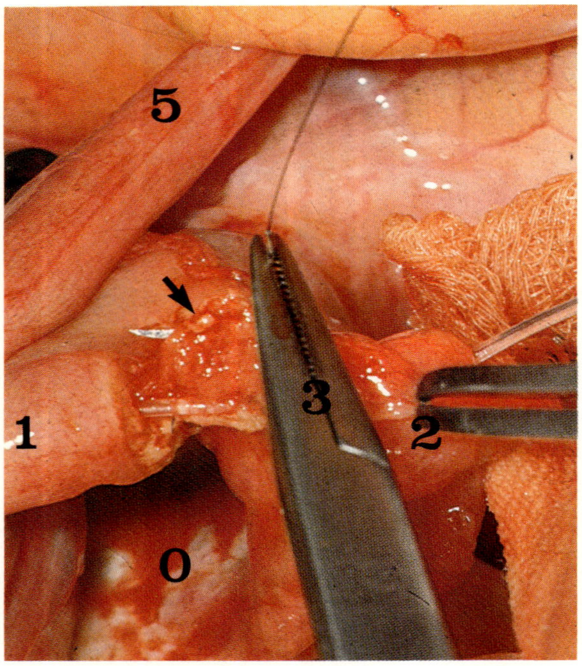

106

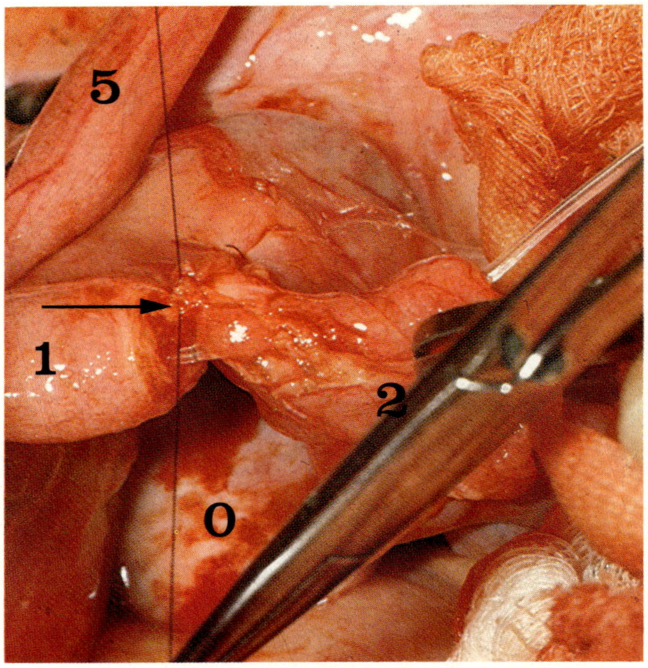

107

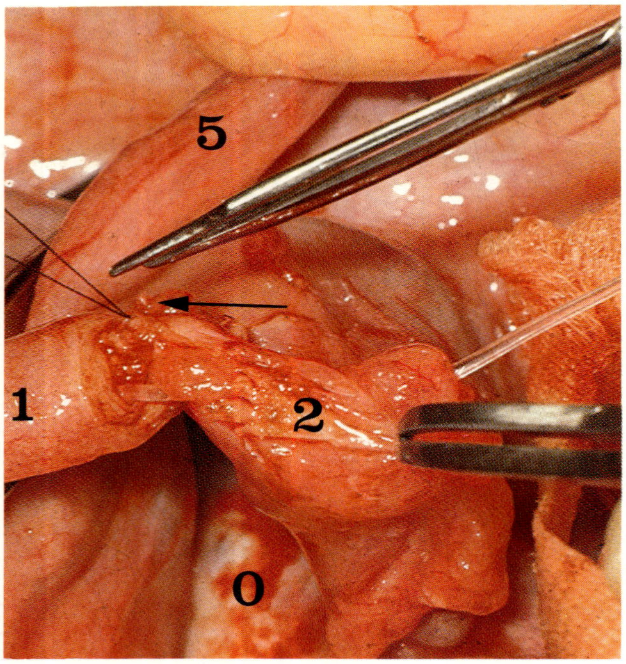

105 to 107 Approximation of ends in 4 o'clock position
The needle transfixes the muscle of the lateral part of the fallopian tube in similar fashion in **Figure 105** (arrowed). The nylon suture is being tied in the 4 o'clock position in **Figure 106** (arrowed) and is about to be cut short (arrowed) in **Figure 107**. Note how the mesenteric halves of the circumference are now in position but the antimesenteric halves lie open with the plastic splint still visible and affording easy access for the insertion of the remaining two sutures.

108

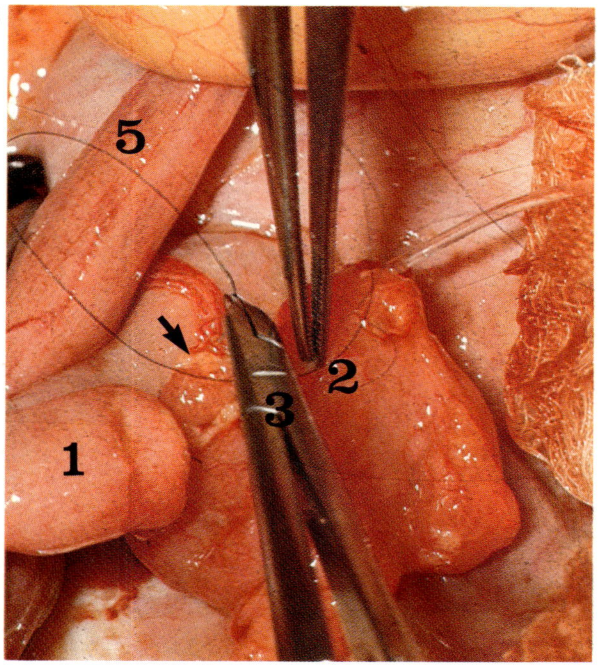

109

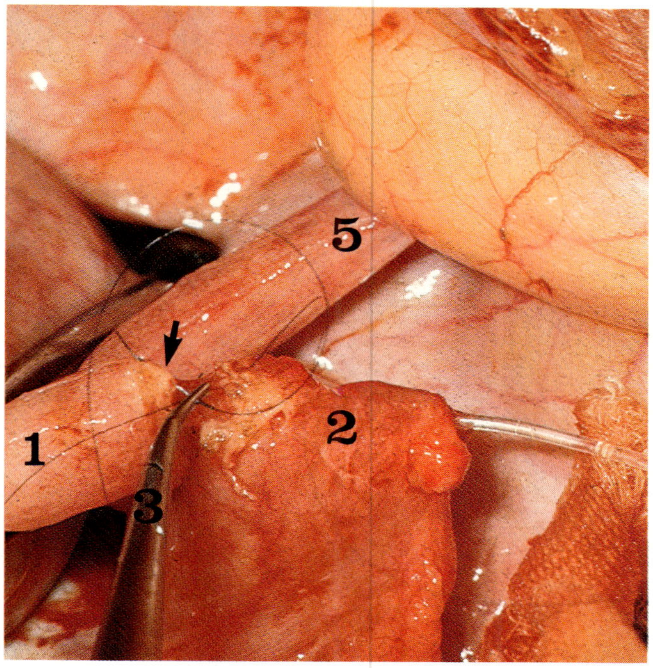

108 to 110 Approximation of tubal ends in 2 o'clock position The needle picks up the muscle of the lateral part of the tube in its antimesenteric half (where arrowed) in **Figure 108** and takes a corresponding bite in the 2 o'clock position on the medial portion (arrowed) in **Figure 109**. The stitch is shown being tied off (where arrowed) in **Figure 110**. The ends of the tube are now beginning to fit together very neatly.

110

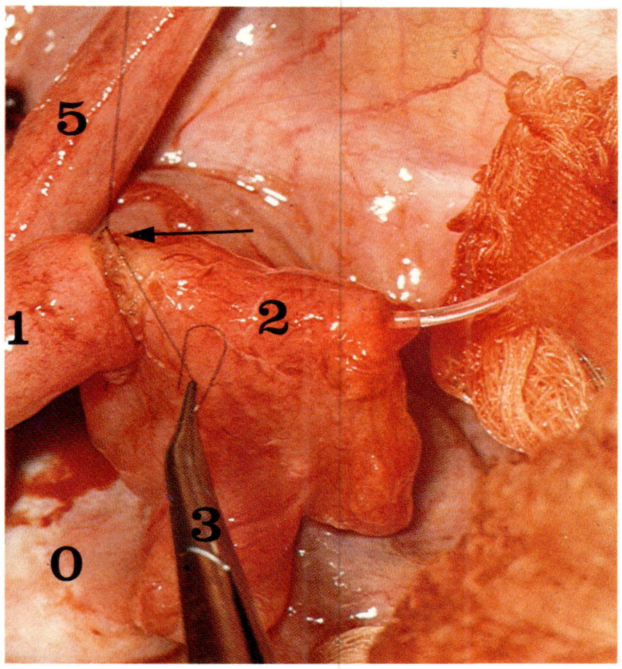

111

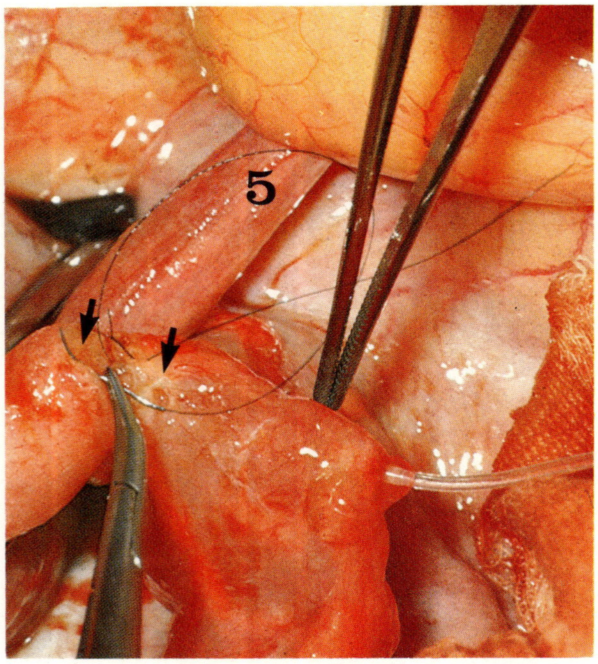

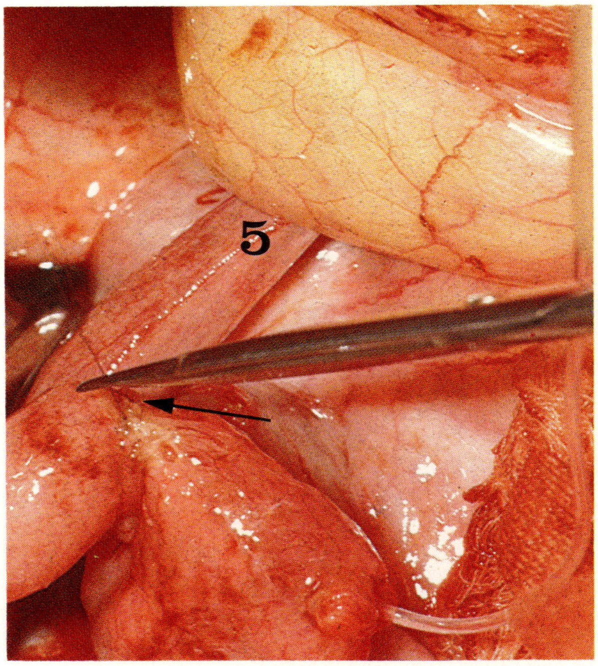

112

111 and 112 Approximation of ends in 10 o'clock position In **Figure 111** the needle has already taken a bite of the muscle in the lateral part of the tube and is seen emerging after taking a corresponding bite of the medial muscle layer in the 10 o'clock position (arrowed). The suture has been tied off and is being cut short (arrowed) in **Figure 112**. To aid orientation at the various stages of this operation the round ligament is numbered (5) and the ovary (0) when these structures are visible in the photograph.

Stage IV: Suture of serosal layer of right fallopian tube

113

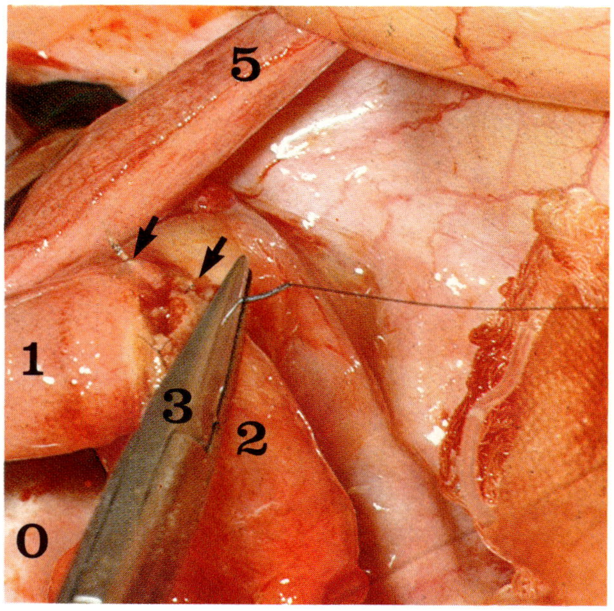

114

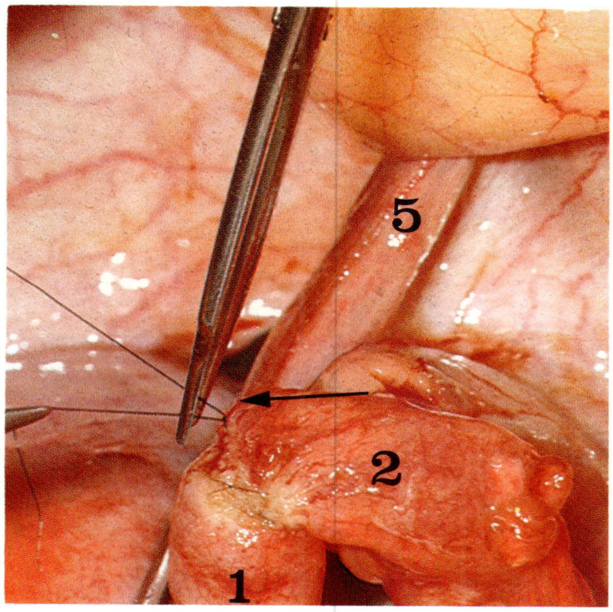

113 and 114 Closure on anterior aspect

Reference was made to the fact that approximation of the serosal coat should not only be neat and precise but that it should extend on to the mesosalpinx to ensure a smooth anastomosis and eliminate any possible area of adhesion. In **Figure 113** the needle is seen to have picked up the two edges well down on the anterior aspect of the mesosalpinx (arrowed) and overlapping the apex of the 'V' previously referred to. The succeeding stitch being cut short in **Figure 114** is on the anterior aspect of the tube itself and the process continues towards the antimesenteric border and then on to the posterior aspect of the tube as seen in illustrations that follow. The actual serosal stitch is a seromuscular one which enters the serosa 3 or 4 mm from the cut edge and includes within it about the same depth of tubal muscle. As it is tied the peritoneum is rolled inwards slightly to give a Lembert effect. This is more likely to give a watertight joint besides being neat and discouraging adhesions.

115

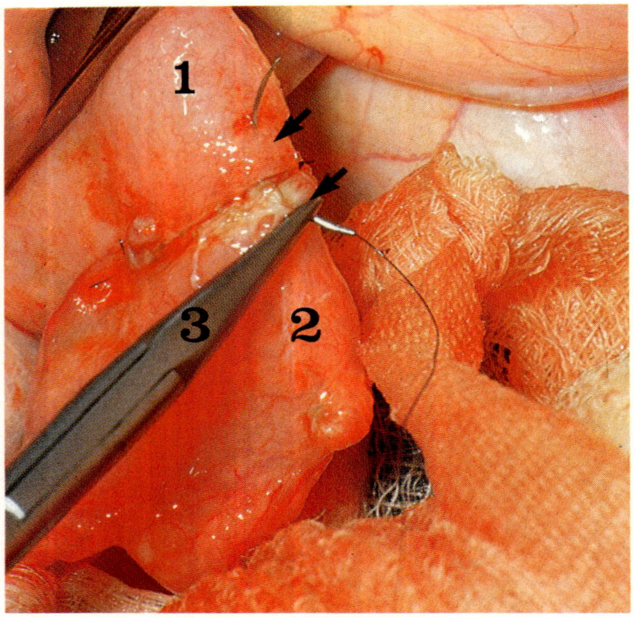

116

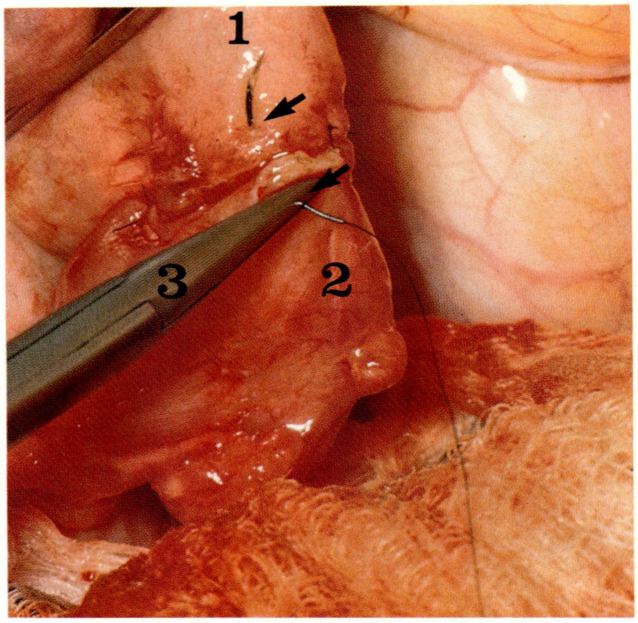

117

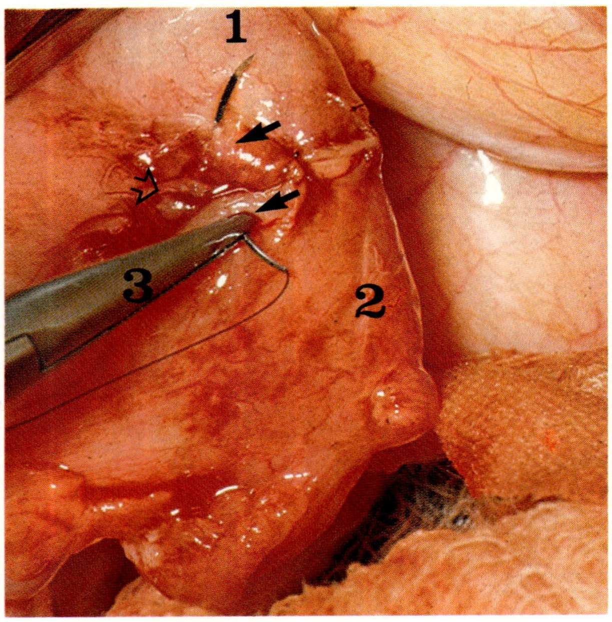

115 to 117 Closure on posterior aspect
Suture continues in the manner described with **Figure 115** showing the insertion of a stitch on the antimesenteric border. The needle pierces the serosa (arrowed) at a distance of 3 mm from the edge and penetrates the muscle to the same depth. A further stitch is being placed in **Figure 116** and in **Figure 117** the peritoneal closure is being carried on to the mesosalpinx posteriorly. One further similar suture is required in the region of the apex of the 'V' (open arrow) to make the surface quite smooth.

Stage V: Appraisal of right tubal reconstruction

118

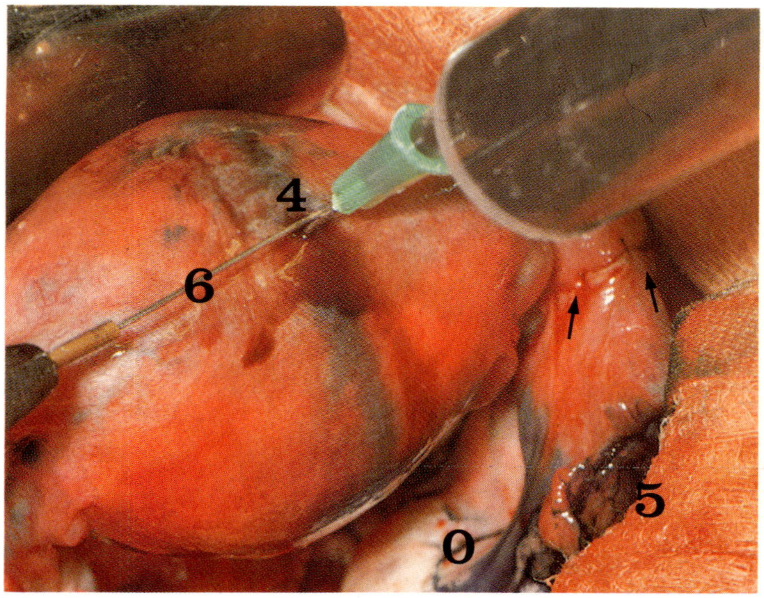

119

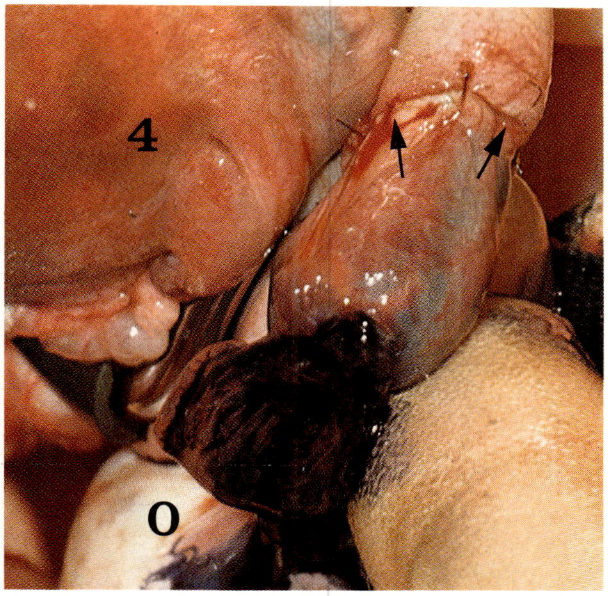

118 and 119 Testing security of suture line and patency of tube

Methylene blue dye is injected into the uterine cavity through the fundus at (4) and can be seen escaping through the fimbrial end of the tube at (5). The suture line (arrowed) is intact. As the syringe is withdrawn the needle is touched with the diathermy point (6) to seal off any bleeding points in its track. The dye is injected under pressure and there is apt to be some leakage of dye from the needle site for a short time. **Figure 119** is a more localised photograph to show the suture line and the escape of dye from the fimbrial end. The uterus is numbered (4) and the ovary (0).

Anastomosis of left fallopian tube

Selected illustrations to emphasise important points.

Stage I: Excision of occluded segment and preparation of tube for anastomosis

120

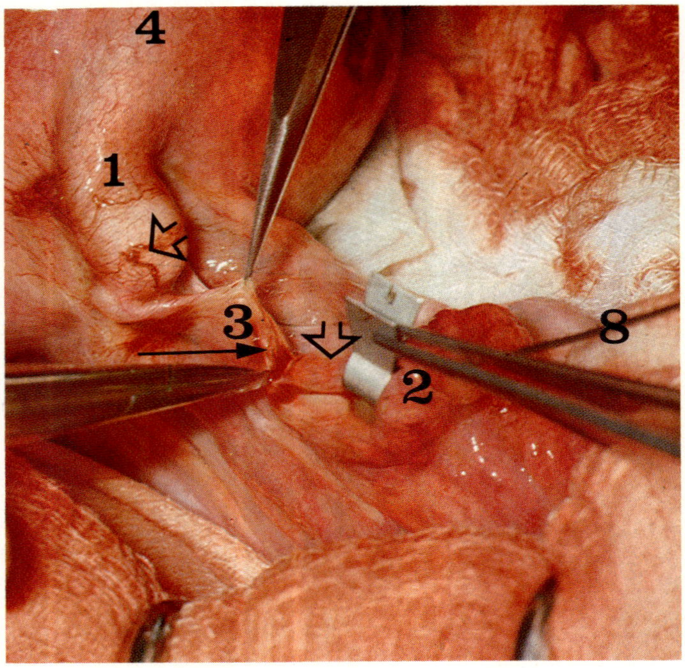

121

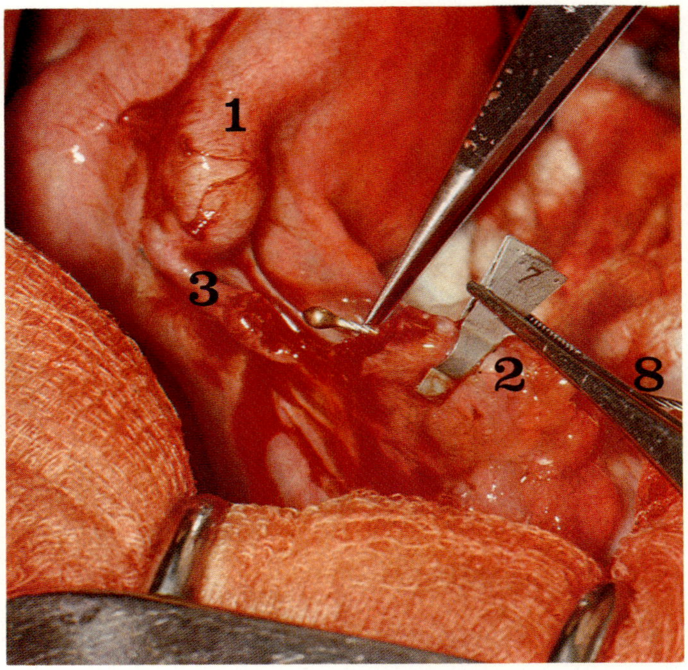

122

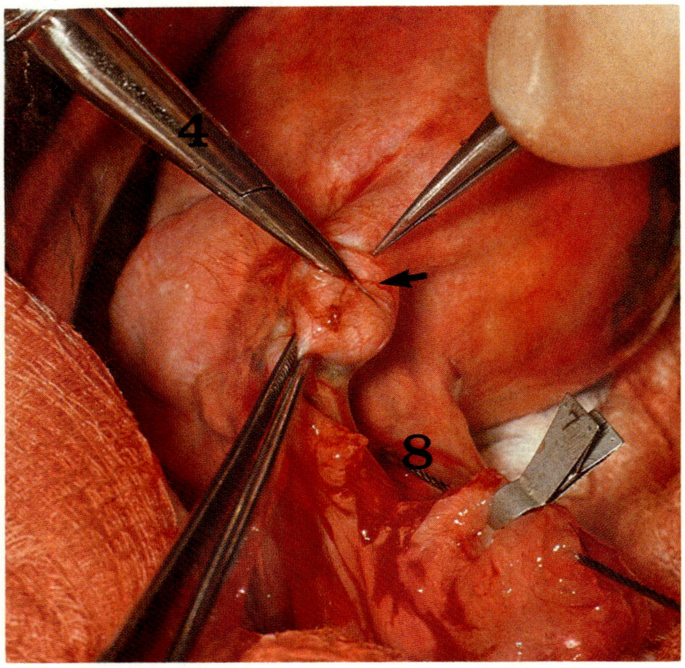

120
A considerable length of the left tube is destroyed (3) and the length between the open arrows will have to be excised. Fortunately there is very little fibrous tissue to excise. The upper border of the mesosalpinx is opened where arrowed and the wire probe is estimating the medial extent of the tubal lumen. The microclip supporting the lateral aspect of the tube is often useful in anastomosis and is shown being used on this side. The numerals are as previously; the wire probe is designated (8).

121
The probe has now defined the medial end of the lateral part of the tube. The mesosalpinx is not invaded any more deeply than necessary to remove the atrophic piece of tube (3).

122
The closed end of the medial part of the tube is relatively avascular and the microscalpel (4) incises it well laterally (arrowed) in seeking the lumen of the tube. There is an obvious shortage of tubal length and every available millimetre must be preserved.

123

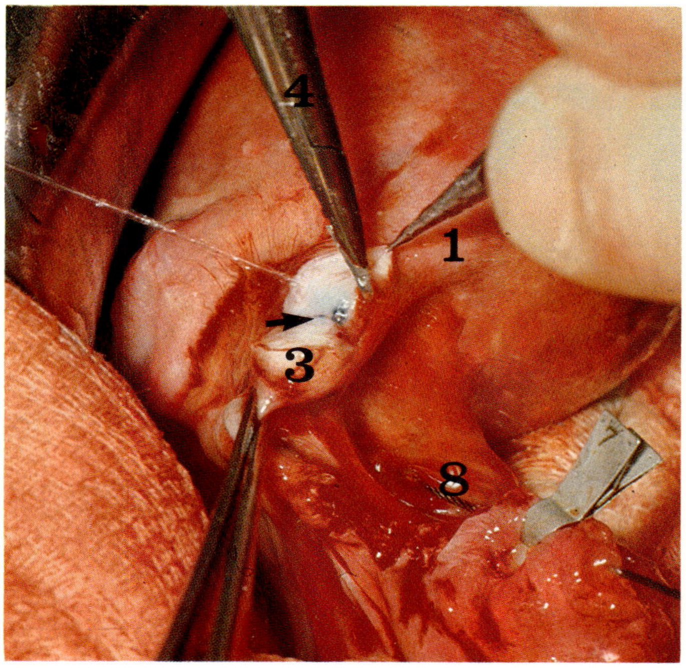

124

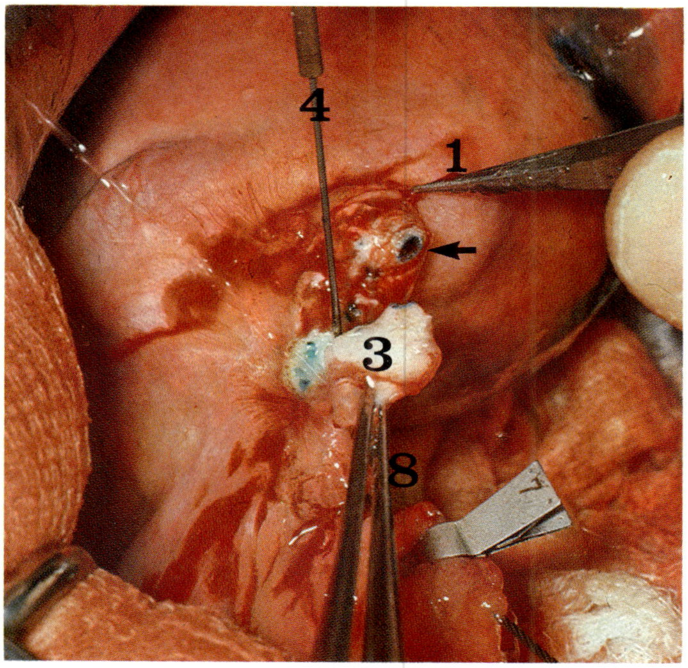

123
The microscalpel encounters a narrow tubal lumen where indicated by the blue dye (arrowed). Thin sections are shaved off the tube, working towards the uterus, until an adequate lumen is revealed. A jet of Ringer's solution is used to keep the area free of blood.

124
The lumen of the tube has now been exposed and the dye is seen escaping from its end (arrowed). The destroyed segment of tube is held in forceps and detached gradually and carefully with the fine diathermy needle (4) which has replaced the microscalpel. The Ringer's solution jet is still being used.

125
A further stage of the same manoeuvre is seen, with the occluded portion of the tube about to be detached with the diathermy. Note that there is very little intrusion into the mesosalpinx; the Ringer's solution jet is of great help at this stage.

125

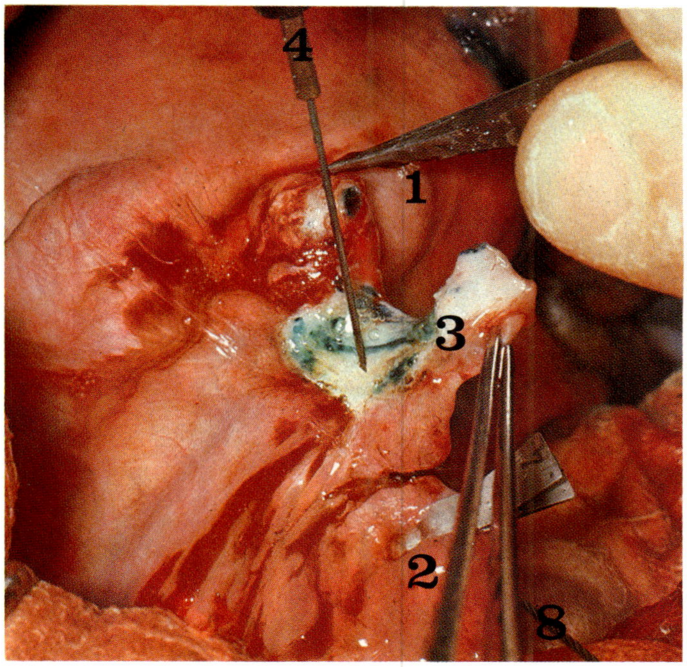

Stage II: Suture of mesosalpinx – left fallopian tube

126

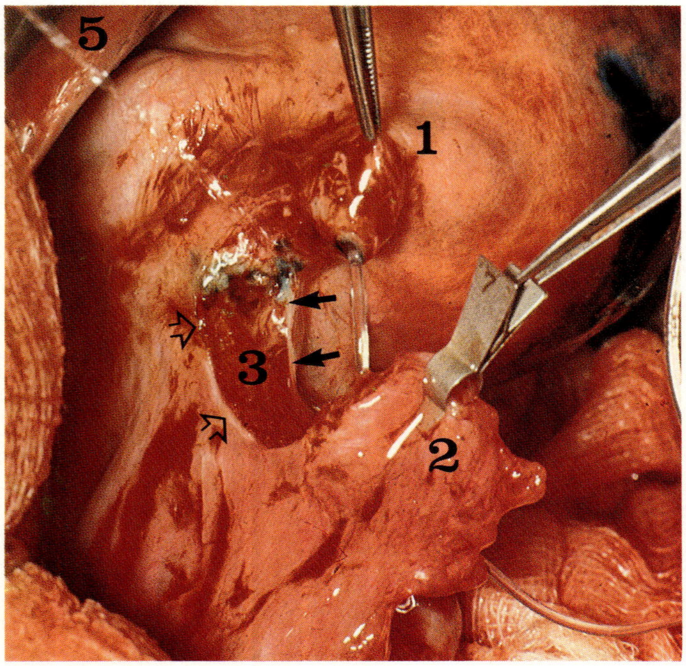

127

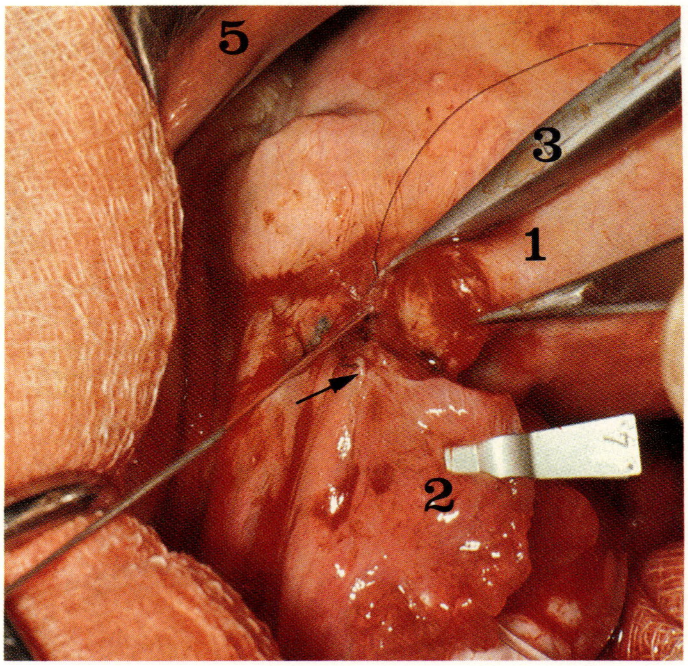

126 and 127
In **Figure 126** the two ends of the tube for anastomosis are splinted on the plastic tube. The open mesosalpinx is seen at (3) with the upper anterior border indicated by fine open arrows and the upper posterior border by fine solid arrows. In **Figure 127** the anterior layer of the mesosalpinx is being closed by the suture carried on a needle holder (3). The medial anterior edge has been picked up on the needle whose point is emerging through the lateral edge where arrowed. A jet of Ringer's solution is playing on the site of suture. Similar sutures are placed anteriorly and posteriorly and when tied off and complete will 'set up' the tube for suture of the muscle layer.

128

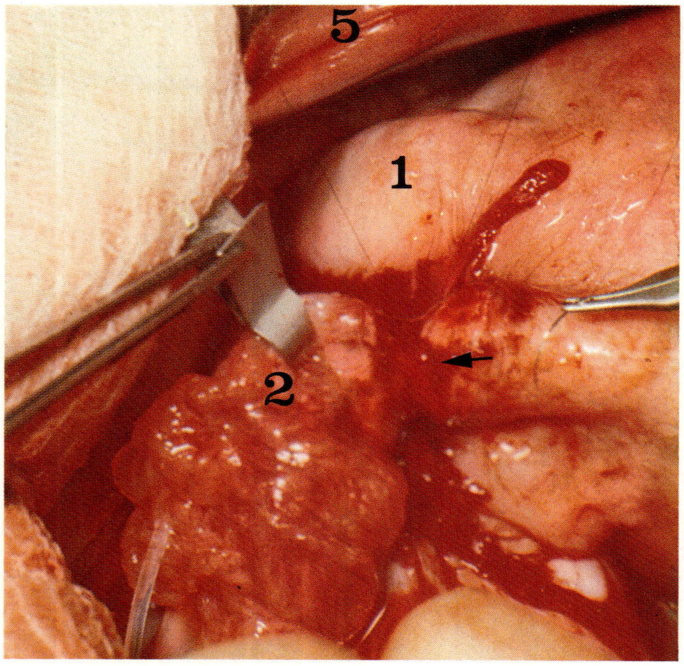

Stage III: Suture of muscle layer of left fallopian tube

128
The tube is viewed from the posterior aspect in this case and the first of the four muscle sutures has been taken through the muscle layers (where arrowed) in the 8 o'clock position and therefore in the mesenteric half of the tubal circumference. The two segments are already opposed by the sutures in the mesosalpinx and when the muscle suture is tied they will come together very neatly.

129

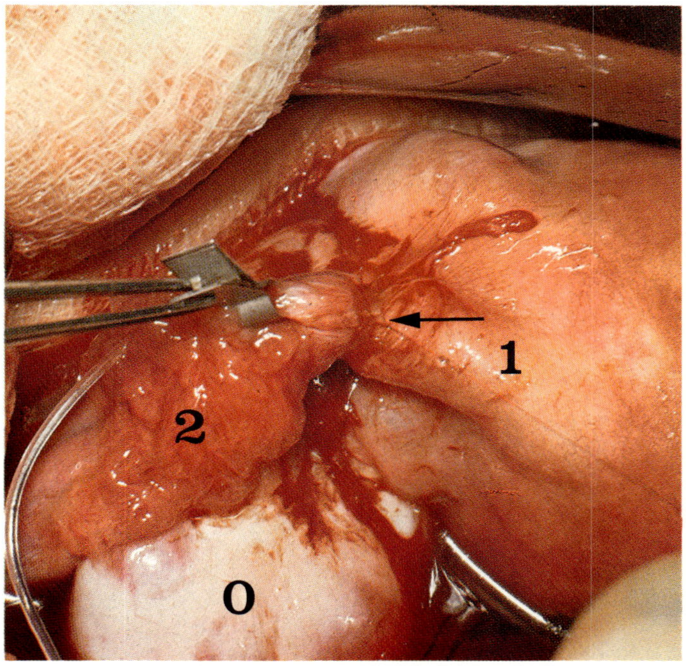

130

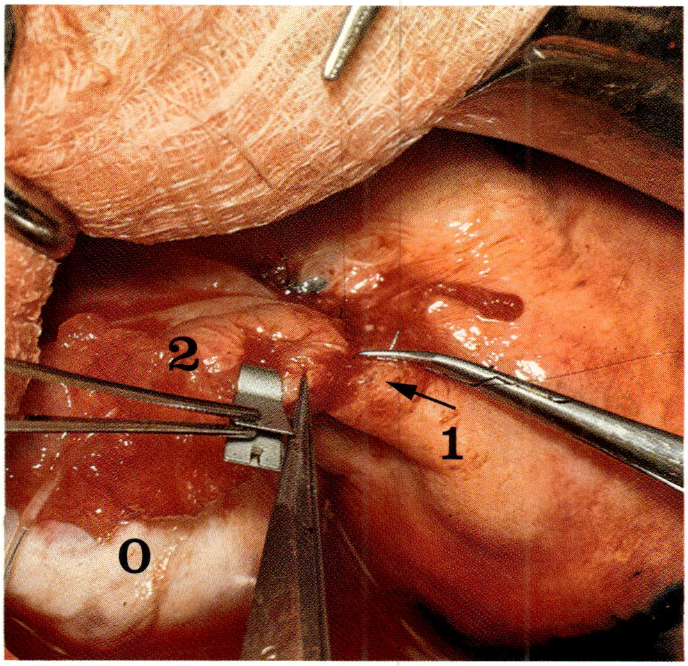

129 to 131

In **Figure 129** the second suture in the mesenteric half of the tubal circumference at the 4 o'clock position is being tied off (arrowed). **Figure 130** shows the first muscle bite in the placing of the 10 o'clock suture (arrowed) and in **Figure 131** the fourth and final stitch in the 2 o'clock position is being tied off (arrowed).

131

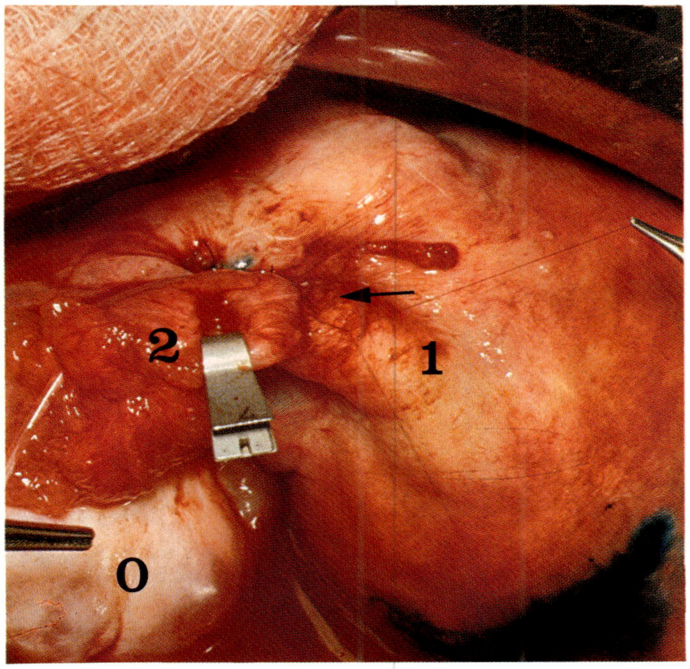

Stage IV: Suture of serosal layer of left fallopian tube

132

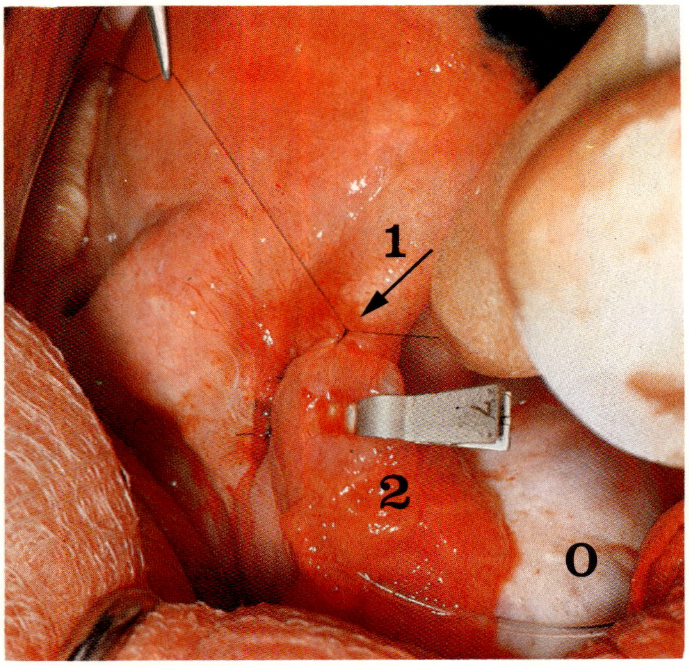

133

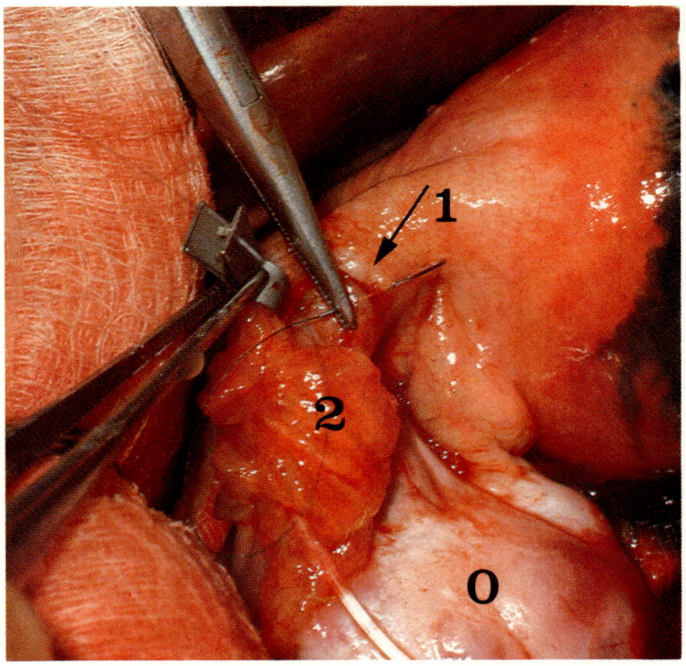

134

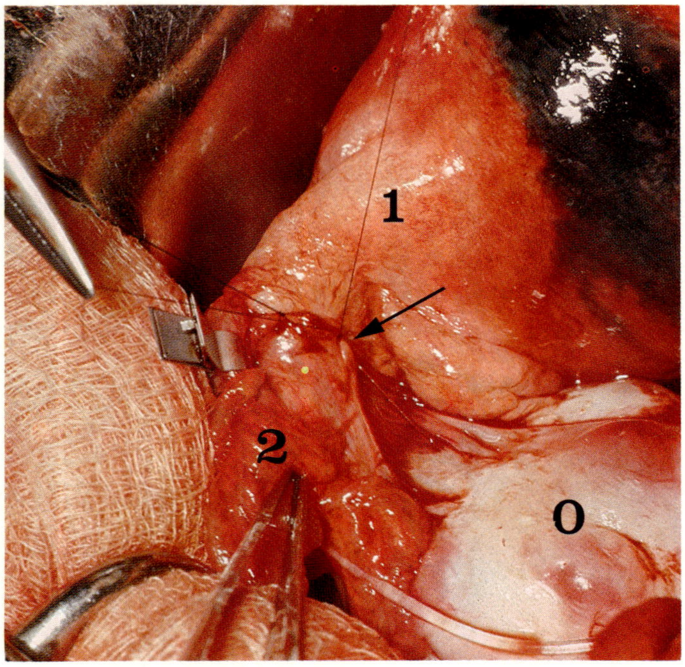

132 to 134
A serosal suture on the anterior aspect of the tube is being tied off to give a smooth Lembert effect in **Figure 132**. A similar suture is being placed on the posterior aspect of the tube in **Figure 133** and this shows very clearly the amount of serosa and muscle included in it. It also demonstrates the desired inversion of the edges. In **Figure 134** the posterior serosal suture is carried on to the posterior surface of the mesosalpinx (arrowed) and as previously discussed. A further similar stitch is required to completely iron out the surface in that area.

Stage V: Appraisal of left tubal anastomosis

135 and 136
Figure 135 shows the anastomosis complete with a smooth surface at the suture line. Dye has been injected from the uterus at (4) and is seen escaping from the fimbrial end (5). There is no leakage at the suture line. **Figure 136** gives a view of both anastomosed tubes with evidence of patency and intact suture lines. The dye tends to escape from the fundal injection site and gives an untidy appearance. The tubes are shorter than one would wish but the essential requirements must have been satisfied because this patient quickly became pregnant.

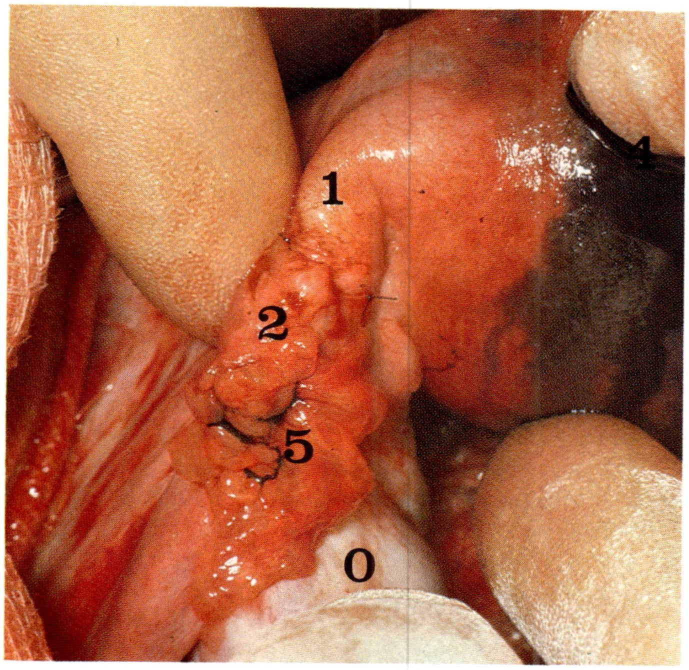

135

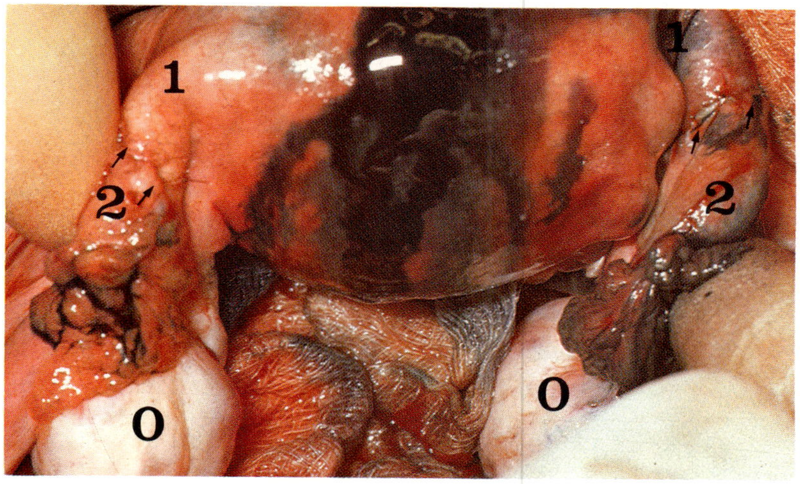

136

Results of anastomosis of the fallopian tube

The results of tubal anastomosis must obviously be greatly influenced by the many factors that the surgeon has or should have taken into account before performing the operation. These include the length of the tube remaining, the site of the blockage, the degree of fibrosis and many others. The question of the shortened tube is an important one and there is general agreement that it is an adverse factor that may lead to continuing infertility, abortion or ectopic gestation. Ampullary deficiency is accepted as more serious than isthmal (Winston 1978) and the ampulla is often partially destroyed in the sterilising operations which precede the management under discussion here. In the purely technical field also, anastomosis of the relatively thin-walled ampullary tube is bound to be less satisfactory. Results in any series may be vitiated by the fact that the more skilled and expert surgeon will tackle some less favourable prospects and thereby reduce his success rate.

Siegler (1978) evaluated the available results and took term pregnancy as the only satisfactory criterion of success. He estimated a 30 per cent success rate with macroscopic and 60 per cent with microscopic surgery. The ectopic pregnancy incidence he considered to be about 10 per cent.

Williams (1978) reported the high figure of 72 per cent from macroscopic methods. He also refers to an assembled ongoing series in which he and collaborators are using his same methods and attaining pregnancy rates of 60–70 per cent. The ectopic pregnancy rate in this larger series is about 6 per cent.

Winston (1978) discussing the prospects when using microsurgical techniques reported a 58 per cent success rate in women who sometimes had extensively destroyed tubes. He considered that reversal of clip sterilisations was particularly straightforward and all the cases he had operated on had a successful pregnancy. He added that microsurgery for sterilisation reversal had a very low incidence of ectopic gestation; there was only one instance in a personal series of 60 cases.

Winston and Margara (1980a, b) subsequently published results of sterilisation operations on 126 patients where the overall percentage of pregnancies was 58 per cent. The figures were broken down according to the site of the anastomosis; an isthmo-isthmal group of 16 patients had a pregnancy rate of 75 per cent with no ectopics, 26 ampullo-cornual cases had a rate of 54 per cent with one ectopic and in 19 ampullary anastomoses the rate fell to 42 per cent but there were no ectopics. The results are in line with what one would expect and emphasise that the thin-walled ampullary portion of the tube presents problems for the surgeon (see table below).

TABLE 1

RESULTS OF TUBAL ANASTOMOSIS FOR REVERSAL OF STERILISATION*

	Cornu-isthmus	Isthmus-isthmus	Cornu-ampulla	Isthmus-ampulla	Ampulla-ampulla	Miscellaneous†	Total
No. of operations	17	16	26	27	19	21	126
No. of pregnancies	12	12	14	17	8	10	73
No. of ectopic pregnancies			1	2		(1)	3
Pregnancy rate	71%	75%	54%	63%	42%	48%	58%

*Operations were classified according to the site of anatomosis. When the sterilisation was asymmetric the operation was classified according to the site of the anastomosis in the longer tube.

†'Miscellaneous' refers to different sites in tubes of similar length, to double anastomoses, and to implantation on one side combined with cornual anastomosis on the other. The figure in parentheses indicates one tubal gestation which occurred in an implanted tube; the cornual anastomosis on the other side was patent.

from Winston and Margara (1980b)

10: Microsurgery for infertility

The status of tubal surgery and its practice remains problematic. What is the place of the microscope and the specialised infertility surgeon? To what extent is microsurgery likely to improve the results of infertility surgery?

The answer to these questions largely remains a matter of personal philosophy, but there is increasing evidence that microsurgery, properly employed, limits tissue damage (Swolin 1967), results in improved pelvic healing and is associated with superior tubal patency (Winston 1980a) and pregnancy rates (Siegler and Kontopoulos 1979). Results seem to be better with the microscope rather than with loupes – certainly the microscope is easier to use and much more versatile. The use of magnifying loupes is tiring and the resolution they provide is really not adequate for the accurate identification of pathologic areas or the placement of fine sutures. It has been suggested that the microscope is costly and cumbersome. Cost should not be a problem as the colposcope is merely an operating microscope mounted in an inverted position on a short stand. For a few hundred pounds it is possible to modify the existing stand and to change the microscope mounting. Indeed, the author uses such a system for a large number of his cases and finds it simple and highly satisfactory. In any case, any reasonably sized hospital should certainly have at least one or two operating microscopes in the operating theatres as microsurgery has increasingly expanded in other surgical disciplines.

The principles of microsurgical technique are aimed at reducing iatrogenic surgical damage to a minimum and have the object of leaving the tissues in the best condition to maintain tubal patency and freedom from adhesions. The use of these principles should unquestionably apply to all infertility surgery, even though the microscope may not be always necessary. For example, it clearly is pointless to use the microscope for myomectomy or a metroplasty, but it is highly pertinent to ensure that the closure of the uterine peritoneum is made with as fine a non-reactive suture as possible and in such a way to avoid adhesion formation postoperatively. Indeed, the same principles should apply to all conservative surgery in the young female patient who may be left infertile by careless ovarian cystectomy or uterine surgery. There is now incontrovertible evidence (Eddy, Asch and Balmaceda 1980) that the use of 3/0 or 4/0 catgut sutures in the repair of the ovarian capsule causes adhesions and that these can be avoided if fine nylon or prolene 6/0 or 8/0 sutures are used.

The use of the microscope

Before using the operating microscope in the clinical situation it is absolutely essential that the surgeon is completely familiar with it. He should be able to make minor alterations to it quickly and easily and should be familiar with its mechanical performance and its optical adjustments. It is vital to know how to clean it, to change objective lenses and to be able to provide its basic service requirements. Unless the surgical team understands how to set the microscope up for clinical surgery, it will become a cumbersome nuisance. The surgeon must have had some previous experience of microsurgery and clearly this is gained privately in the laboratory rather than in the operating room.

Most gynaecological surgeons will be more familiar with the Carl Zeiss (Oberkochen) type of microscope than any other, so the following comments apply to this microscope. The principles, however, apply to all microscopes. Abdominal microsurgery will be greatly facilitated if the following equipment is available:

(1) A 250 mm or 300 mm objective lens. Most colposcopists will be familiar with a working distance of 200 mm. This is too close for most tubal surgery and longer focal length lens should be acquired.

(2) A geared angled coupling between the microscope carriage arm and the body (Zeiss catalogue No. K120/76). This enables the microscope to be swung from side to side while it is mounted in an oblique axis.

(3) Some form of extension arm between the microscope coupling and the microscope stand. This will give greater mobility and flexibility as the microscope stand will be further away from the abdominal wound.

(4) Sterilisable rubber cups which slide over the control knobs on the microscope body. This is simpler and safer than using elaborate drapes to 'bag' the microscope.

Unless there is going to be an exceptionally heavy case load in a training centre, we recommend the use of a single-man microscope rather than a two-man microscope. The diploscope is more difficult to use and more expensive.

The principles of gynaecologic microsurgery

(1) Approach with good exposure. The use of a large incision is really important. To struggle to achieve a good view through an inadequate incision is to court tissue damage and will increase the chance of poor healing. We routinely employ a Pfannenstiel incision, unless of course the patient already has a midline surgical scar. It is important that the transverse suprapubic incision is made large enough and we generally extend it to include the oblique abdominal wall muscles.

(2) Avoidance of peritoneal abrasions. The handling of the genital tract tissues should be gentle and minimal. We prefer to use glass rods or smooth instruments rather than fingers wherever possible and never clamps or forceps.

(3) Constant irrigation with warmed isotonic fluids. Drying of the peritoneal surfaces and the ovary capsule should be avoided. We use Ringer lactate solution for all irrigation and for soaking laparotomy pads. Sterile water is not appropriate as it sucks salts out of the tissues.

(4) The use of fine, low energy diathermy for haemostasis and dissection. Blended diathermy delivered through a very fine needle point is ideal as it causes very limited damage. Conventional surgical diathermy machines are not suitable for this kind of dissection as their power output is too great. Most of the time we use an output of 5–15 watts such as is achievable with the instruments made by Valleylab and Siemens (Winston 1980b).

(5) The use of few, simple microsurgical instruments. Ophthalmic instruments are by no means ideal for work in the pelvis. Better by far is a custom-built needle holder, forceps and scissors designed specifically for this surgery. A highly satisfactory range is supplied by Spingler-Tritt of West Germany.

(6) Sutures should be atraumatic and fine. We very rarely use any suture thicker than 5/0 prolene (which can be handled with the naked eye) and prefer 6/0. For tubal anastomosis, salpingostomy and some ovarian surgery we use 8/0 or 9/0 nylon which gives superb plastic results. Some authors recommend Vicryl and Dexon – but all absorbable sutures require the mobilisation of the inflammatory reactive process for their absorption and we therefore prefer inert non-absorbable sutures.

(7) Adequate peritoneal coverage on abdominal closure. Raw areas should be covered, where possible, by mobilising the serosal coat of the damaged organ. Where the raw areas are too great then the best management seems to be the use of split peritoneal grafts. This peritoneum can be taken from the upper abdomen and all fat and connective tissue must be cleaned from its visceral surface before being sutured into position. Omental grafts are generally unsatisfactory and seem to increase rather than diminish adhesions.

(8) Proper abdominal closure. Careless closure of the abdominal peritoneum leads to unwanted adhesions. A good technique is to use everting mattress sutures which leave an excellent suture line. 3/0 polyglycolic acid sutures are certainly thick enough for this purpose.

Comparison of macro and microsurgical results

Reference has been made in the preceding chapter to the results that can be obtained using macrosurgery for the treatment of tubal and peritubal disease. In Table 1 a summary of 14 series is presented in which macrosurgery was employed in the treatment of patients with *complete* occlusion of the terminal part of the tube. Comparison can therefore be made with two sets of series in Tables 2 and 3 of published and unpublished results on similar groups of women with terminally occluded tubes in whom microsurgery was used to produce a salpingostomy. Results from the usage of both techniques in tubal anastomosis has already been given on page 130.

TABLE 1

PUBLISHED RESULTS OF SALPINGOSTOMY BY MACROSURGERY

Author	Patients	Term Pregnancy	Patent Tubes	Tubal Pregnancy	Abortions
Boyd & Holt (1972)	77	5 (6.5%)	n.a.	2	2
Clyman, M.J. (1968)	27	5 (18%)	74%	n.s.	n.s.
Crane & Woodruff (1968)	34	2 (6%)	57%	2	4
Fjallbrant, B. (1975)	35	6 (17%)	n.a.	3	2
Foix, A. (1974)	12	1 (8%)	n.a.	1	0
Hanton *et al.* (1964)	32	1 (3%)	50%	1	4
Jessen, H. (1971)	25	5 (20%)	n.a.	3	5
Lamb & Moscovitz (1972)	35	2 (6%)	n.a.	3	n.s.
Mroueh *et al.* (1968)	60	1 (2%)	n.a.	0	0
Mulligan, W.J. (1966)	66	11 (17%)	53%	6	3
Ozäras, H. (1968)	106	2 (2%)	n.a.	0	n.s.
Rock *et al.* (1978)	99	16 (16%)	n.a.	6	n.s.
Siegler, A.M. (1969)	27	2 (7%)	n.a.	0	0
Young *et al.* (1970)	18	3 (17%)	n.a.	3	0
Total	653	62 (9.5%)	54%	30	20

n.a. = not assessed.
n.s. = not stated.

References to Table 1
Boyd, I.E. and Holt, E.M. (1972). *J. Obstet. Gynaec. Brit. Commonw.* **80**, 142.
Clyman, M.J. (1968). *Fertil. Steril.* **19**, 537.
Crane, M. and Woodruff, J.D. (1968). *Fertil. Steril.* **19**, 810.
Fjallbrant, B. (1975). *Acta Obstet. Gynecol. Scand.* **54**, 563.
Foix, A. (1974). In Esterilidad Conjugal, Panamericana, Buenos Aires.
Hanton, E.M., Pratt, J.H. and Banner, E.A. (1964). *Am. J. Obstet. Gynecol.* **89**, 934.
Jessen, H. (1971). *Acta Obstet. Gynecol. Scand.* **50**, 105.
Lamb, E.J. and Moscovitz, W. (1972). *Int. J. Fertil.* **17**, 53.
Mroueh, A. and Hajj, S.N. (1969). *Int. J. Fertil.* **13**, 215.
Mulligan, W.J. (1966). *Int. J. Fertil.* **11**, 424.
Ozäras, H. (1968). *Acta Obstet. Gynecol. Scand.* **47**, 489.
Rock, J.A. *et al.* (1978). *Am. J. Obstet. Gynecol.* **52**, 591.
Siegler, A.M. (1969). *Obstet. Gynecol.* **34**, 339.
Young, P.E. *et al.* (1970). *Am. J. Obstet. Gynecol.* **108**, 1092.

TABLE 2

PUBLISHED RESULTS OF SALPINGOSTOMY BY MICROSURGERY

Author	Patients	Term Pregnancy	Tubal Pregnancy	Abortions
Gomel (1978)	50*	11 (22%)	10%	4%
Swolin (1975)	33	8 (24%)	18%	
Winston (1980)	241	42 (17.5%)	9.5%	7.5%
Total	324	61 (18.8%)		

*Note that of these 50 patients, nine were lost to follow-up or excluded from the reported series for other reasons.

References to Table 2
Gomel, V (1978). *Fertil. Steril.* **29**, 380.
Swolin, K. (1975). *Am. J. Obstet. Gynecol.* **121**, 418.
Winston, R.M.L. (1980). *Fertil. Steril.* **34**, 521.

TABLE 3

UNPUBLISHED RESULTS OF MICROSURGICAL SALPINGOSTOMY, LEUVEN SYMPOSIUM, BELGIUM, 1980

Author	Patients	Term Pregnancy	Tubal Pregnancy	Abortions
Beyth	36	2 (6%)	2	1
Boer	72	12 (17%)	10	3
Frantzen	11	2 (18%)	1	1
Gordts	79	18 (23%)	n.a.	–
Hedon	30	2 (7%)	1	0
Rock	87	19 (22%)	5	5
Sarris	18	2 (11%)	0	3
Total	333	57 (17%)	(19)	(13)

(Personal communications)

Preparation for microsurgery

Adequate preparation before using the microscope is vital. The basic essential is to ensure that the surgeon is comfortable. It is quite impossible to perform accurate microsurgery unless one is relaxed and working in a comfortable position. We prefer to be seated whenever possible. To improve comfort a padded stool with a square seat is best. Round hard stools cause sciatic nerve pressure and become very tiring – particularly if the surgeon is using his feet to operate a diathermy pedal or the remote controls of an electrically driven microscope. The position of the body is important and is seen clearly in **Figure 1**. The back is straight and the surgeon's eyes naturally meet the eye-pieces of the microscope without straining. Note how the microscope is angled to achieve this position. The arms are extended and the surgeon's wrists are supported on the wound edge in front of him. In order to achieve this ideal body position, the surgeon can adjust the height of the microscope on its column, the operating table on its hydraulic base, and his stool. Generally one needs to have the operating table lowered as far as it will go. In order to increase the comfort of the surgeon's sitting position, we usually place an extension flap on the foot end of the operating table. This allows us to have the patient positioned further down the table with her thorax over the central column and her pelvis over the free end. This allows space so that the surgeon can sit with his knees under the table and still be in position to operate in the pelvis.

From **Figure 1**, note that the surgeon wears his eye-glasses whilst using the microscope. It is a mistake to remove one's spectacles when using the microscope because normal vision is required as well. Sterility is maintained by wearing the surgical mask properly over the bridge of the nose (it is not necessary to slip the mask down), by draping the microscope column (at 1), and by the use of autoclavable rubber cups on the controls (at 2). The extension bar to the micro-scope carriage arm is at (3). The television camera (at 4) is valuable because it allows the scrub nurse and any assistants a clear view of the operative field.

1

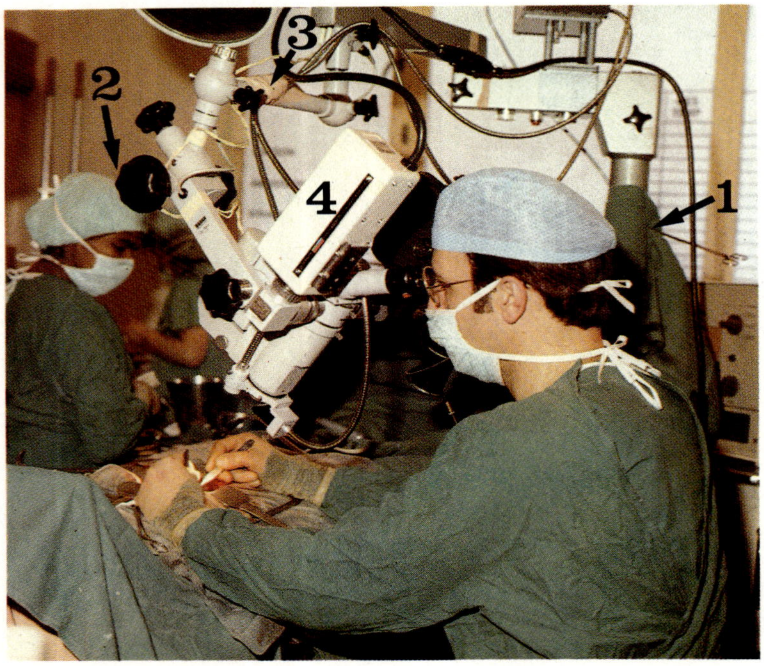

2

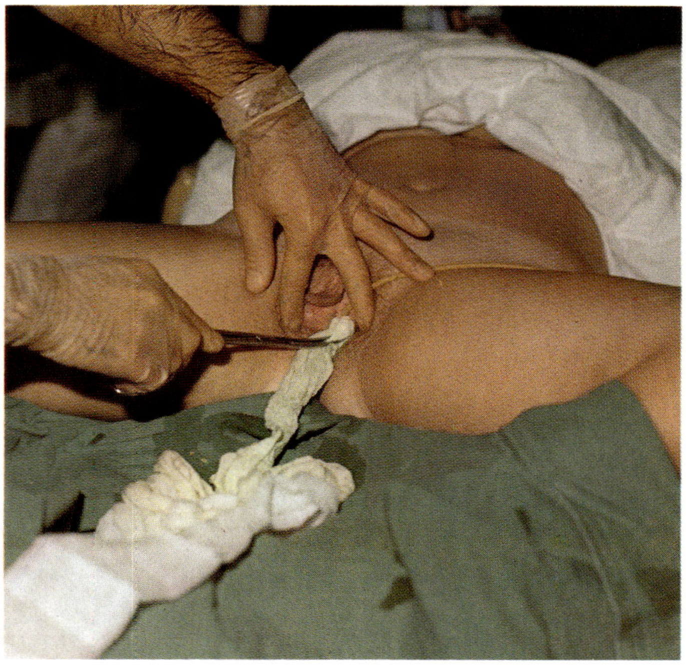

2 Packing the vagina

A key aspect of microsurgery is to support the tissues in a fixed focal plane so that they do not pop in and out of focus continually. For this reason we make a platform in the pelvic cavity. Before preparing the abdominal skin we leave a Foley catheter in the bladder and place it on continuous drainage. This prevents the bladder getting in the way if the operation takes a long time.

The vagina is very thoroughly cleaned and sterilised as far as possible. A 4 inch ribbon gauze is now placed in the vagina, and placed high up in the posterior and anterior fornix. A pair of Bozemann's forceps are helpful for this. Packing should be continued until the uterine cervix is elevated as far as possible. The tail of the pack is left between the patient's legs so that it can be easily pulled out if necessary. We generally employ packing routinely for reversal of sterilisation operations or if there are few pelvic adhesions. Packing is less helpful if the uterus is retroverted by many adhesions or if performing cornual anastomosis.

3

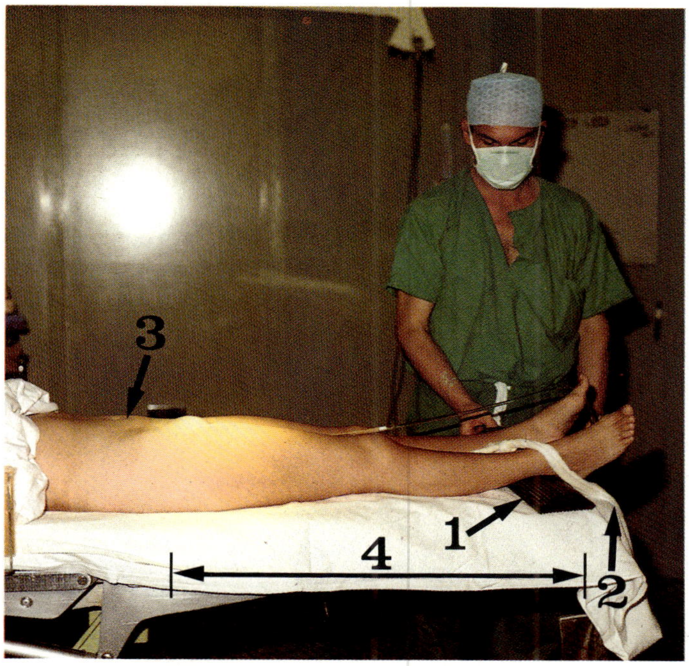

3 Positioning the patient

This should be checked by the surgeon himself or a senior assistant. Microsurgical cases can take two hours or more and so care must be taken to ensure that there are as few pressure areas as possible. We employ an ankle support pad (1) which relieves calf pressure. Note that the tail of the vaginal pack (2) hangs over the edge of the table where it can be easily retrieved if the pack needs to be removed during the procedure. The dome-shaped abdominal wall (3) is caused by the uterine fundus which has been elevated out of the pelvis by the pack.

In addition to ensuring that the patient's position is satisfactory, the surgeon should confirm that the catheter tubing is free of drag. Relatively slight pressure in the urethra from pulling on the catheter can cause marked urinary urgency and even stranguary immediately post-operatively. It is also vital to ascertain that the diathermy pad is fitted closely to the patient's skin, otherwise burning can occur. In **Figure 3**, the table extension is seen at (4). In our case, this is a home-made aluminium metal flap which slots into the foot end of the table.

4

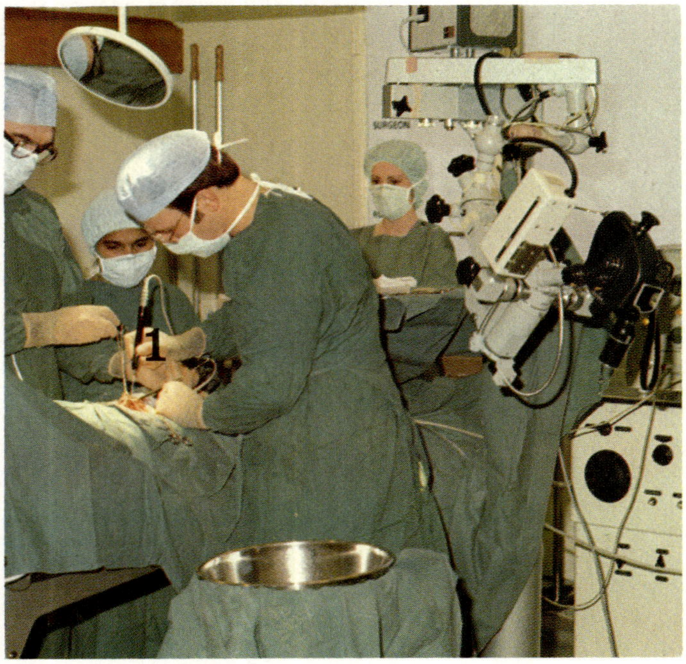

5

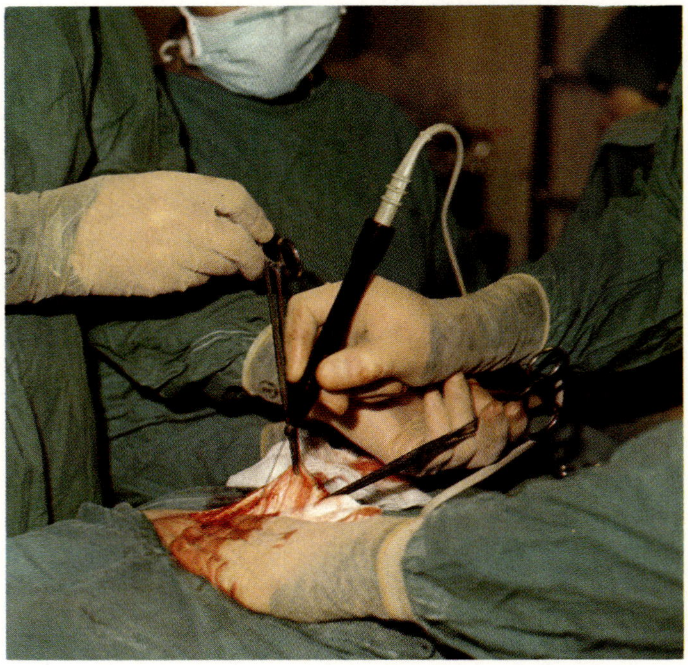

6

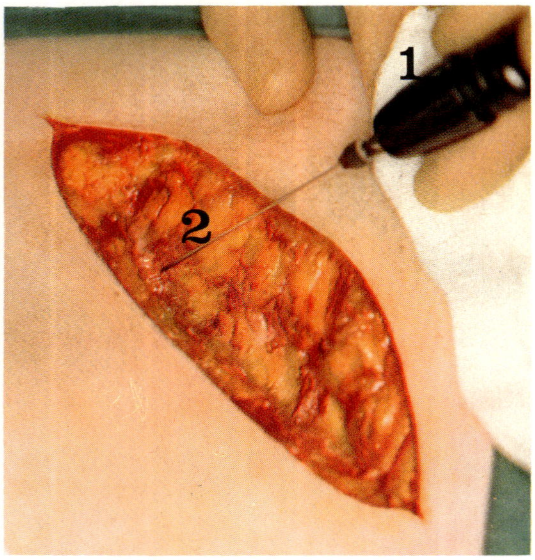

4 to 6 Making the abdominal incision
A Pfannenstiel incision is made but only the skin is incised. The incision is made transversely at the superior margin of the pubic hair line. Note that the microscope stands ready in **Figure 4** in its folded position. The body merely needs to be swung across – the height is already adjusted. The column has already been draped.

Once the skin is incised, cutting diathermy is used for the fat and deeper layers. This gives the best haemostasis. This is important because unnecessary bleeding into the peritoneal cavity mars the view through the microscope.

The electrode handle (1) being used is the bakelite diathermy handle of Siemens. It has a fingertip control button. **Figure 6** shows the electrode at (2). This electrode is actually a standard cutting skin needle taken from a Davis and Geck skin suture. When using this form of diathermy approach to the peritoneum, it is very important not to hurry but to allow time for small vessels to be coagulated by the action of diathermy needle. Generally only the tip should be employed otherwise there is too much current dispersed.

7

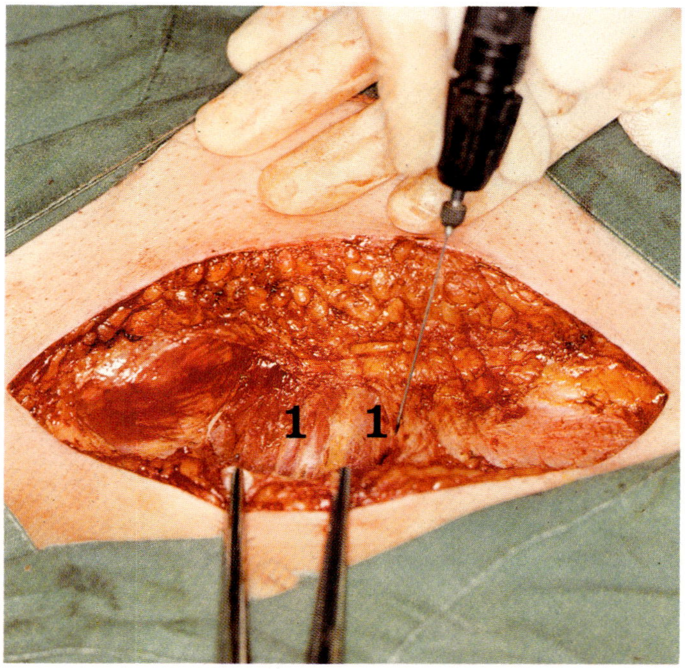

8

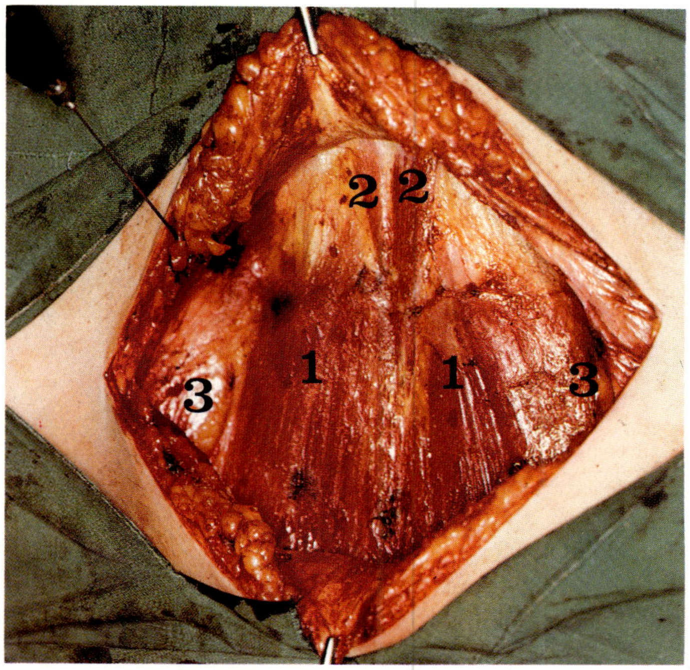

7 and 8 Incision and dissection of the rectus sheath
(The symphysis pubis is at the top of the picture.) The rectus sheath is incised transversely in the midline. Its upper edge is held with two Kochers forceps. Note that incision of the aponeurosis is carried further laterally than is usual, to increase exposure. Dissection under the rectus sheath should continue up to the umbilicus above and down to pubic symphysis. Rectus muscles are at (1), pyramidalis at (2) and peritoneum can be seen laterally at (3). The rectus muscle can now be separated in the midline to expose the peritoneum.

9

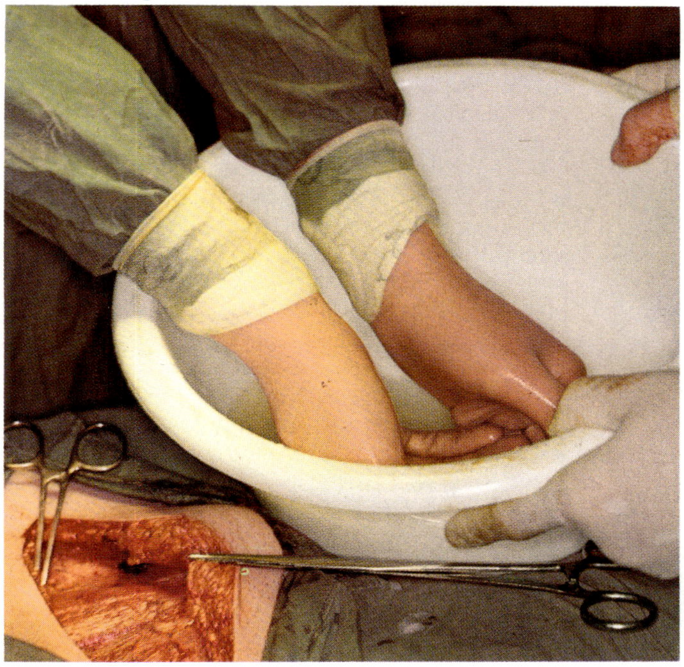

9 Removal of glove powder
Once the peritoneum is exposed, the surgeon, his assistant and the scrub nurse must carefully clean their gloves in a splash bowl of Ringer lactate. This is to remove any talc or odd pieces of lint and to diminish the chance of foreign material being unnecessarily left in the peritoneal cavity. Once this work has been completed, gloves should be dried with a damp pack and both the splash bowl and the pack discarded.

10

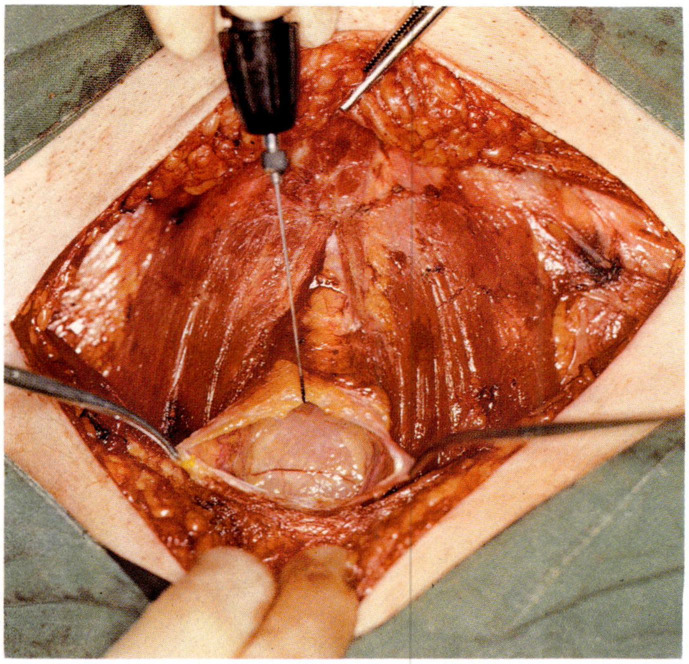

10 Incision of the abdominal peritoneum
This can be conveniently made bloodless if diathermy is employed. Diathermy should be avoided here if laparoscopy has shown that there are adhesions to the anterior abdominal wall. The peritoneal incision is taken down to the tip of the bladder peritoneum and this is best seen by transillumination.

11

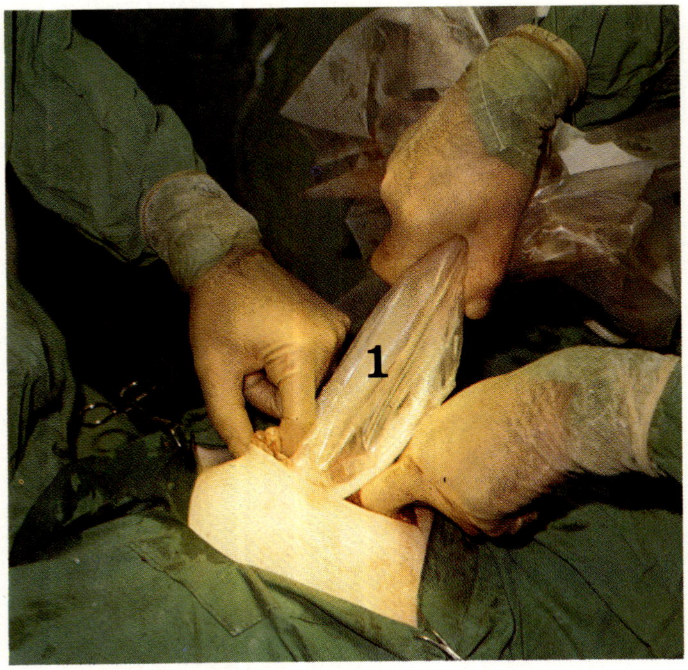

12

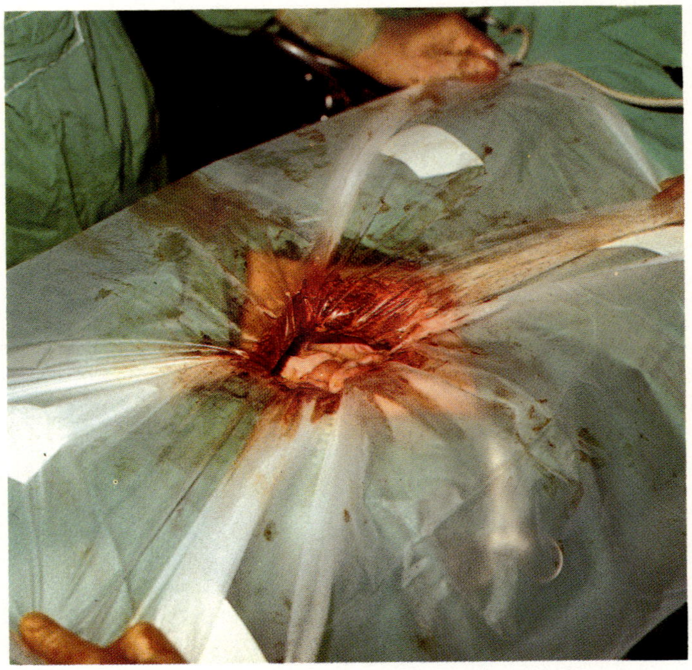

11 and 12 Insertion of the plastic drape
A plastic drape on a 7 inch ring (1) (3 M) is now inserted into the peritoneum. This can be stretched out as in **Figure 12**. This drape keeps the wound edge uncontaminated and prevents oozing into the abdominal cavity. Moreover, it protects the peritoneal edge from drying and damage.

13

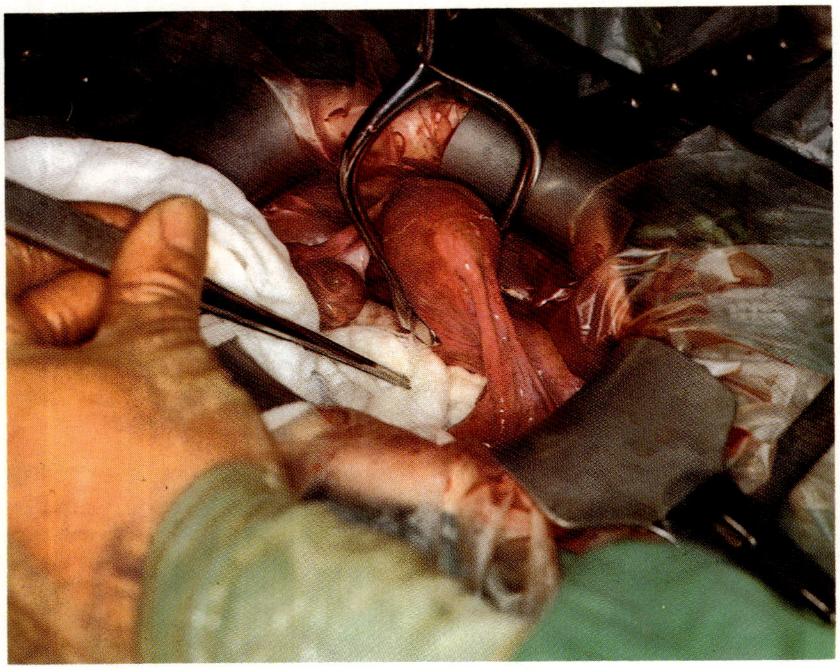

13 Packing the pouch of Douglas
A Kirschner four-bladed retractor is now put in position with the bigger pair of blades on the lateral margins of the wound. A Shirodkar or Buxton clamp is placed across the supravaginal cervix and the uterus is pulled upwards in the direction of the broad arrow. A damp gauze pack is pushed well into the pouch of Douglas so that the uterosacral ligaments will be on stretch. This pack elevates the uterus and will eventually provide the base for a platform in the pelvis on which the appendages will rest. Note that this stage of the procedure cannot proceed unless the appendages are free of adhesions. If they are adherent to the pelvic side wall or the broad ligament, they must be liberated first. It may be an advantage to use magnifying loupes for this.

14 Final exposure
Once the pouch of Douglas pack is in position a silastic pad (made by Spingler-Tritt) (1) can be put in place. This pad has slits for each appendage and fills the brim of the pelvis comfortably. It provides an ideal, non-abrasive background which is smooth and glare free. Blood clots will not readily form on it. Note how stable each appendage is. The Shirodkar clamp is in position and methylene blue dye has just been injected transfundally to test tubal patency. This patient has bilateral hydrosalpinges with mild ovarian adhesions.

14

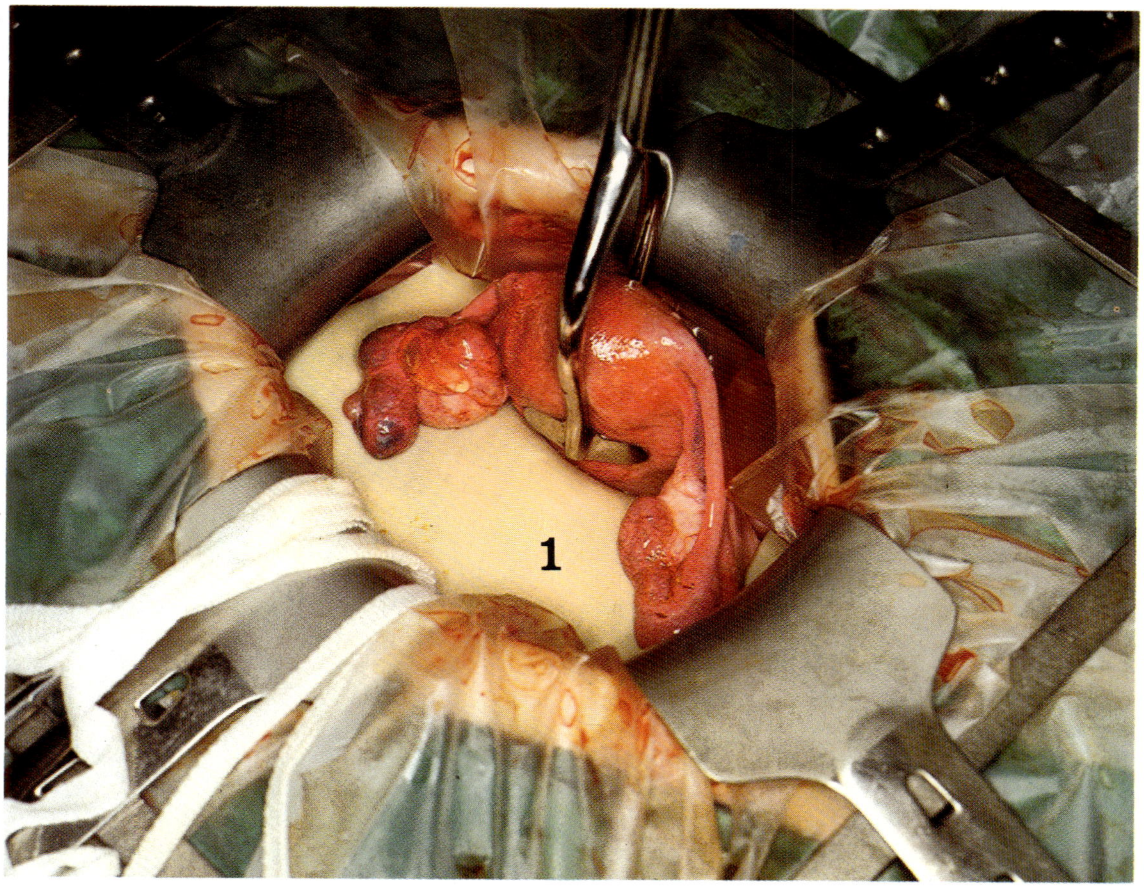

15

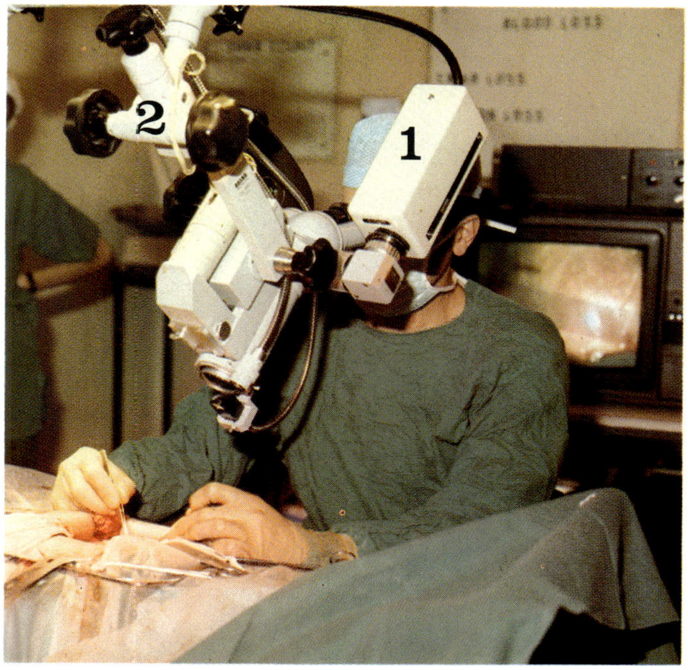

16

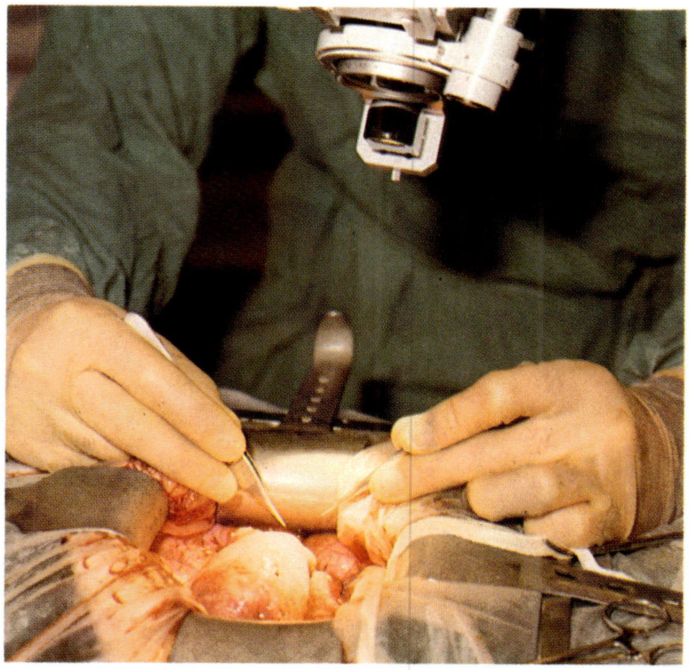

15 Position of the surgeon for salpingostomy
The operating table has been tilted laterally towards the surgeon. The television camera is at (1) and the monitor screen can be clearly seen by the scrub nurse. The geared angled coupling is at (2). When operating for salpingostomy the surgeon sits on the opposite side to the table on which he is working, i.e. he works on the right tube from the patient's left side and vice versa. This will give the best view of the fimbrial-ovarian relationship.

16 Position for tubal anastomosis
Here it is generally an advantage for the surgeon to work from the lateral side of the tube so that he sits on the same side on which he is working. In this case he is doing a right cornual anastomosis, seated on the patient's right side. Note the excellent hand support the retractor and the firm wound edge give him.

Salpingolysis and salpingostomy

Salpingolysis and oophorolysis may be justifiable procedures on their own or they may precede salpingostomy or fimbrioplasty. It is very important that all tubal and ovarian adhesions are freed before attempts are made to perform delicate surgery on the tubal ends, otherwise it will be impossible to restore a good anatomical relationship between the fimbria and the ovary.

In general we try to avoid operating merely to divide minor adhesions, as the evidence in favour of this improving fertility is debatable. When the tubes are patent and the fimbrial ends are relatively free, it is doubtful whether division of pelvic adhesions will substantially improve matters and it may even make them worse. However, recent experimental work (Margara 1980) has demonstrated that relatively flimsy ovarian adhesions are associated with poor ovulation and lowered fertility and that when these adhesions are removed microsurgically, fertility is improved. For this reason we are inclined to be rather more aggressive in the treatment of adhesions than was the case formerly.

The published results following salpingolysis vary enormously and probably greatly depend on the selection of cases. Nevertheless technique is important and microsurgeons feel that recurrence of adhesions after properly performed adhesiolysis should be an unusual sequel. Pregnancy rates vary considerably after salpingolysis but figures of between 40–65 per cent have been recorded following a microsurgical approach (Diamond 1979; and Caspi, Halperin and Bukovsky 1979). There is also an increased likelihood of ectopic pregnancy following these operations but this is almost certainly because of the pre-existing epithelial damage which tends to be the sequel of any pelvic inflammatory disease.

If there are pelvic omental adhesions it will be necessary to divide these first. The microsurgical diathermy is ideal for this. Partial omentectomy may be helpful and we often employ this when adhesions are extensive. There is clinical and experimental evidence that this avoids recurrent adhesions. The first stage in liberation of the adnexa is to free and elevate the ovary where it is adherent in the ovarian fossa. This must be done before the pouch of Douglas is packed and before the microscope is in position. If a raw area is left in the broad ligament or on the pelvic side wall we generally prefer to close this just before closure of the abdomen at the end of the procedure.

Whilst hysterosalpingography is vital to delineate mucosal pathology in hydrosalpinges before surgery, laparoscopy is indispensible too. **Figures 17** and **18** demonstrate the laparoscopic appearance of hydrosalpinges in the patient illustrated in the following pages. Note that a second puncture is always employed for all diagnostic laparoscopy and that for this we generally employ the Verres needle. We photograph the right and left tube separately in all patients for clinical record purposes. We never proceed to laparotomy immediately after laparoscopy in the elective situation. We allow two to three weeks to elapse so that adjunctive treatment can be started when necessary and so that the peritoneum has a chance to recover from exposure to carbonic acid. Moreover, it is absolutely essential to discuss one's laparoscopic finding at length and in detail with both husband and wife so they have a clear idea of the prognosis. Many of the psychological problems associated with tubal surgery occur because the surgeon has not discussed the situation in detail or because the patient and her husband have not assimilated and evaluated the information given to them.

17

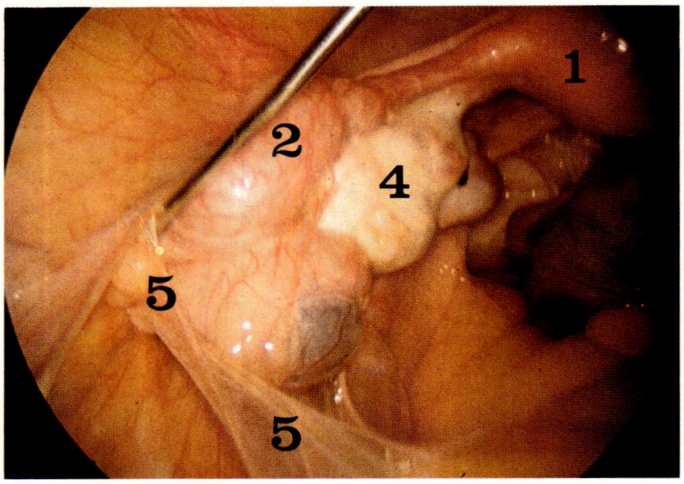

18

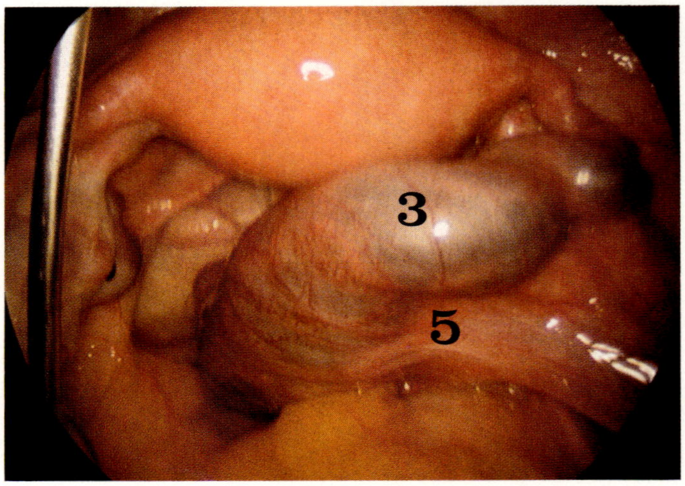

17 and 18 Left and right hydrosalpinges respectively (laparoscope view)

These hydrosalpinges carry a relatively good prognosis in tubal surgical terms. They are free of the ovarian capsule, the adhesions around them are flimsy and not fibrotic or vascular. The tube wall is thin and not cystic and its vascular pattern is still predominantly circular in the ampullary portion. The isthmus on either side is not expanded or fibrotic, there is no cornual hold-up of dye and no adhesions at this point. The ovarian surface is moderately clean and the ovaries are only lightly tethered in the ovarian fossa. Two follicles and an old corpus albicans can be seen in the right ovary, suggesting that it is normally active. The uterus is at (1), the left tube (2), the right tube (3), the left ovary (4). Adhesions are at (5).

19

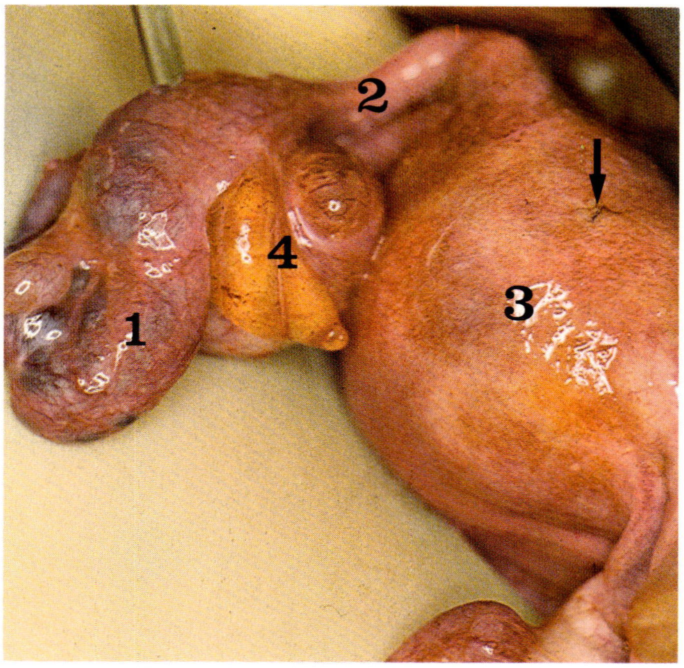

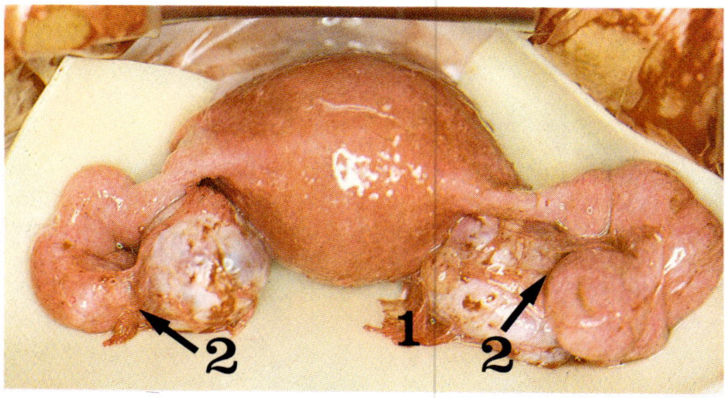

21

19 to 21 Salpingo-oophorolysis before salpingostomy
Both appendages have been dissected free from the lateral pelvic wall and laid on the silastic platform. In **Figure 19** the left ampulla is at (1) and the left isthmus at (2). The uterus is at (3). A fine arrow denotes where dye has been injected transfundally to test tubal permeability. The left tube has filled but there is no spill. The medial upper surface of the left ovary is still covered with adhesions at (4) and these will be removed and the ampulla freed before any attempt at salpingostomy is made.

In **Figure 20**, adhesions are being elevated by glass rods (1), and divided using low intensity diathermy delivered with a fine needle (thin arrow). When dividing such adhesions they should be cut short on the tubal serosa but care should be taken to avoid leaving a raw area on the tube. Magnification is valuable for this. The adhesions can be left long on the ovarian capsule and removed subsequently when they can be cut flush with the tunica albuginea of the ovary using microsurgical scissors to avoid burning the ovary.

Figure 21 shows this dissection almost completed. The adhesions have been left long on the ovary (1) but the ampulla is relatively free. The most lateral part (2) of the tube is still adherent to the ovary and this will need to be dissected free before the salpingostomy is started. Note that the peritoneum is glistening and moist from frequent irrigation and that the operative field is free of blood.

20

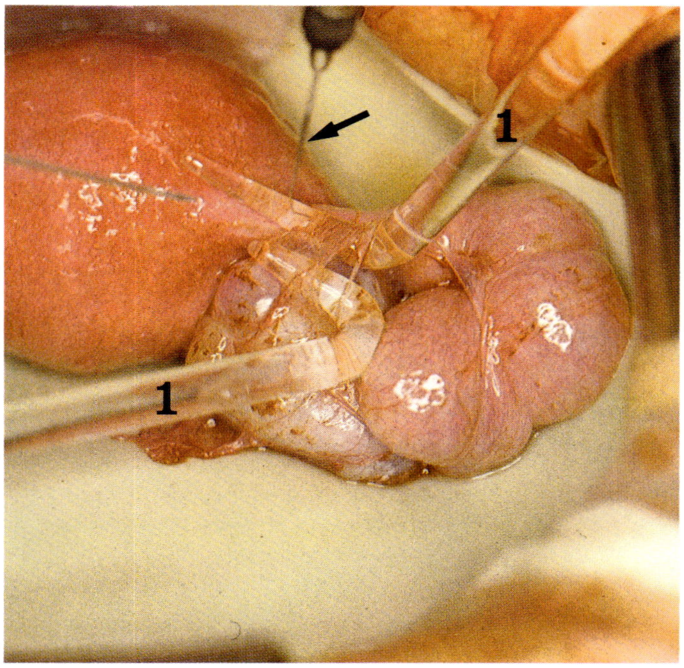

22 to 24 Identification of the terminal point of the tube *(Magnification factor at bottom right corner.)* The ampulla is seen at (1) and the obliterated fimbrial ovarian ligament at (2). Glass rods are (3) and the diathermy needle (4). The background is the silastic platform. It is a major error to open the tube at its thinnest part (seen at 5). The tube must be opened at its most terminal point. Failure to do this will result in a linear salpingostomy in the tube wall. Such a salpingostomy frequently tends to reocclude immediately postoperatively by a process of natural healing (Israel 1951). The microscope should be utilised to identify the terminal point which is usually represented by a line of fibrous scar tissue (6). The tubal blood vessels invariably tend to converge at this point, making identification relatively simple. Failure to identify this point will make it difficult to re-establish a proper fimbria ovarica.

Using the finest diathermy needle an incision about 1–2 mm in length is made at the terminal point (6) **Figure 24**. This incision is made down to and including mucosa and the methylene blue dye is allowed to leak out of the tube.

22

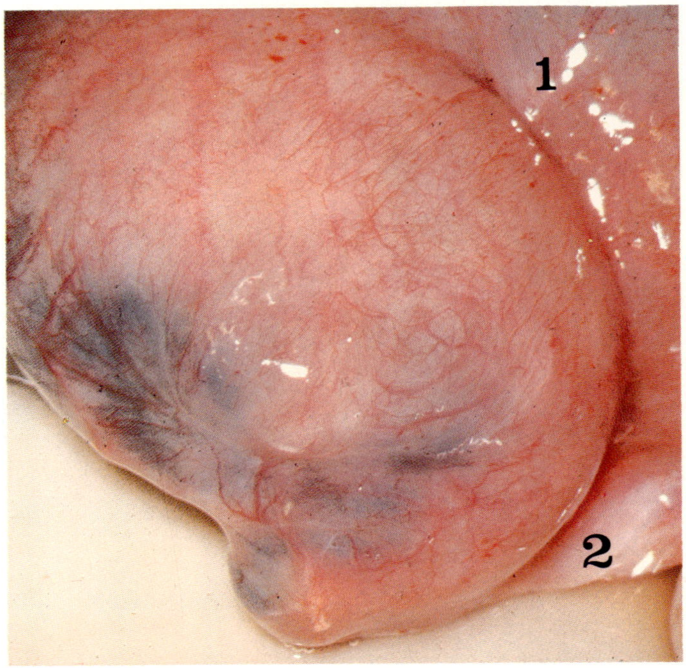

x 3

23

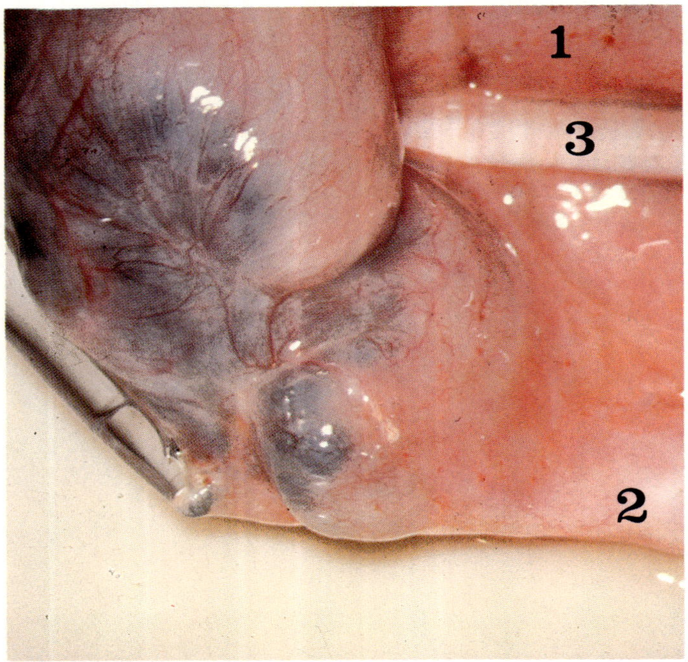

x 3

24

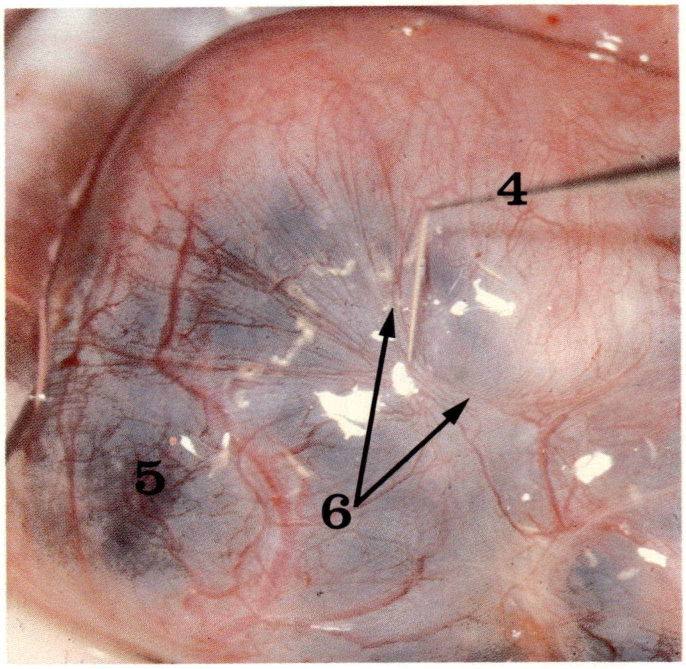

x 4

25

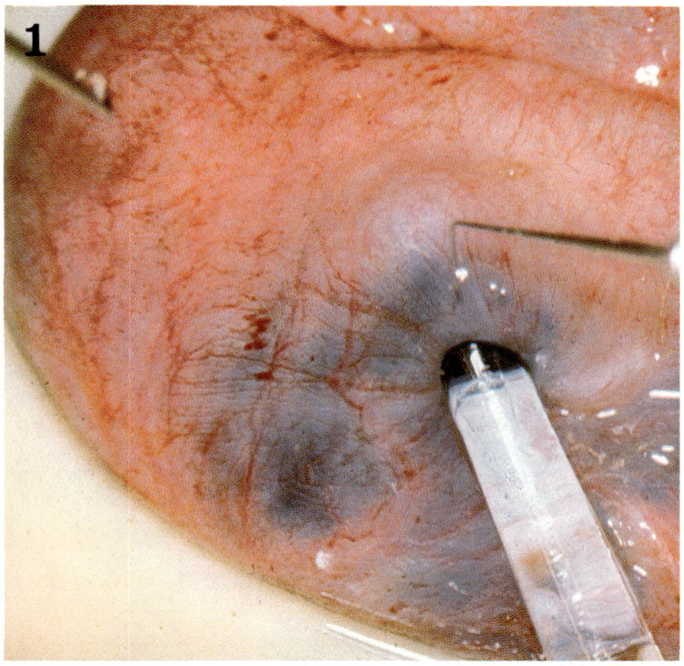

x 4

25 to 28 Enlarging initial tubal incision
The tip of a glass rod is inserted into the hole in the tube. It is elevated to stretch the tube wall to expose the lumen and examine the musculature. The tube has now lost its turgor (**Figure 25**) as the dye escapes. Constant irrigation is provided by the assistant's needle (1).

26

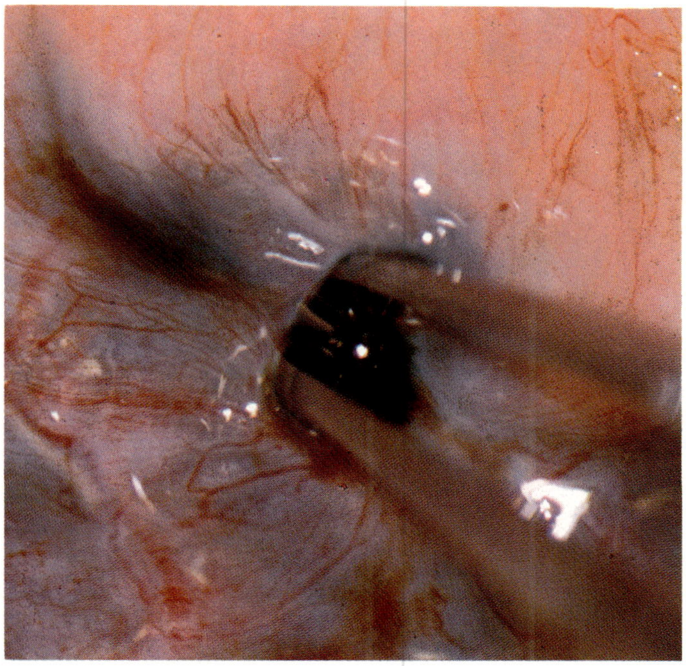

x 10

26. Once a small hole has been made a fine pair of microsurgical forceps may be inserted into the terminal hole and the mucosal folds (if present) examined. It is a considerable advantage to know in which direction the folds run, so as to avoid cutting across them.

27

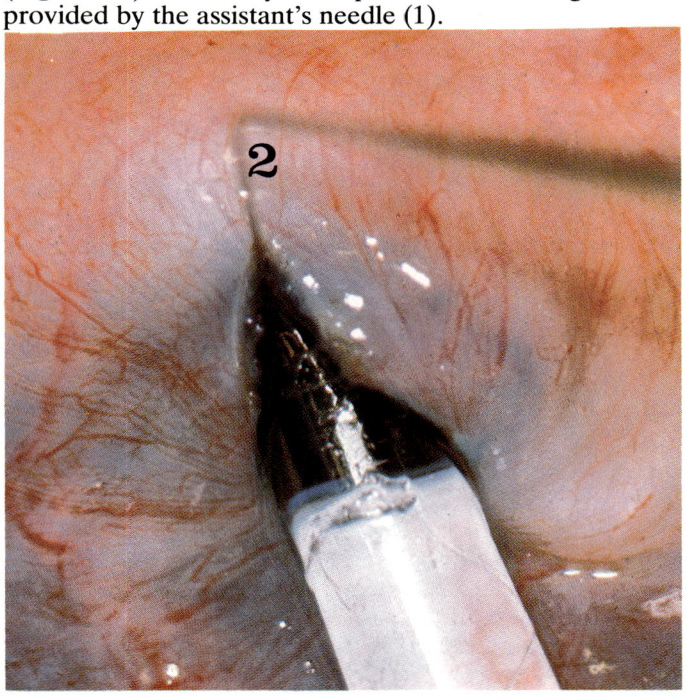

x 12

27. The glass rod is reinserted and the tubal wall elevated. Small radial cuts are made with diathermy (2) in the wall along the glass rod. These cuts should be between blood vessels and parallel to the mucosal folds.

28

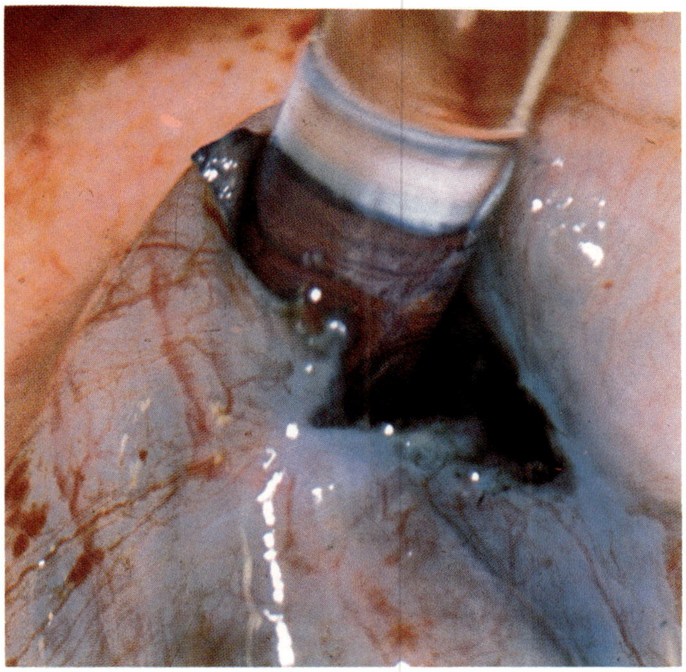

x 16

28. Small multiple cuts are made and the tube gradually opens out. Note that there should be no bleeding if this is done properly. If one of the radial cuts causes marked bleeding it generally implies that the incision is too far from the terminal margin of the tube (i.e. that one has cut into the tubal wall rather than across scar tissue).

29

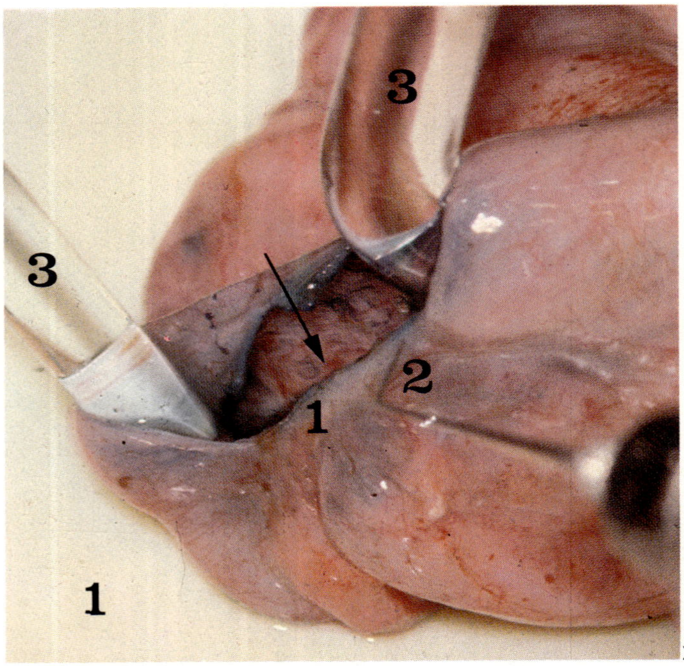

x 4

30

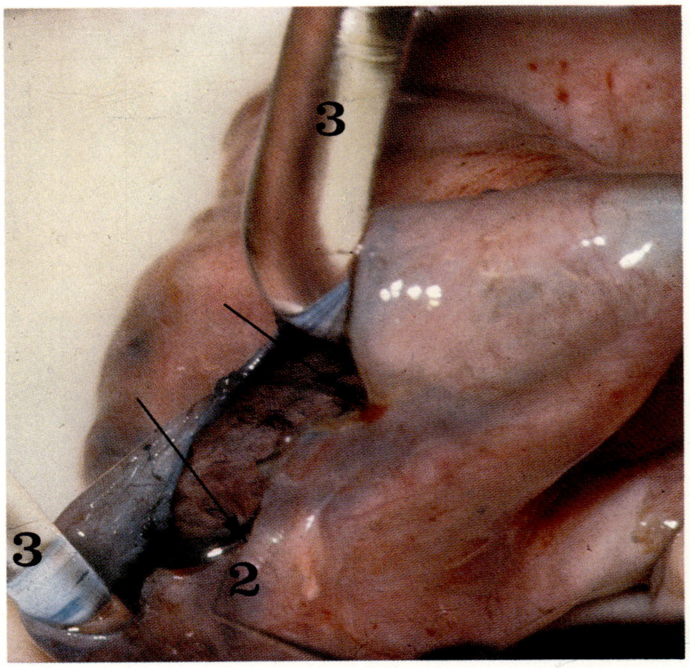

x 4

31

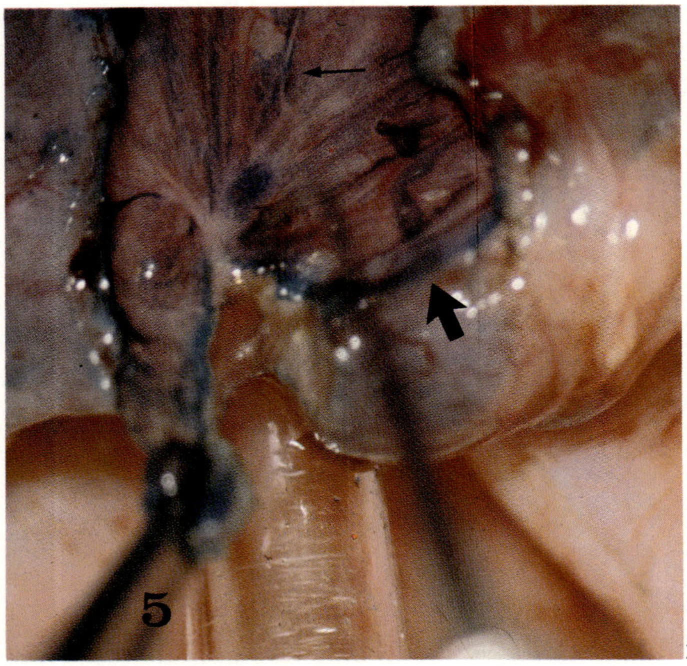

x 16

29. Sometimes when there is marked fibrosis (1) of the ostial rim it is helpful to insert two glass rods (3) and pull the ostium open. Diathermy (2) can now be applied to the fibrotic rim and further incisions made along the line of the blood vessels. The diseased and atrophic tubal epithelium can now be clearly seen through the hole (arrow). Note that the most severely diseased areas do not stain readily with dye.

30 shows how two further cuts (arrows) are made in the fibrotic area to open the tube little by little. The upper of the two cuts is bleeding slightly at its apex and so it has almost certainly been extended far enough. Eventually one of these incisions will need to be carried some distance towards the fimbrial ovarian ligament so as to evert the mucosa in the region of the fimbria ovarica.

31. A major area of fibrosis on the inferior tip of the ostium is encountered. This is being incised with the diathermy needle. Fine toothed forceps (5) are used to pick up the worst of the fibrotic tissue to facilitate its excision. In general, one should avoid excising tubal tissue unless it is absolutely unavoidable – small areas of fibrosis like this have no useful purpose and prevent good eversion of the ostial edge. The thin arrow indicates a very atrophic mucosal fold. Thick arrows indicate the edge of the cut tubal peritoneum.

32

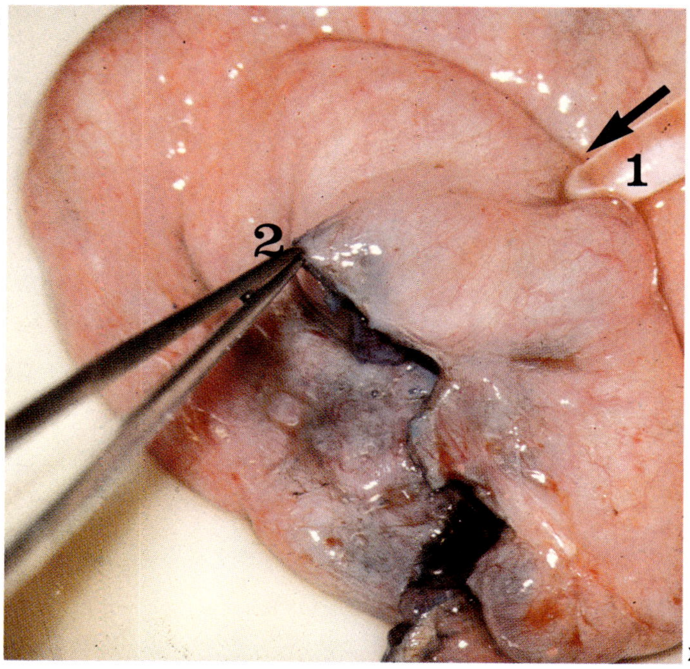

x 4

33

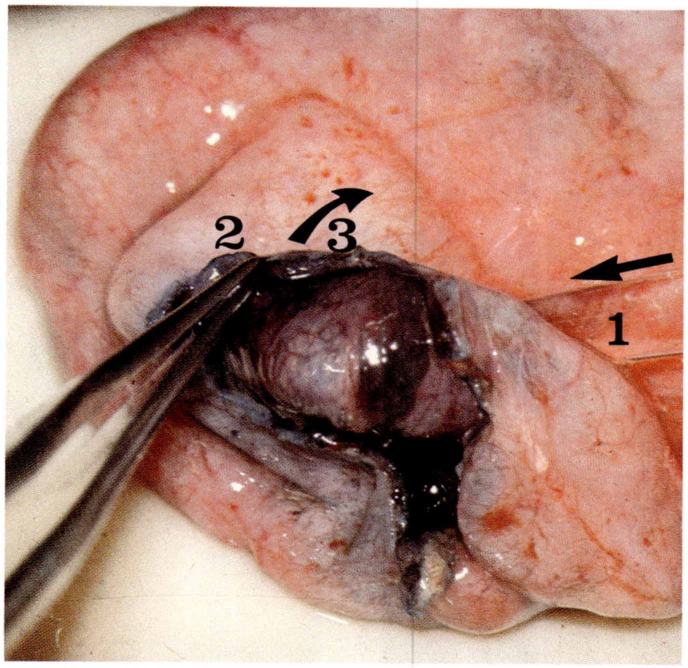

x 4

32 to 35 Eversion of the tubal edge
The tubal ostium is now big enough and the surgeon prepares to evert the tubal mucosa. A glass rod is pressed against the serosal surface (1) in the direction of the arrow whilst the toothed forceps (2), held in the left hand, hold the ostial edge. The edge is pushed over the advancing tip of the glass rod and the upper edge (3) of the ostium is easily everted (**Figure 33**). At this point any residual muscle tone of the tube itself may help to aid the eversion.

34

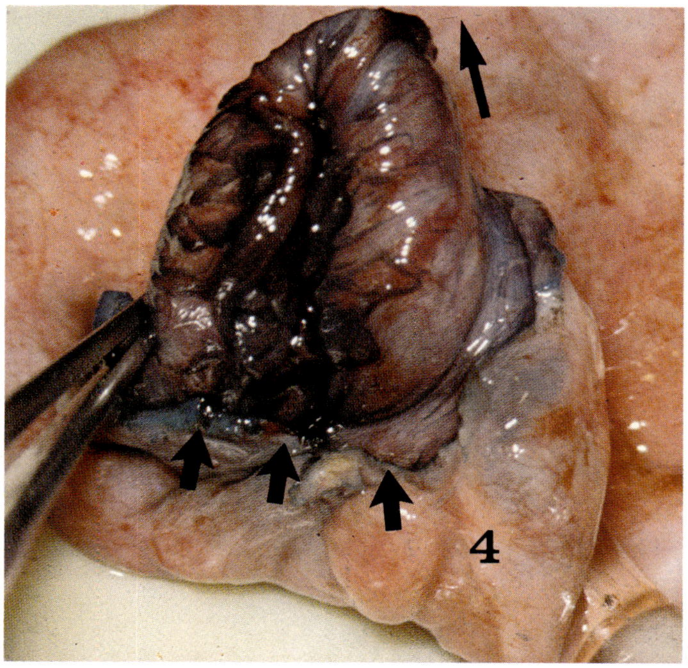

x 4

35

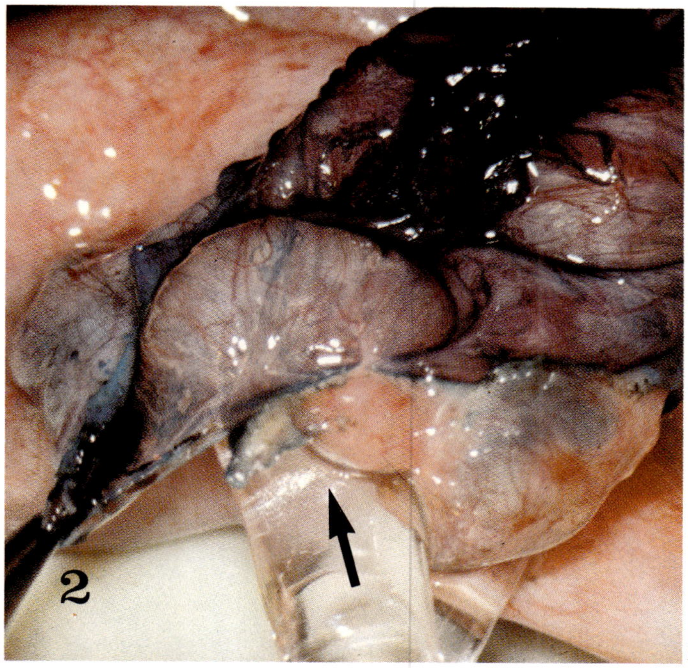

x 4

34. The upper edge of the ostium is now completely everted by the advancing tip of the glass rod (direction indicated by the arrow). When the glass rod is withdrawn the mucosa will stay in this everted position. Attention is now turned to the posterior ostial tip (broad arrows). At the end of the procedure the fibrotic fimbria ovarica (4) will be incised.

35. Leaving the upper ostial edge everted, the glass rod is used to evert the lower edge. The arrow denotes the direction of thrust. The tooth forceps at (2) are used to pull the mucosal edge down over the glass rod.

36

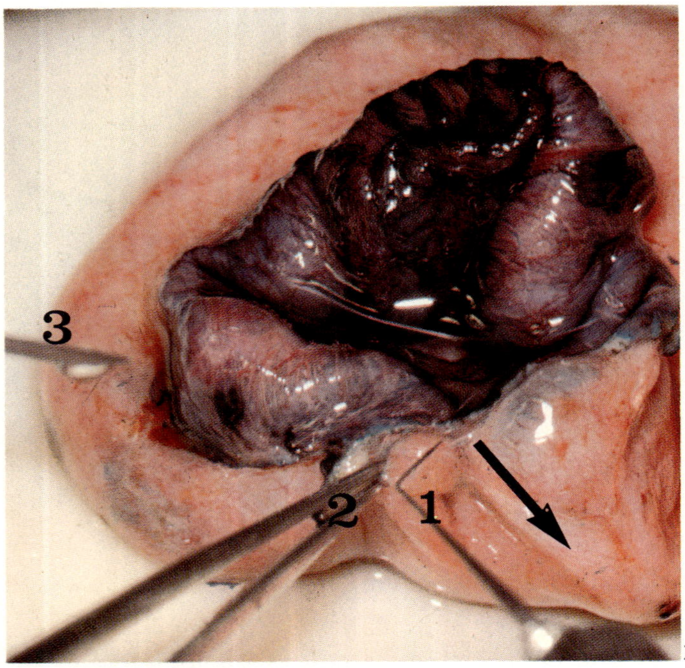

x 4

36 to 42 Fashioning and suturing the ostium
The serosa and muscle over the fimbrial-ovarian ligament (**Figure 36**) is incised using diathermy (1). The arrow denotes the direction of this incision. This will open the ostium so that it faces the ovary. The toothed forceps (2) are used to steady the ostial edge. Irrigation needle is at (3).

37

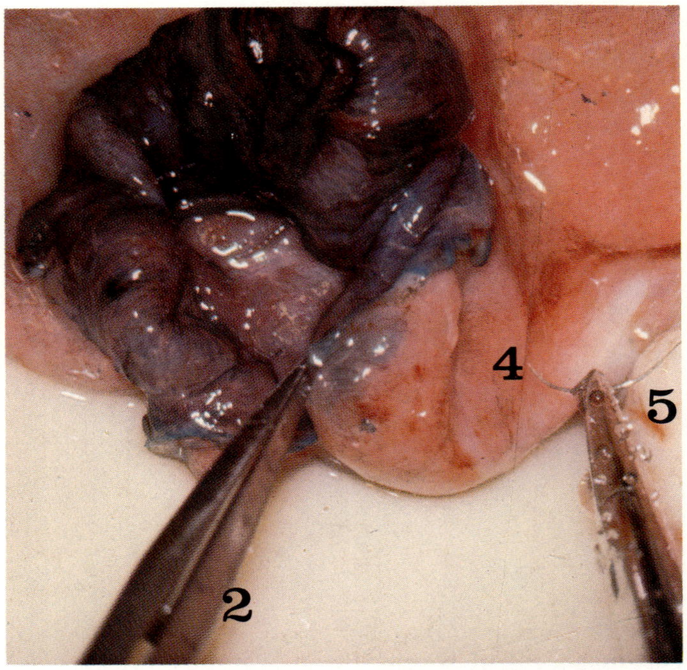

x 4

37 and 38. The ostium is completely fashioned and no further incision is needed. Muscle tone may hold this tube open in inversion but to make certain of this a few peripheral fine sutures are placed at strategic points. The most important sutures are those to the lateral edge of the fimbria ovarica, placed first – one on either side. 8/0 nylon

38

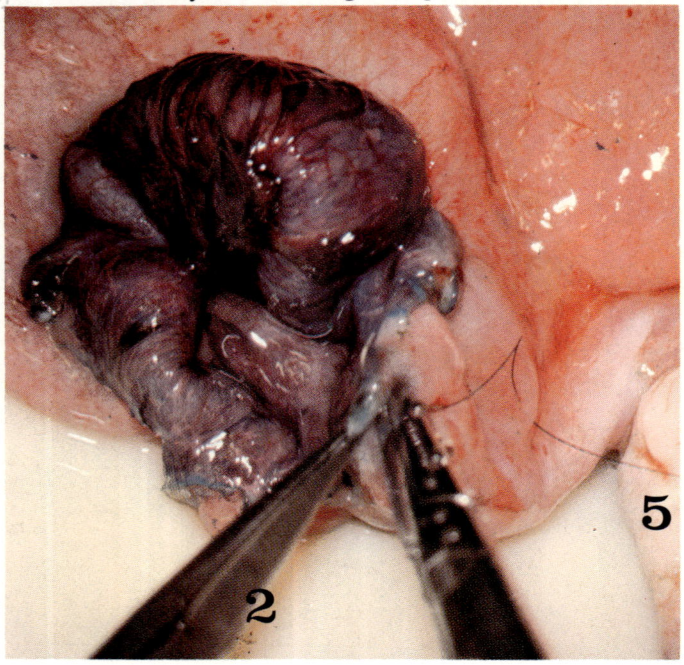

x 4

is used and a bite is taken of the serosa (4) and then of the edge of the mucosa; no raw area is left. The edge of the ovary (which must be left free of tubal sutures wherever possible) is at (5).

39

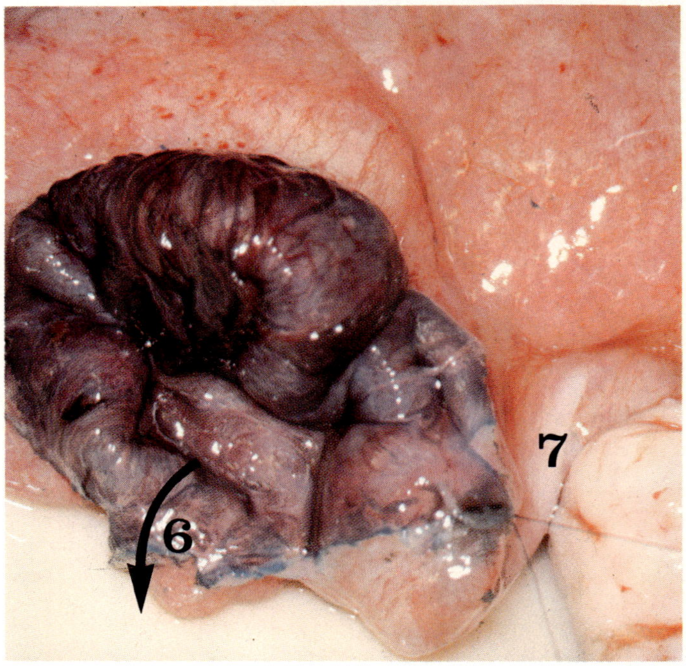

x 4

39. The sutures are tied and cut short. A similar stitch should now be placed in the opposite edge of the re-fashioned fimbria ovarica (6) so that the edge will be everted in the direction of the arrow. It is very important that these sutures do not interfere with the base of the fimbrial ligament (7) so as to avoid fimbrial blood supply, which runs in this ligament.

40

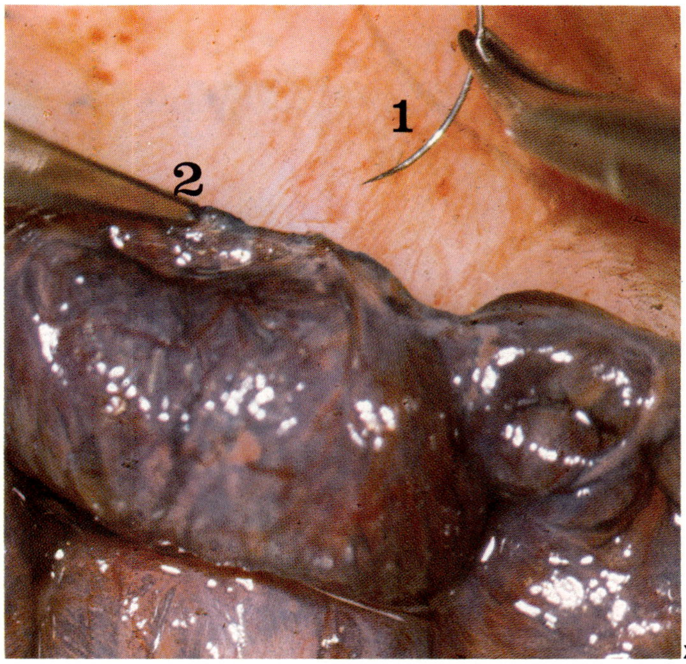

x 16

41

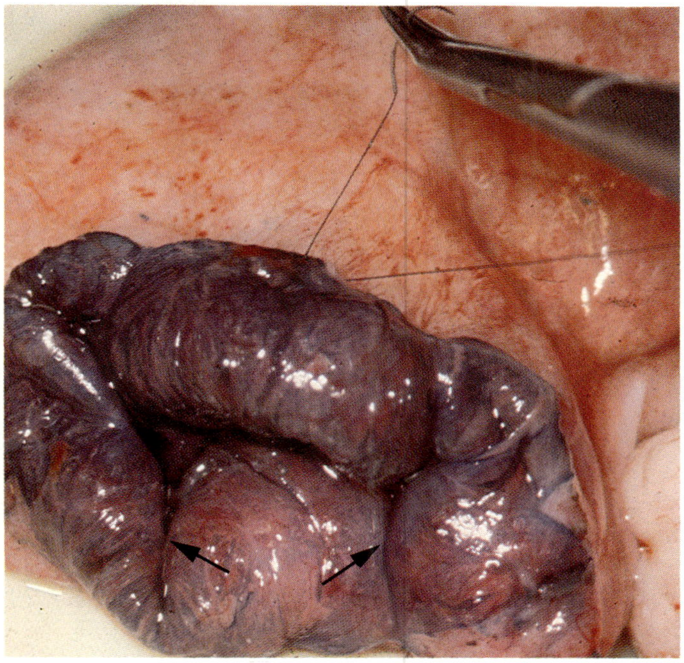

x 6

40 to 42 Final peripheral sutures

The 8/0 nylon on a round-bodied needle (1) is now used to suture the edge of the mucosa in situ. Note that the microsurgical needle is held half-way along its curvature and that the curve of the jaws of the needle-holder points away from the direction of travel. Notice also that the merest edge of the mucosa is held in the forceps at (2). Crushing injury must be kept to a bare minimum otherwise adhesions are very likely. These peripheral sutures are placed so as to minimise raw areas. It is very important, too, that the mucosal edge is not over-everted; if it is, obstruction to the epithelial blood supply will occur with poor venous drainage and necrosis. Note also that the tubal ostium is not too large (**Figures 41** and **42**). By limiting the size of the ostium, we have managed to achieve some 'folding' of the mucosa (arrows). This will oppose the mucosal surfaces, and hopefully the ciliated cells may be able to transport the gamete more effectively between the two surfaces. This mucosa is flattened and very atrophic.

42

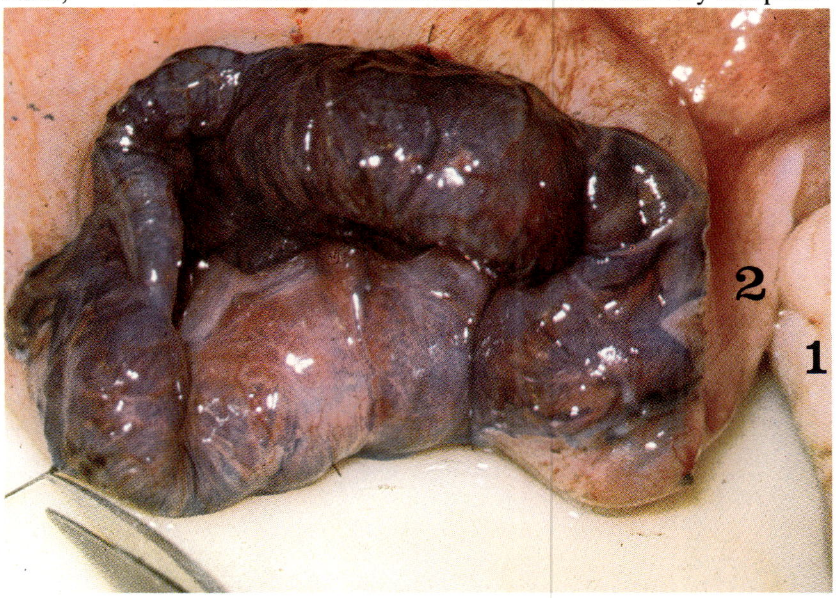

x 6

42. The final result shows a good mobile ostium. There has been very little bleeding. The ostium has been constructed in such a way that it can ride over the entire surface of the ovary (1). This has been possible because of careful dissection at the start of the procedure (before commencing the actual salpingostomy) and because the fimbrial ligament (2) has been left intact.

43

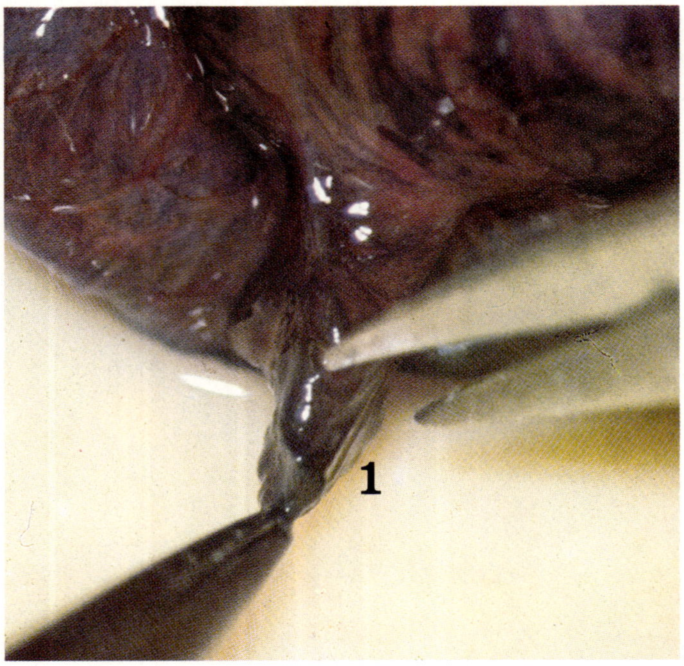

x 20

44

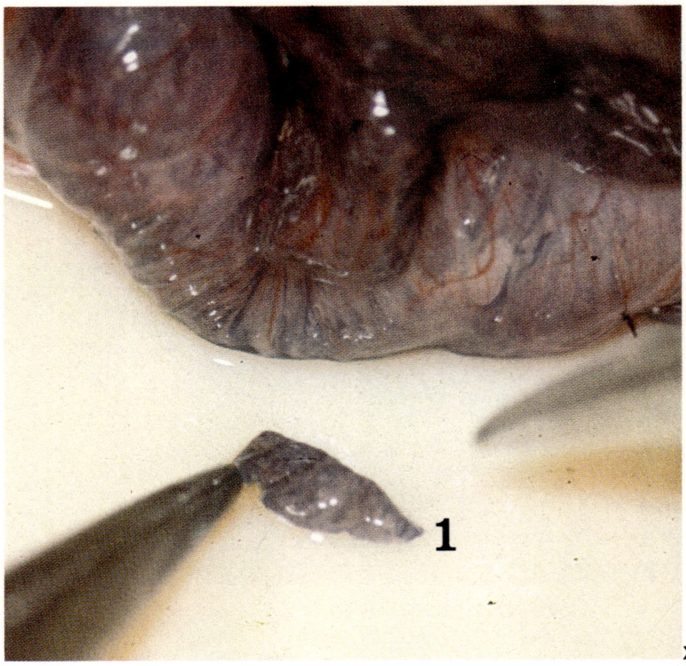

x 20

43 and 44 Removal of mucosal microbiopsies
Before completing the procedure, the mucosa is carefully examined under the microscope and two or three biopsies are taken from representative areas of the ostium. Whenever possible, a small piece of mucosal fold is included in such a biopsy. These biopsies can be taken at the end of the operation, or preferably as soon as the mucosa is exposed. It is very important that they are fixed within 5 seconds of removal so that accurate cell counts can be made on electron microscopy (page 149). In general, we have found a correlation between successful outcome and the number of ciliated cells in these biopsies (1).

45

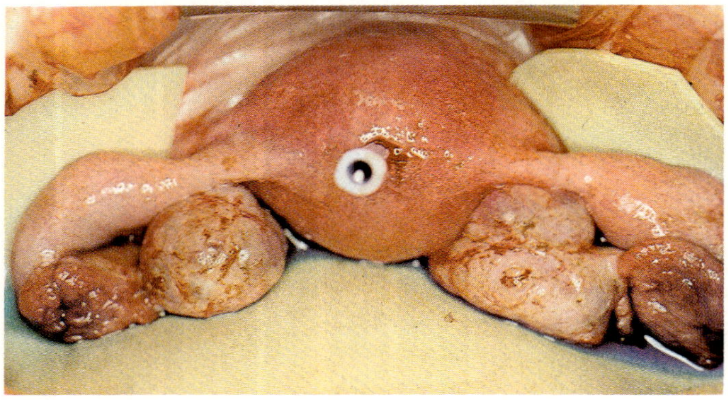

45 and 46 The final result
Dye has been injected through the fundus and there is good spill. The ovaries are free and both tubes completely mobile. The fimbria ovarica has been satisfactorily reconstructed on either side and there is complete haemostasis.

46

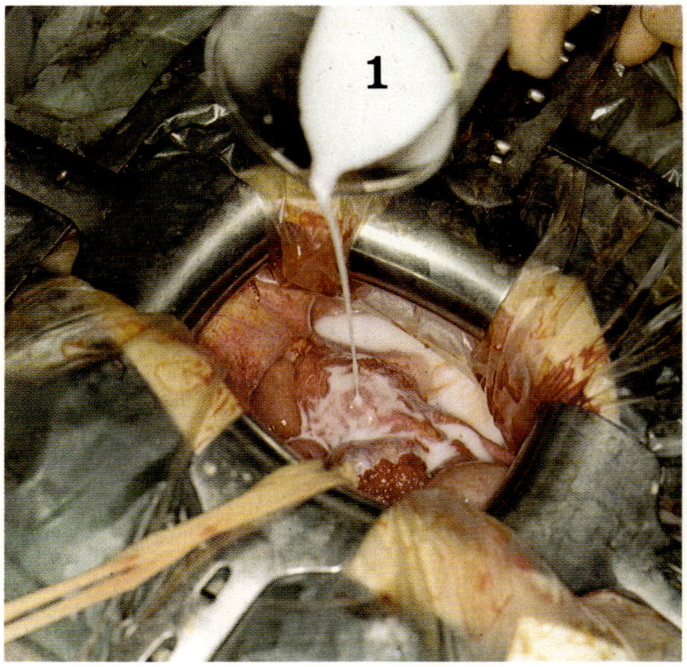

46. After removal of the vaginal pack and immediately before abdominal closure the pelvis is washed clean. When indicated, 1.5 g of hydrocortisone acetate is left in the pelvis. This is poured in from a beaker (1), care being taken not to spill this fluid into the wound edge for fear of delaying wound healing. Hydrocortisone acetate is insoluble and will remain in the pelvis for 3–10 days. It may help to diminish adhesion formation.

47 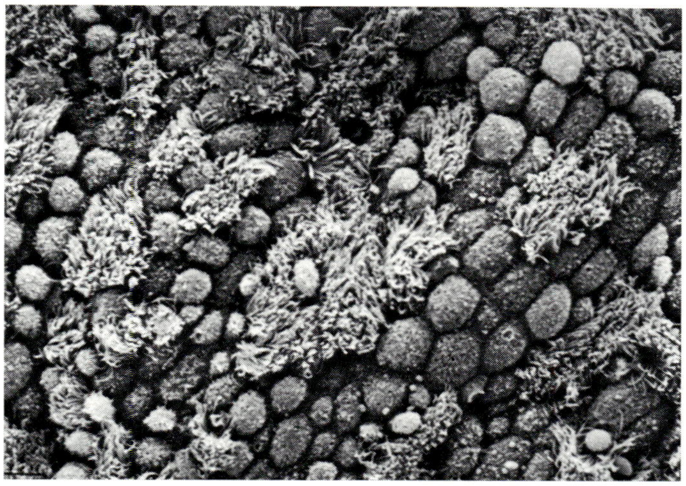

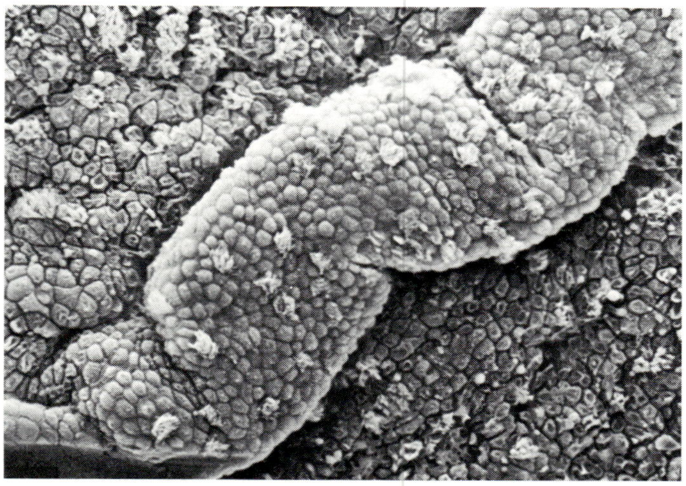 48

47 and 48 Scanning electron microscopy
Scanning electron microscopy of the epithelial surface and planimetric cell counts seem to be of help in determining a patient's progress following surgery (Vasquez, Boeckx, Winston and Brosens 1980). The normal human ciliated cell count is around 62 per cent in fimbrial biopsies, irrespective of the time of the menstrual cycle. This count falls markedly following inflammation and especially following tubal obstruction. It seems probable that the longer-standing the hydrosalpinx, the more depressed the ciliated cell count, the poorer the prognosis and possibly the poorer the chance of regeneration. Associated with this loss of ciliated cells is a change in secretory cells – the most marked being a general flattening, loss of microvilli and cell desquamation. On conventional light microscopy the normally columnar epithelium becomes flattened and cuboidal and strips very easily.

Figure 47 shows a typically normal human ampullary microbiopsy ×1600. The ciliated cells are plentiful and sited uniformly over the surface of a mucosal fold. Occasional blebs of secretion can be seen on the apices of the cells. For comparison **Figure 48** shows the epithelium from a hydrosalpinx ×900. There is considerable loss of ciliated cells and the mucosal fold running diagonally across the picture is attenuated. The problem with such biopsies is that they can only be taken at the time of tubal surgery and they would therefore seem to have a very limited value in deciding which patients should have operation.

Laparoscopic division of adhesions

49 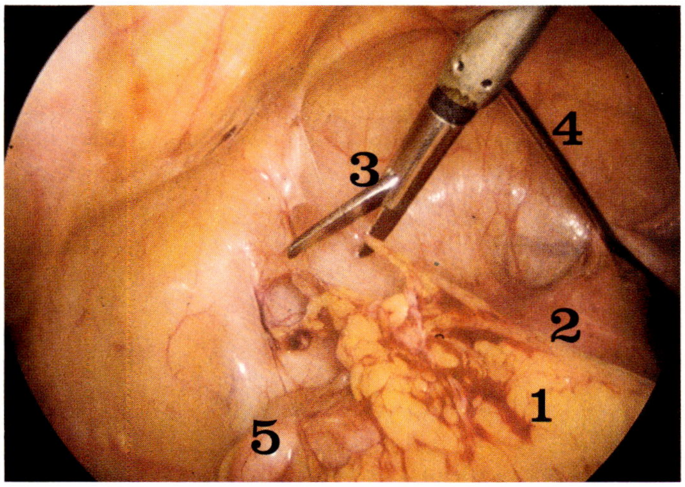

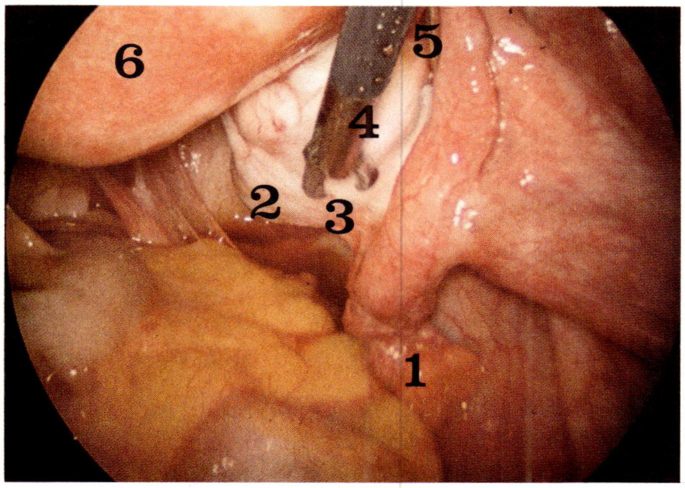 50

49 and 50 Laparoscopic division of adhesions
In **Figure 49** the omentum (1) is adherent to the bladder peritoneum and the uterine fundus (2) and left uterine cornu. The laparoscopic scissors (3) are used to cut adhesions and to improve access and visibility. Note the use of a third puncture instrument (usually desirable in such procedures) at (4). The sigmoid is at (5). The third instrument is used to elevate the right cornu and to stretch the adhesions. This pelvis, which initially looked quite unsuitable for surgery, showed good tubes after this procedure.

In **Figure 50** adhesiolysis has already started – initially the fimbria (1) were adherent to the lower pole of the ovary (2). There are still ampullary adhesions (3) to the ovarian capsule which will be divided by scissors (4). The tube is being retracted laterally by the third puncture instrument (5) to place the adhesion on stretch. The uterus is at (6) and is about to be elevated out of the pelvis.

51
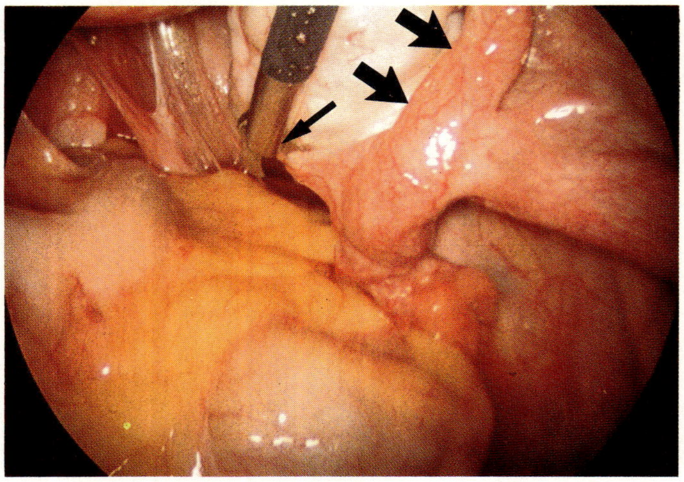

52
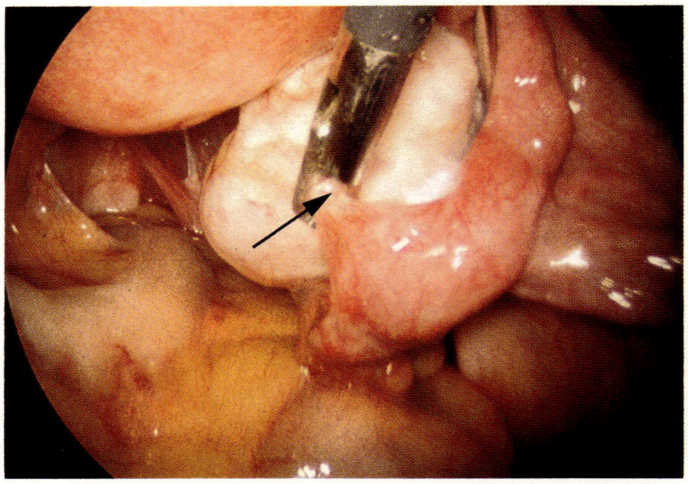

51. The uterine fundus is pushed up well out of the pelvis by an assistant and adhesiolysis can continue. One blade of the scissors (arrow) is hooked under the adhesion and the tube (broad arrows) is placed on stretch.

52. Taking extreme care that no other organ is touching the electrically active end of the scissors, limited diathermy is applied and the tissue turns slightly white (arrow). This diathermy must be minimal and considerable experience is required in its use. The adhesion can now be divided bloodlessly using the same instrument.

53
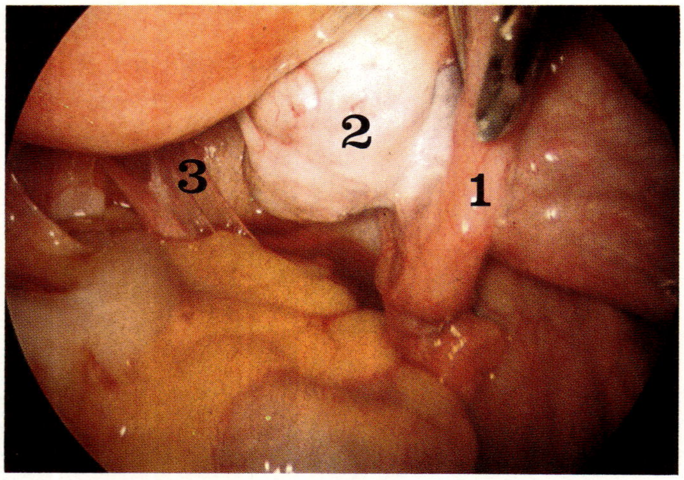

53. The final result. The ampulla of the tube (1) is now free of the ovary (2). There is no bleeding, and most important no raw or large burnt area. Attention will now be turned to the primary adhesions behind the uterus at (3). This patient conceived 2 months after this procedure. She had been infertile for 5½ years.

It must be emphasised that division of adhesions using laparoscopy is a very skilled procedure and must not be attempted by surgeons who are not experienced both in laparoscopy and tubal surgery. There are numerous dangers, especially those of uncontrolled burns or extended peritoneal damage. These operations should be done only when there are facilities to proceed to laparotomy if necessary.

Laparoscopic division of adhesions: indications

Laparoscopic surgery has a place in the treatment of the infertile patient. We use it in two situations. In the first (**Figure 49**) the approach illustrated is useful if the pelvis is obscured by adhesions. Such adhesions can be divided so that a proper view of the appendages and uterus can be obtained and a definitive diagnosis made. This is necessary before operability can be determined and can save the patient an unnecessary 'infertility laparotomy'.

In the second situation (**Figure 50**) we employ division of adhesions under laparoscopic control where there are limited tubal or ovarian adhesions which are splinting or immobilising the fimbria or ampulla, diminishing ovarian mobility or covering the ovary or fimbria and potentially preventing ovum pick-up.

Ovarian surgery with salpingolysis

Figures 54 *et seq.* Infertility may result from the careless surgical treatment of ovarian cysts and endometriosis in young women. Therefore it is preferable that microsurgical techniques be used even though the microscope may not always be required. Occasionally loupes, or even the naked eye, may be quite sufficient. The principles enumerated at the beginning of this chapter are appropriate. Special attention should be taken to avoid raw peritoneal areas and the ovarian capsule, when necessary, should be reconstituted with fine non-absorbable sutures. For this purpose 6/0 prolene is ideal as it can be handled with equal facility either under the microscope or naked eye. It is a cardinal principle that interim appendicectomy should not be combined with these clean procedures; to do so is asking for inflammatory or adhesive damage. Postoperative steroid therapy may be appropriate. The following sequence of photographs shows the need for careful planning of these procedures involved with lysis of the tube and ovary.

54 and 55 A patient with an endometriotic cyst 5 cm in diameter
The tube is adherent (1), along the ampulla. The fimbria ovarica (2) is also adherent. Note that the region of the ampullary-isthmic junction is adherent to the lateral wall of the uterus (3) – these adhesions are fibrotic. Several peritoneal adhesions are already divided (from bowel) – these have been left long on the ovarian capsule until they can be removed flush with the capsular surface (4) at a later time.

Figure 55 shows the first stage of the surgical procedure completed. The first stage must be to liberate the ovary as far as possible – in this case from the uterus. The raw ovarian ligament has been sutured using 6/0 nylon (thin arrow). This has greatly increased ovarian mobility but has left a large raw area on the ovarian capsule (broad arrows).

54

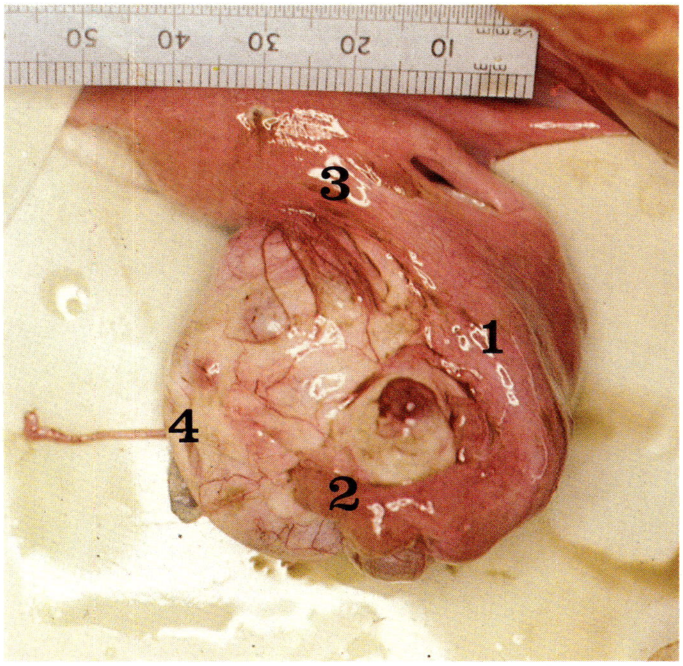

55

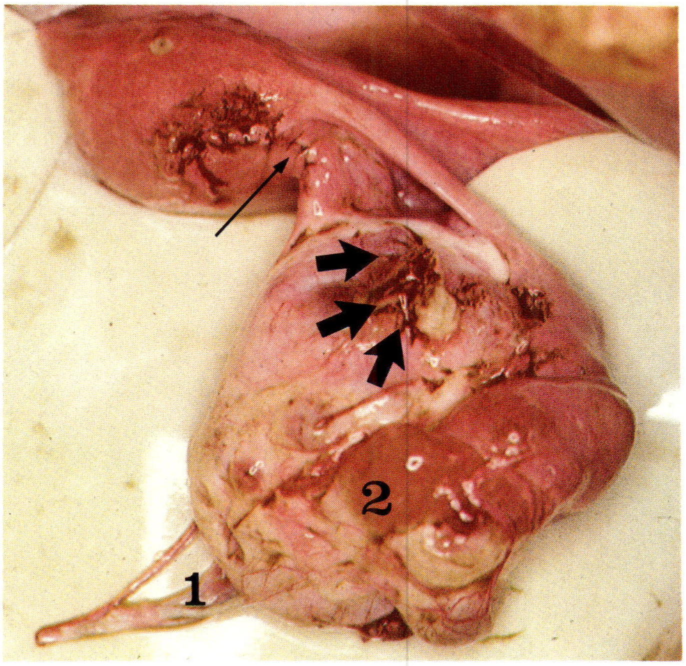

56

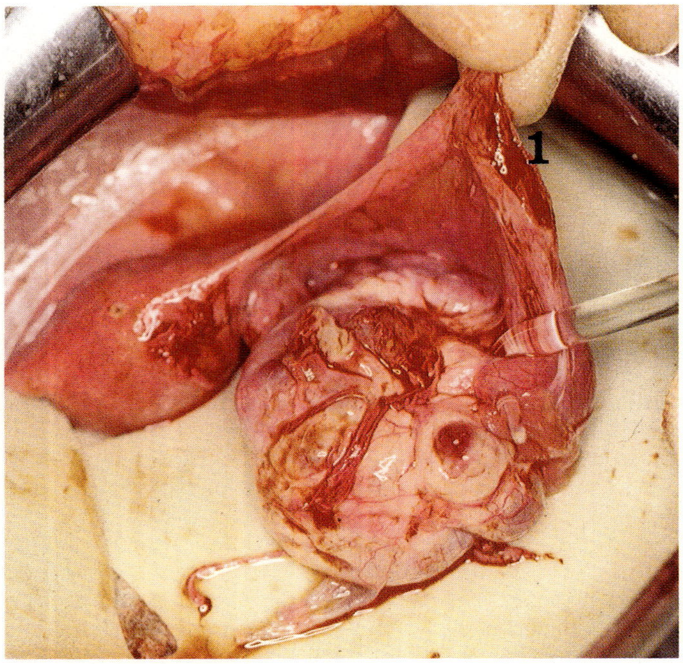

57

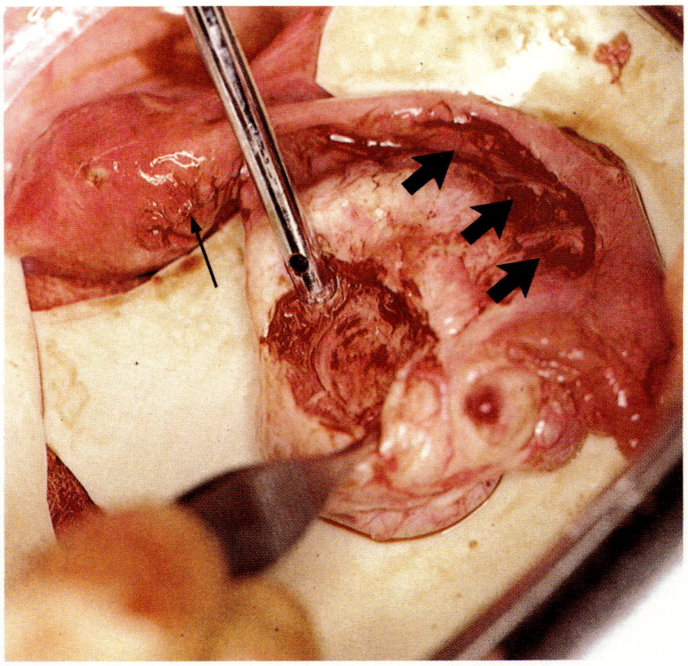

56. The tube can now be completely freed from the ovary so that there is access to the ovarian surface for cystectomy. This is necessary in order to choose the best site for incision into the ovarian capsule to reduce recurrent fimbrial adhesions. The raw area of the ampullary-isthmic junction has been lifted up (1).

57. The fimbria have now been lysed as has the ampulla, leaving a raw area in the mesosalpinx (broad arrows). This is not bleeding and does not require immediate repair. The serosa of the uterus has been closed as it was oozing (thin arrow). Ovarian cystectomy can now be done *through the already damaged capsule* to minimise further disorganisation.

58

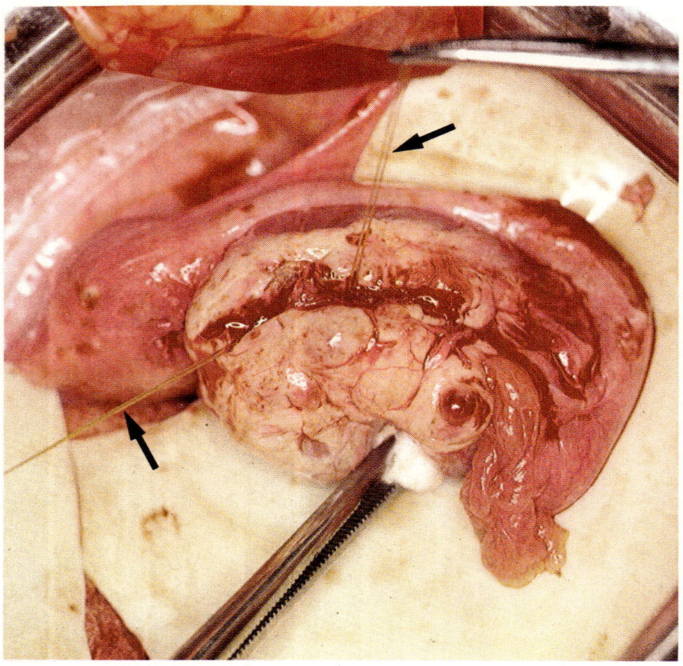

59

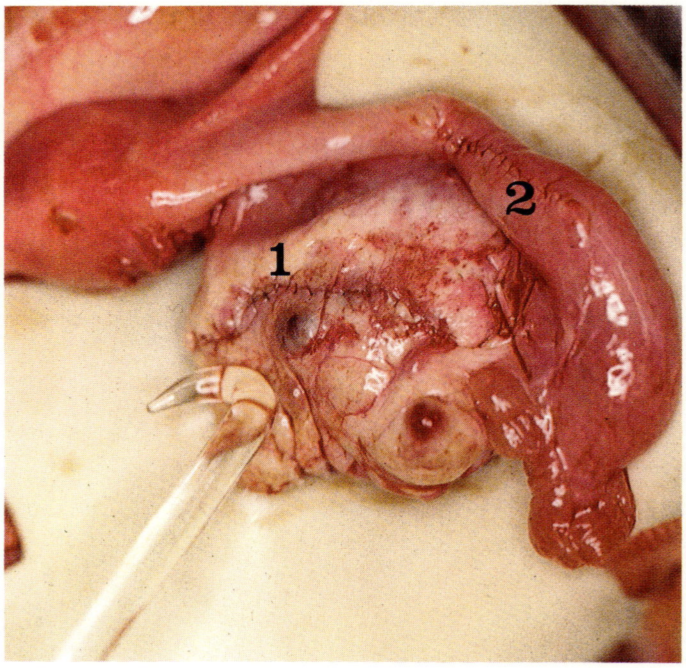

58. Cystectomy is performed routinely using dissection between the cyst wall and ovarian tissue. The stroma is reconstituted with a few 4/0 polyglycolic acid sutures (arrow). Note that the ovary looks larger than it really is due to photographic foreshortening.

59. Final result. The ovarian surface has been cleaned and the capsule sutured with 8/0 nylon (1). Note that the site of the scar has been planned so that the chance of the fimbria adhering to this area subsequently is minimised. The ampulla (2) (and the mesosalpinx which is obscured in the picture) have been sutured with 8/0 nylon. The fimbria are now completely free. A short course of steroids was given; this patient conceived four months after surgery.

Tubal anastomosis

Tubal anastomosis is a procedure which is performed with increasing frequency. This is, of course, partly due to the regrettable rise in the incidence of unwanted sterilisation, but also because organic cornual occlusion due to inflammatory disease is being diagnosed more often. It is possible that the actual incidence of this condition is on the increase and perhaps the frequency of therapeutic abortion has something to do with this.

In the following section, the author has decided to concentrate on anastomosis at the cornual end of the tube because this procedure, which has special diagnostic and surgical problems, serves as an excellent model for microsurgical tubal anastomosis in general. We consider that the microscope is essential for optimal surgical results – in the cornual area the internal diameter of the tube is usually 0.4–0.6 mm and there is good evidence that tubes of this diameter need relatively high magnification for good coaptation (Hedon, Wineman and Winston 1980). In most cases of cornual disease due to inflammation and with nearly all patients following sterilisation, the intramural portion of the tube is relatively free from damage. The object of cornual anastomosis is to identify the healthy intramural portion and to join the

60 The laparoscopic appearance of a patient with inflammatory cornual occlusion
Her x-rays are reproduced overleaf (**Figure 62**). Note the bulbous nodular expansion of the cornu (broad arrows) before the injection of dye; the isthmus immediately beyond this point (thin arrow) is also damaged – it is white and rather rigid and its blood supply is abnormal. The probe (1) is being used to evaluate the flexibility of the isthmus beyond this point, in an attempt to get an approximate idea of the amount of fibrosis and damage. The ovary (2) and the uterus (3) are healthy. When dye was injected into the uterus at this examination, there was no tubal filling but the cornu expanded (suggesting that the intramural portion had partially filled). Subsequently, dye extravasated into the lymphatics of the mesosalpinx. This appearance is consistent with salpingitis isthmica nodosa (in this patient's case, this tentative diagnosis was subsequently confirmed histologically). The appearance may also be seen in tuberculosis, sarcoidosis and adenomyosis of the cornu. Provided the diagnosis is not tuberculosis, cornual anastomosis in this kind of patient gives a 45–55 per cent chance of an intrauterine pregnancy.

60

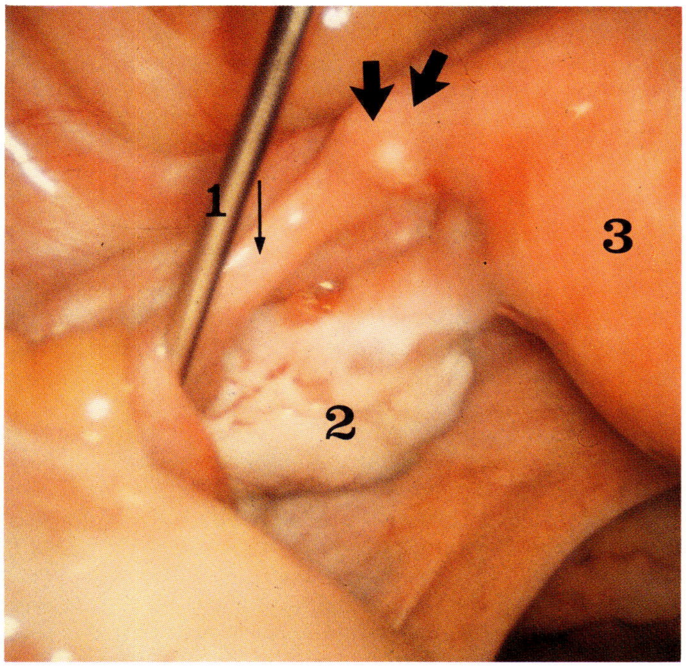

61 A tube following diathermy coagulation for sterilisation
The ampulla (1) and the ovary (2) are completely free of adhesions (which is usually the case following diathermy). Approximately 6 cm of ampulla are healthy and available for reconstruction. The cornu (3) is fibrotic and contains a collection of spider vessels (thin arrow) commonly seen after this injury. The thick arrow denotes the fibrosis at the ampullary end and all the tissue between the two arrows is fibrotic mesosalpinx, a single cornual burn having resulted in complete necrosis of the isthmus. This is the problem with diathermy coagulation which causes very variable and unpredictable damage – in many cases the whole tube seems to necrose, probably because of interference with its blood supply.

61

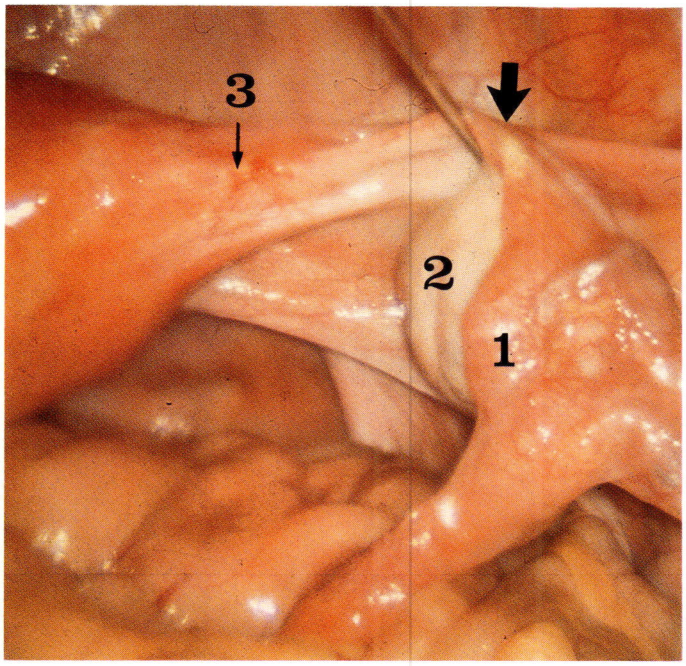

62

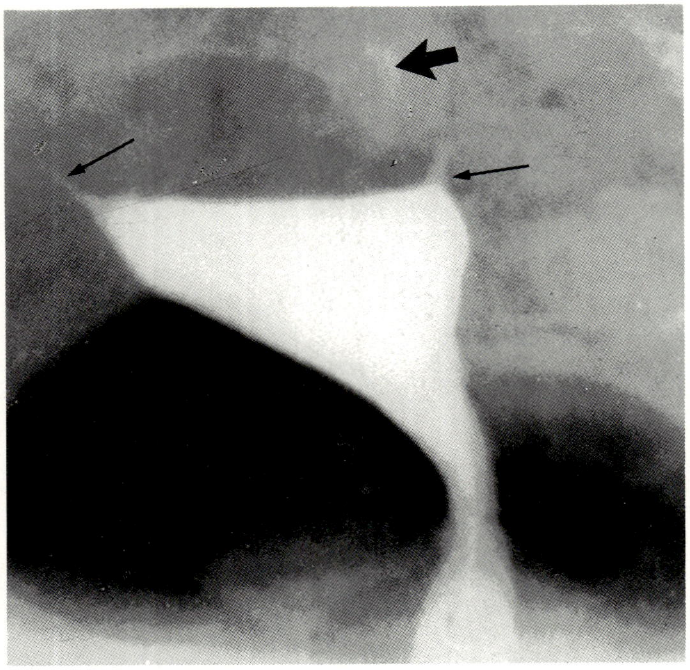

62 A radiograph of the patient seen in Figure 60
There is intramural filling on both sides (arrows) and the outline of the intramural portion is slightly fluffy, an appearance that we associate with inflammatory damage. This appearance is *not* due to 'spasm'. Indeed tubal spasm is a rare event provided that the patient is treated with minimal cervical stimulation and very slow injection of dye (1 ml per minute or less). The broad arrow shows opacification which was not present on the plain x-ray initially – this could represent extravasation or lymphatic filling. This amount of intramural filling suggests that it is very likely (but not certain) that there will be enough intramural portion to perform cornual anastomosis and so avoid tubal implantation. Sometimes x-rays are not absolutely reliable. One may see no cornual filling very occasionally yet some part of the intramural tube is patent. Very infrequently, one may get cornual filling when this portion is so damaged that anastomosis is pointless or not feasible.

63

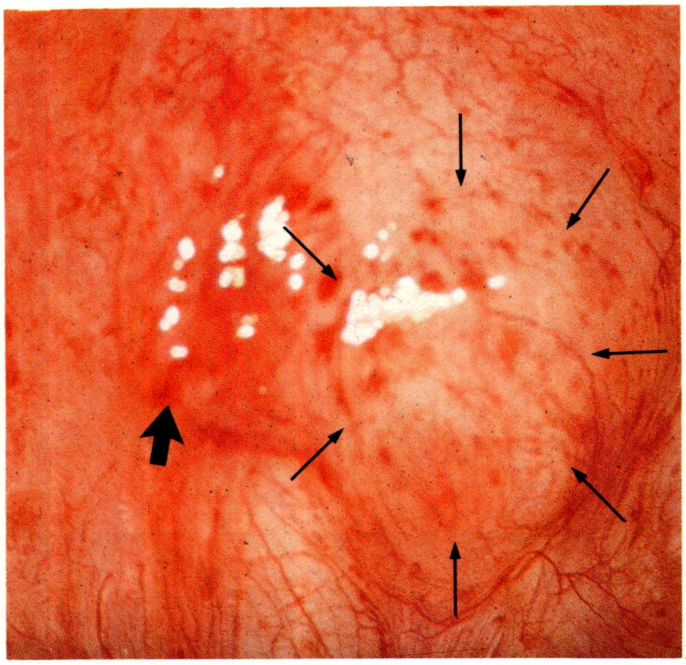
x 10

undamaged lateral part of the tube on to this after removal of the diseased or occluded isthmic segment.

The advantages of tubo-cornual anastomosis over implantation seem to be:

(1) Preservation of the maximum length of tube.
(2) Preservation of a potential sphincter mechanism where the tube meets the cornu.
(3) Minimisation of damage to the vasculature of the cornu.
(4) More accurate joins of the two lumina and therefore less risk of subsequent blockage.
(5) Reduction in damage to the uterine wall and therefore less necessity to deliver the patient by Caesarean section in the event of successful pregnancy.

Both laparoscopy and hysterosalpingography are helpful investigations in the evaluation of the status of the intramural portion, particularly if there is any evidence of inflammatory blockage.

63 View under the microscope
(Magnification bottom right-hand corner). Following diathermy coagulation it can sometimes be quite difficult to decide where to incise the cornu so that the intramural portion can be located. This applies when there is no medial tube attached to the cornu. This picture shows a close-up view of the cornu following fulguration; dye has been injected under pressure into the uterine cavity, to expand the cornu. Following injection the cornu has turned white and is bulging (arrows). Note also that abnormal blood vessels are seen on the left (broad arrow); this gives a rough idea of where to locate the intramural portion. Occasionally one may see a little blue dye within such vessels. This must not be confused with the intramural tube; such dye staining will be diffuse rather than discrete and will track under the serosa.

64

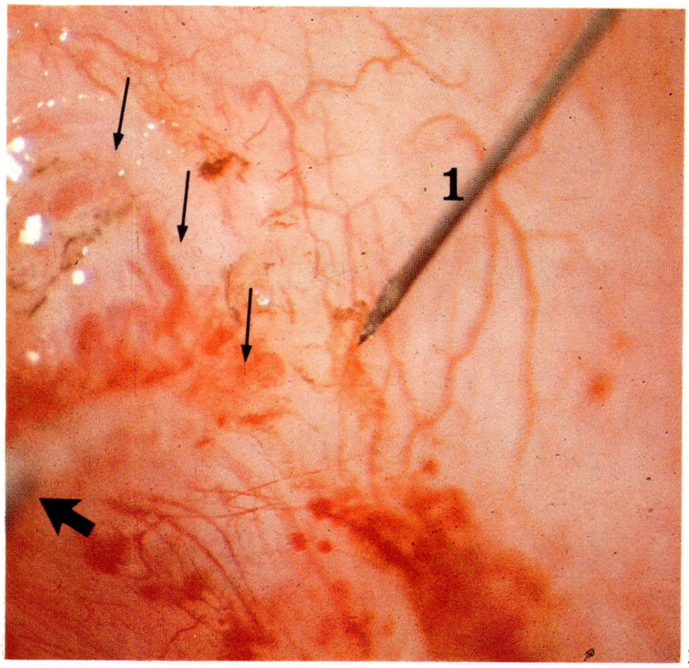

x 16

65

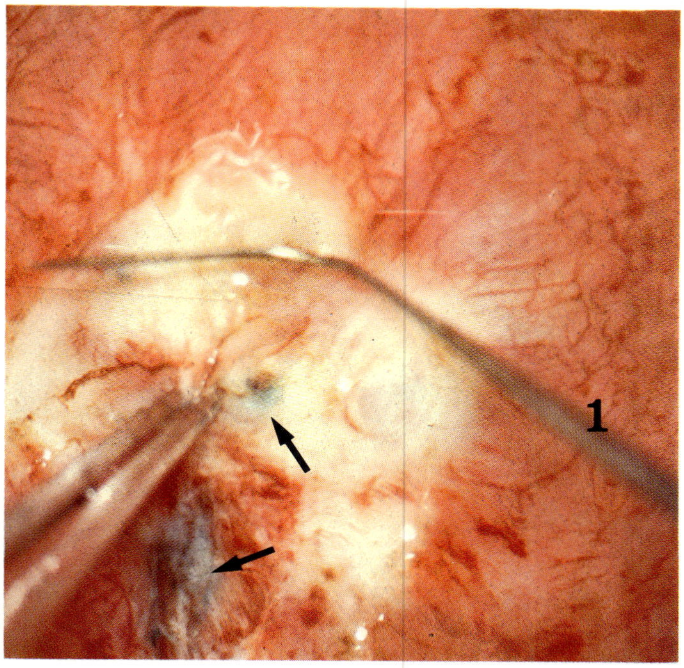

x 10

64 Stripping the serosa from the cornu
The first stage of the procedure is to strip the peritoneum from the uterine muscle in the area of the cornu. This can be achieved by incising the bulging portion of the cornu with a knife or by injecting a little adrenaline in Ringers solution under the serosa and then peeling the peritoneum downwards, towards the broad ligament. In this case the 25 gauge needle (1) has been used to inject adrenaline (to limit bleeding) and the peritoneum has been stripped at the top of the picture (arrows). The forceps pulling the peritoneum off the cornu are just seen (out of focus) at the edge of the picture (broad arrow).

65 Use of the diathermy needle
This shows a common mistake. The diathermy here (1) has been used to cut slices from the cornu, rather than using a knife. The result has been a diffuse over-coagulated area; this can be seen very clearly as a whitish-yellow avascular burn. If diathermy is used at all to cut away tissue at the cornu, it must be used very carefully and at low current to avoid this. Note, too, the extravasation of blue dye in this patient (arrows). This dye is not in the tube but in the vessels and can lead to mistaken identification.

66

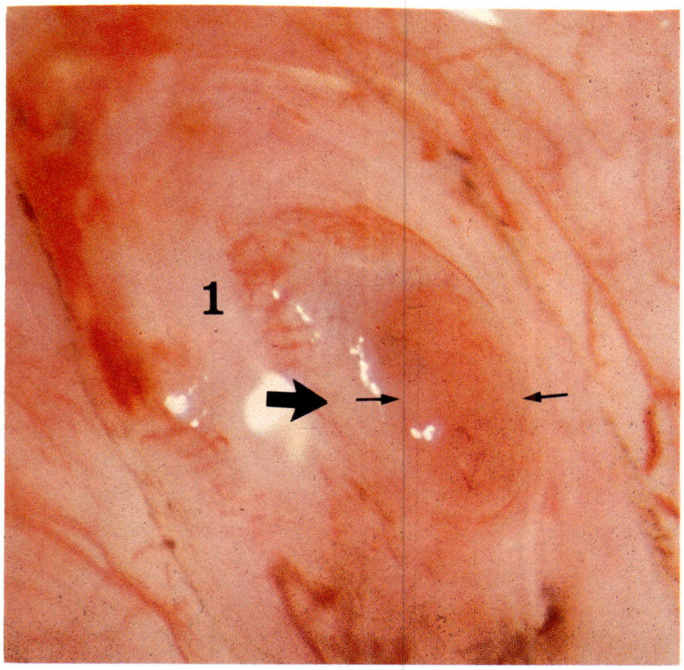

x 40

66 The intramural portion
This shows the intramural tube after transection with a scalpel. It is healthy and the high power microscope view helps in deciding this. Note that no blue dye is present in the lumen; this does not indicate tubal blockage at this point but merely that the most distal part of the healthy intramural point did not fill. The lumen is seen between the arrows. The lamina propria is seen between this margin and the broad arrow. Circular muscle coat is seen (1). Note that signs of health in this case are: pink mucosa with several small vessels; mobile, thin lamina propria; good striations in the circular muscle.

67

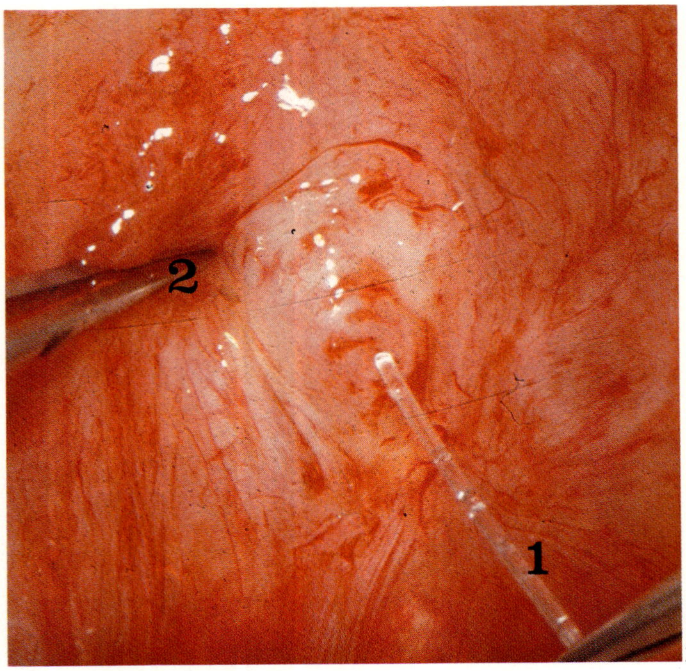

x 10

68

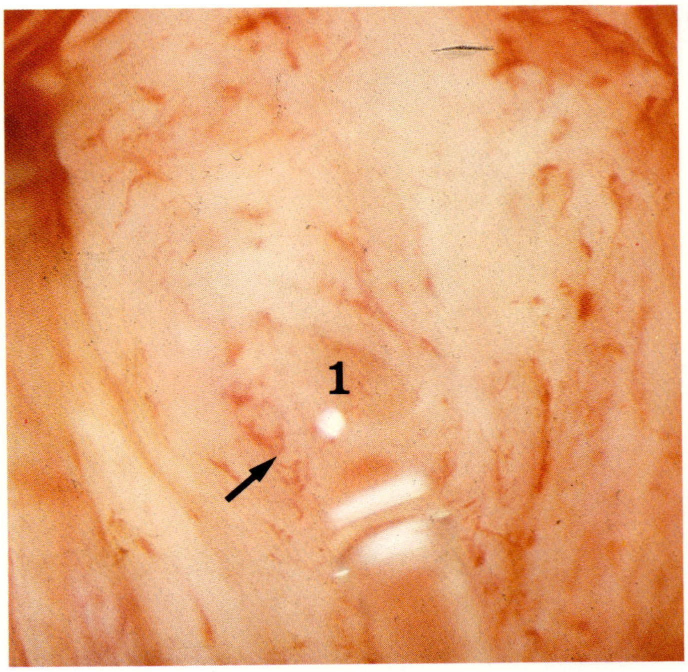

x 25

67 to 69 Insertion of a splint
Whilst we avoid leaving indwelling splints in the tube, we feel that a splint can be an enormous help during the anastomosis itself. Apart from helping to identify the position of the lumen, it promotes stability of the join during suturing. Moreover, as will be seen in later photographs of technique, the splint can be used to retract the mucosal surface from side to side during suturing. The choice of splint is very important. One tendency is to use material which is damaging because it is too thick. One should bear in mind that the lumen is generally 0.45 to 0.6 mm in diameter and clearly this diameter should not be exceeded. Another mistake is to use a nylon suture. Nylon sutures are rigid and can perforate (or even strip) the delicate tubal epithelium – this has been shown in animal models. Because of its inherent rigidity even very thin nylon can be very difficult to insert into the uterine cavity. We recommend low-density polyethylene rod of 0.45 mm diameter. It is very flexible and smooth and can (almost) invariably be inserted with ease through the intramural portion into the uterine cavity. When inserting such a splint it is important to insert in the correct direction, i.e. in the direction that the intramural portion takes. In **Figure 67** the splint (1) is being inserted in a slightly upward direction. By retracting the cornu with closed microsurgical forceps (2) one can easily see what direction the first part of the intramural tube takes.

69

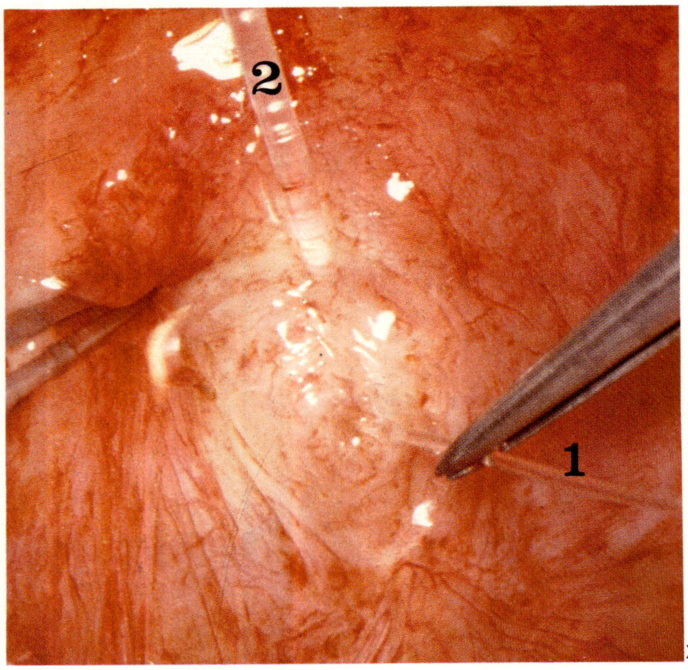

x 10

Figure 68 shows a high power view of the splint in the lumen (1). Note the excellent vascularity of the tubal epithelium at this point (arrow). Fibrous tissue would look solid and yellowish. The splint can be gently moved from side to side to see if the tube is mobile in the cornu at this point.

Figure 69 shows the splint now being inserted in a slightly backwards and downwards direction (1). The outer part of the cornu has been transversed and the uterine end of the tube and the uterus will be entered easily in this manner. The column (2) is, in fact, a jet of Ringer lactate squirted by the assistant to keep the tissues moist and clean.

Once all pathological tissue has been removed from the cornu there is bound to be a certain amount of bleeding from the freshly cut uterine tissue. This can be partly controlled with the systemic injection of 20 units of syntocinon and the application of a little local adrenaline. We prefer not to use more than minimal diathermy for fear of causing fibrosis; the aim must be to perform the anastomosis fairly quickly, for as soon as the two ends are brought together, the bleeding will cease.

70
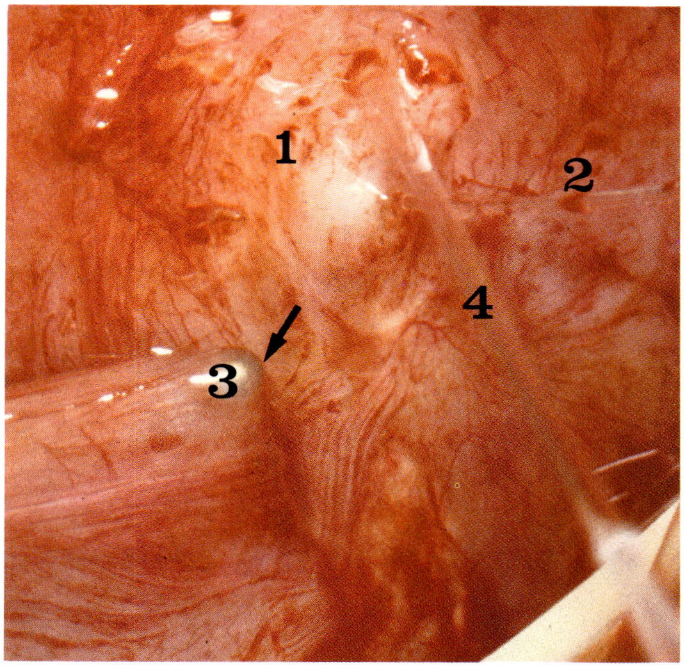

71
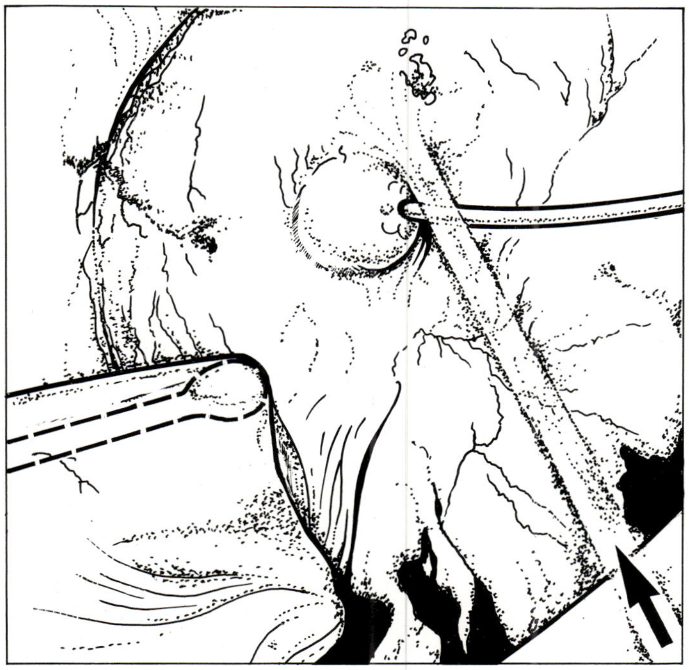

70 to 74 Overcoming luminal disparity
One major problem with cornual anastomosis, particularly following sterilisation, is that there is commonly a long mid-segment of tube missing. Consequently when joining ampullary end to cornu, the surgeon encounters difficulties because the internal diameter of the ampullary end is much bigger than the lumen of the cornual portion. One way to overcome this luminal disparity is to avoid transecting the ampullary portion of tube completely, but rather to fashion a small hole in it which is about the same size as the diameter of the cornual lumen and then to join the two segments at this point.

A grooved probe (from Spingler-Tritt), with a bulbous tip about 1 mm across, is used. The probe is passed through the fimbrial ostium and on into the ampulla. The tip of the probe is directed into the closed blind end of the ampullary segment. **Figures 70** and **71** show the cornu (1), the splint (2), the blind-ending ampulla (3) with the bulbous end of the probe distending it (arrow). An irrigation jet is seen (4).

72
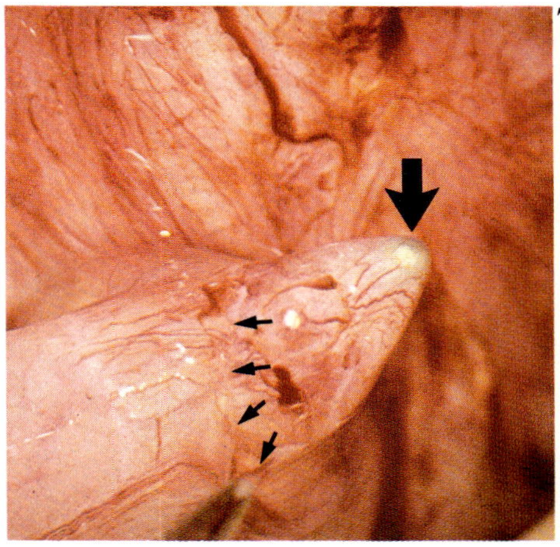

73
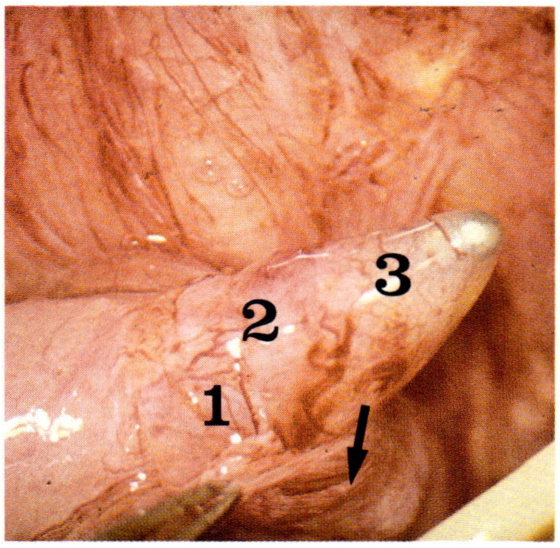

74
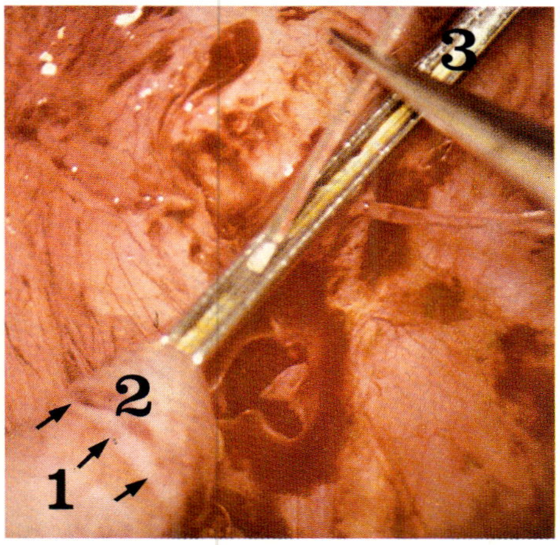

The next stage of the procedure is to strip the serosa off the blind end of the ampullary portion, keeping the mucosa and muscle intact (**Figure 72**). Here the peritoneal coat has been circumcised – the cut edge is marked with thin arrows and the tip of the probe in the blind end with a broad arrow. Note that the peritoneum contains some abnormal blood vessels but that the muscularis is mobile and free of fibrosis.

In **Figure 73** the cut edge of the serosal coat (1) is grasped with forceps and stripped back towards the mesosalpinx (arrow). Note that the muscle coat (2) is healthy and intact and that the mucosa (3) is distended by the tip of the probe. When the very end of the tube is transected the surgeon will have, in effect, prepared three layers which he can suture during anastomosis – namely serosa, circular muscle and mucosa.

In **Figure 74** the very tip of ampullary segment has been cut right across and the end of the probe (3) advanced through the hole so created. The tubal serosa is at (1) and its cut edge marked with arrows. The muscularis is at (2). The integral groove in the probe is ready to receive the outer end of the polyethylene splint. This is fixed in the groove and the probe can now be withdrawn back into the ampulla and out through the fimbria. The splint will follow and thus the whole length of the tube can be very simply cannulated without trauma.

75

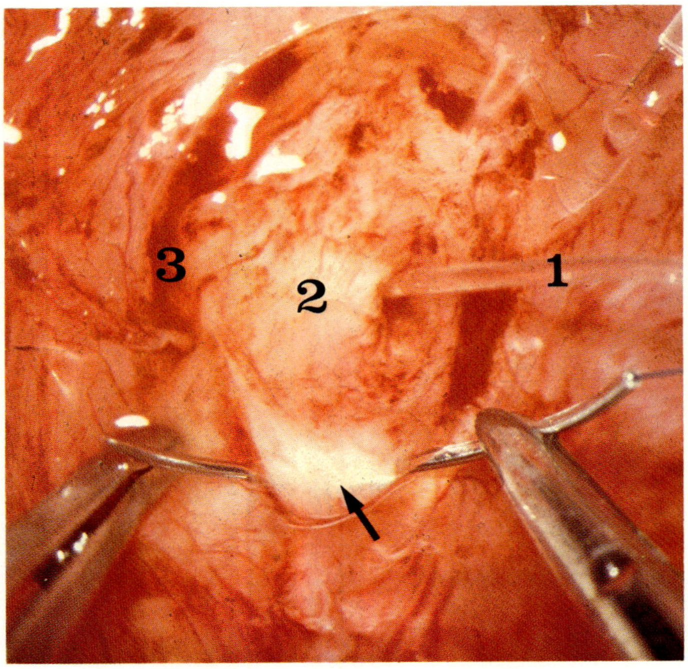

x 10

76

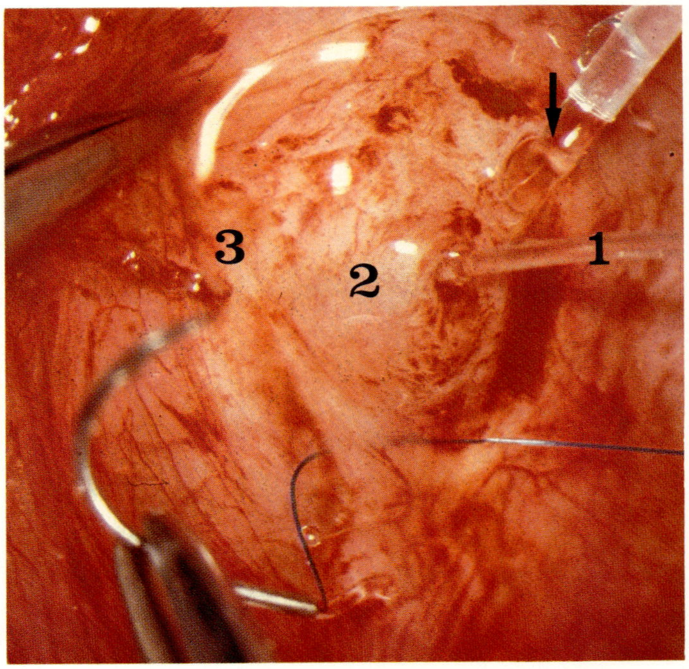

x 10

75 to 78 Placing a stay suture in the mesosalpinx

A cardinal principle of tubal anastomosis is to avoid tension at the join. This is especially important in microsurgery as the sutures used for the actual join are so fine. The best way to reduce tension is to approximate the two ends of the tube by inserting a stay suture in the mesosalpinx, just below the join.

Figure 75 demonstrates the beginning of the insertion of this suture of 6/0 prolene. The splint is (1), the circular muscle of the cornu (2), the edge of the uterine peritoneum (3). Note that the needle is placed in the connective tissue below the circular muscle coat (arrow) not in the tube itself.

Figure 76. The prolene suture is now pulled through the tissue a little way. Note the constant irrigation with Ringer's solution (arrow). Numbering is as for **Figure 75**.

77

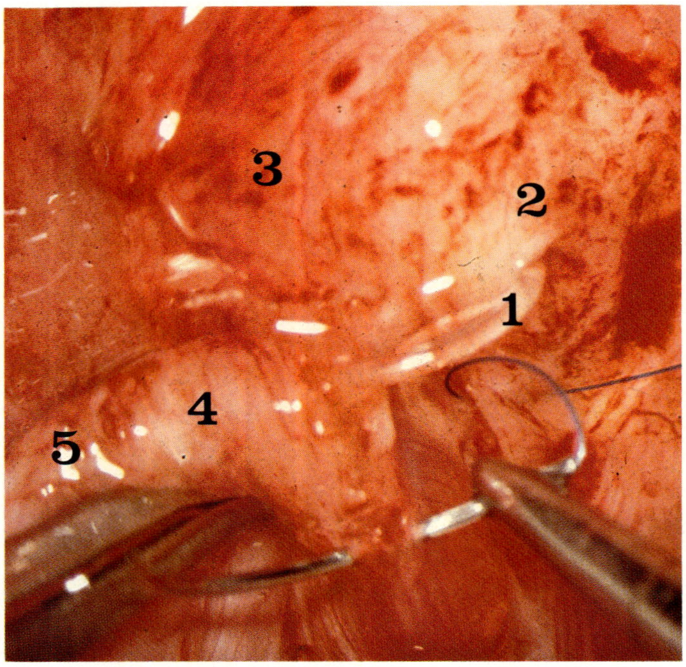

x 10

78

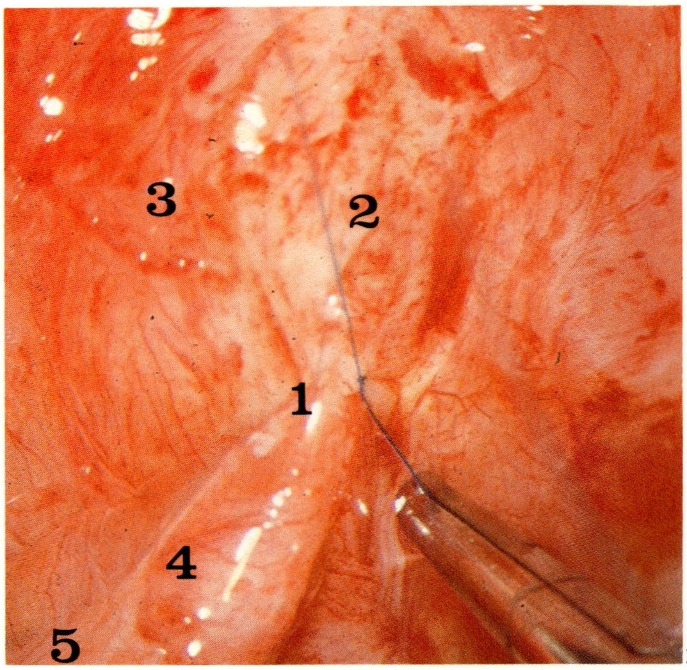

x 10

Figure 77. The ampullary end of the tube is brought into the field of view and a bite of the tissue *just beneath* the tube is taken. Note that this bite lies exactly the same distance away from the lumen as it did on the cornual side. Splint is marked (1), cornual muscle (2), uterine serosa (3), ampullary muscle (4), ampullary serosa (5). Note that the forceps on the left are not used to grasp tissue but only to steady or retract it.

Figure 78. An instrument tie is made. This manoeuvre should not be attempted until it has been repeatedly practised in the laboratory. Usually a double throw should be placed in the first knot to overcome tension. In this photograph the mucosa of the ampulla can be seen underneath the splint (1); numbering is as for **Figure 77.**

79

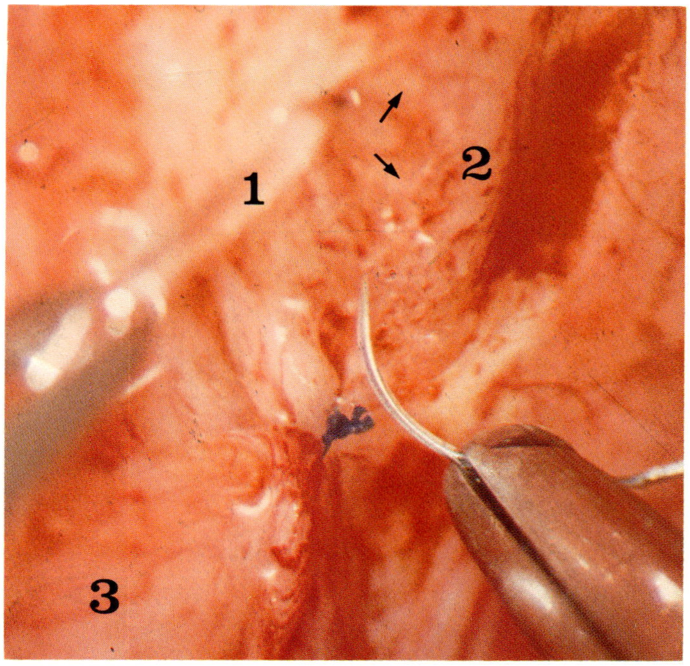

x 16

80

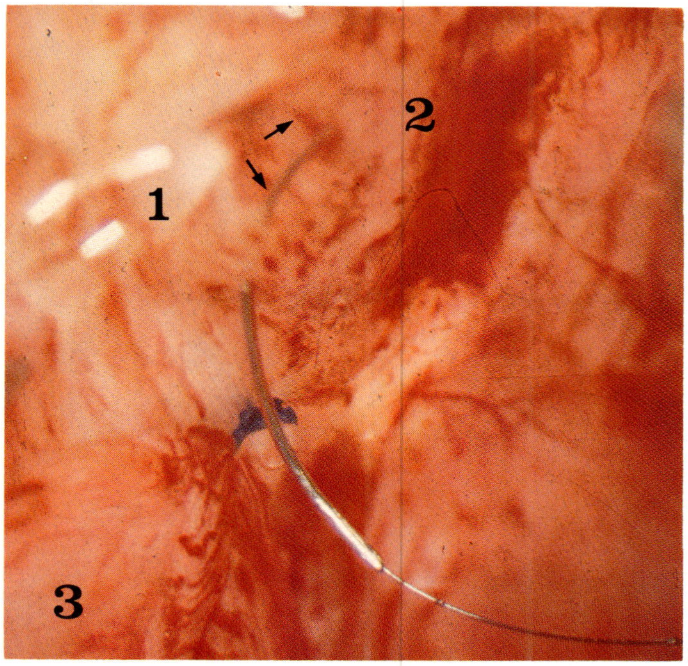

x 16

79 to 82 Placing the first anastomotic stitch
A 3 mm curved needle on 8/0 nylon (Spingler-Tritt) is now used for the tubal anastomosis. It is essential that the first stitch is at the base of the join, above the stay suture, in the 6 o'clock position. If this stitch is omitted at this stage it will be found difficult, if not impossible, to place it later. Note that these photographs are taken at the actual working magnification and consequently the depth of focus is very shallow, only fractions of a millimetre.

Figures 79 and **80** show how a bite of the cornual muscle is first taken. Note that the needle is passed upwards through the muscle towards the lumen on the cornual side (**Figures 79** and **80**). In these photographs the splint is at (1), the cornual musculature (2), the ampullary musculature (3). The blue stitch in the centre is the stay suture and the thin arrows delineate the edge of the cornual epithelium.

81

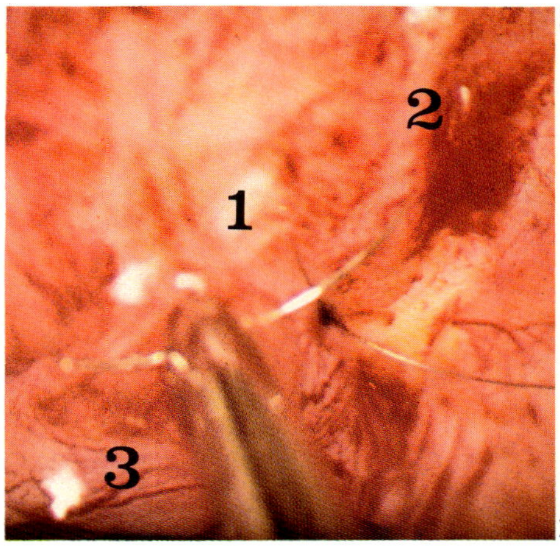

x 8

82

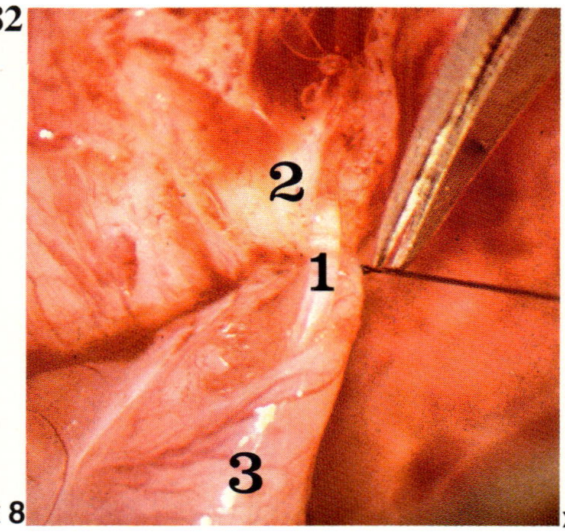

x 8

83

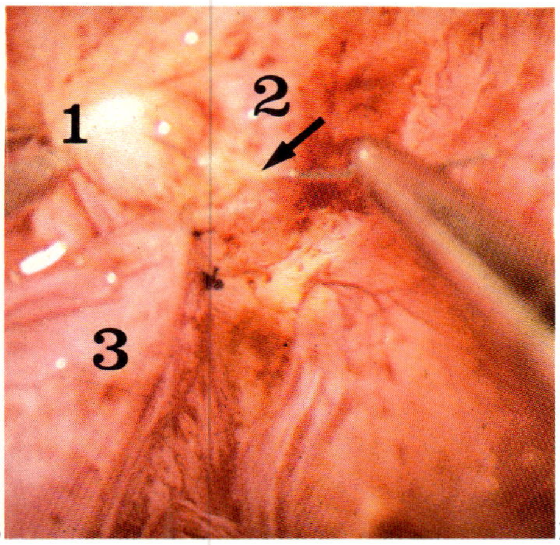

x 8

Figure 81 shows how the needle is reversed away from the lumen on the ampullary side. This is so that the knot will be tied away from the epithelial surface. Wherever possible the suture is passed through muscle but the epithelium is not included in the bite as there is evidence that healing may be better.

In **Figure 82** the microscissors are used to cut the first anastomotic stitch very short. The suture has been tied using instruments in the standard microsurgical fashion. In **Figure 83** the second anastomotic suture has been started at the 4 o'clock position, cornual side first (arrow).

84
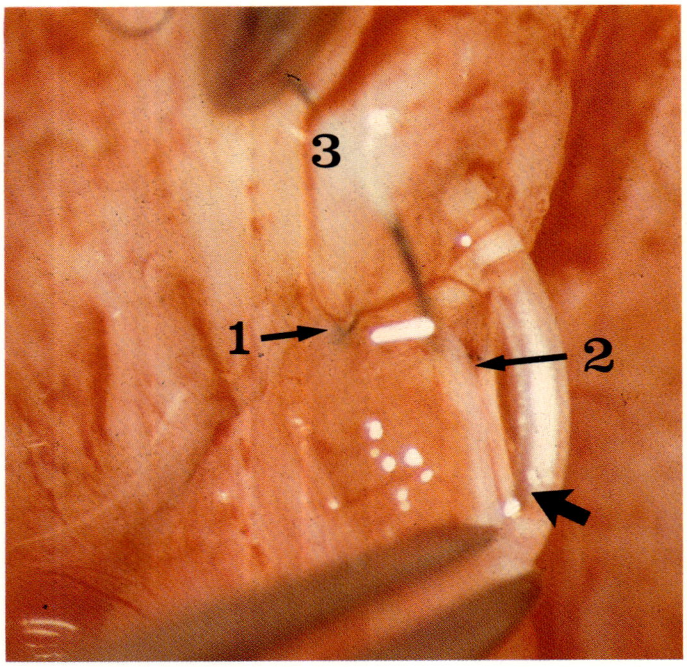

x 25

85
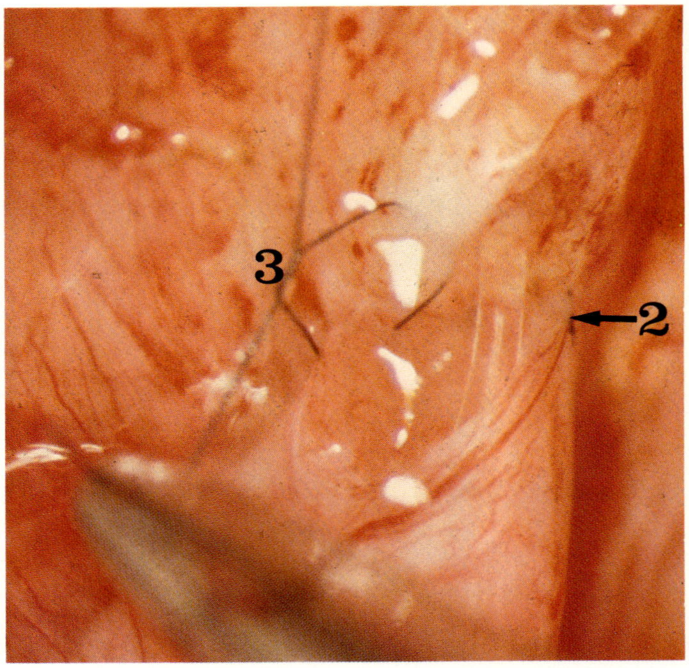

x 25

84 to 87 Third and fourth anastomotic sutures
In **Figure 84** the first suture at 6 o'clock is arrowed at (1) and the second at (2). The third suture is now placed on the medial side of the anastomosis at about the 9 o'clock position (3). Note that the bite of cornual muscle does not include any mucosa. The value of the plastic splint (broad arrow) is clearly seen in these photographs. Firstly it shows much more clearly where the two tubal edges really are and secondly it can be used as a retractor. In **Figures 84** and **86** the surgeon is grasping the splint with the forceps rather than crushing the tissues. By grasping the splint he gets adequate purchase to take properly divided bites of the tubal tissues.

In **Figure 85** the suture at 9 o'clock is being tied. A square knot is used here as the tension is now minimal. Some surgeons like to tie all knots at the end after the stitches are

86
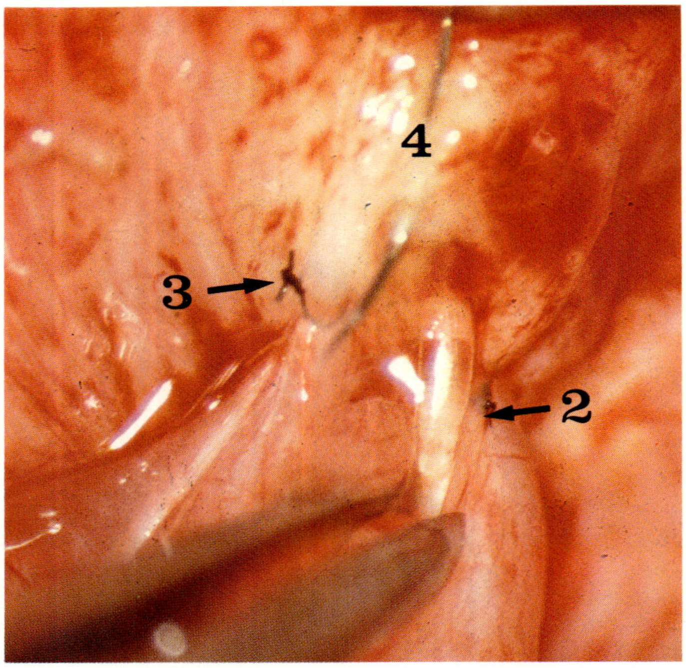

x 25

87
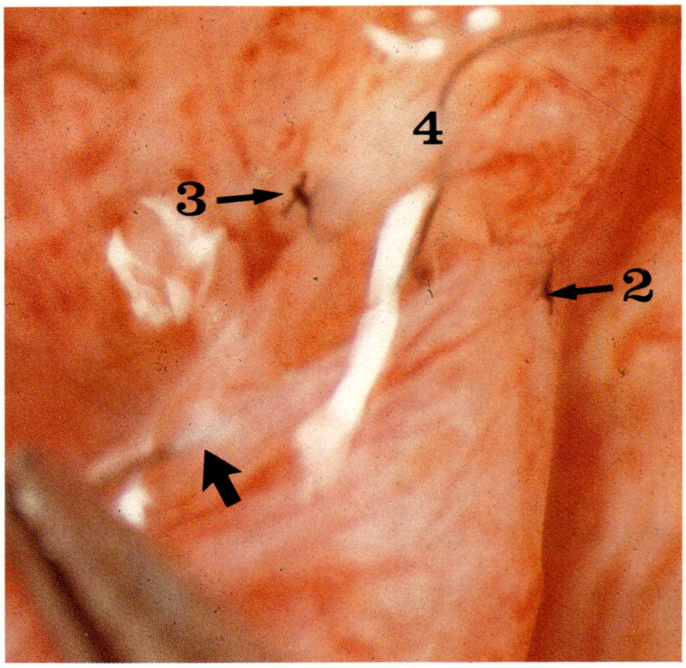

x 25

in place. Generally, we prefer to tie each suture in turn as it is inserted.

Figure 86 shows the fourth suture being placed (4). This stitch is almost in the 12 o'clock position. Stitches No. 2 and No. 3 are arrowed (2) and (3). It is now relatively easy to avoid placing the suture through mucosa as the tissues are stabilised by the earlier sutures. Note that each stitch is still commenced on the uterine side and is tied away from the lumen.

In **Figure 87** the fourth anastomotic suture (4) is now taken through the ampullary side of the anastomosis (broad arrow) and is seen in situ.

88

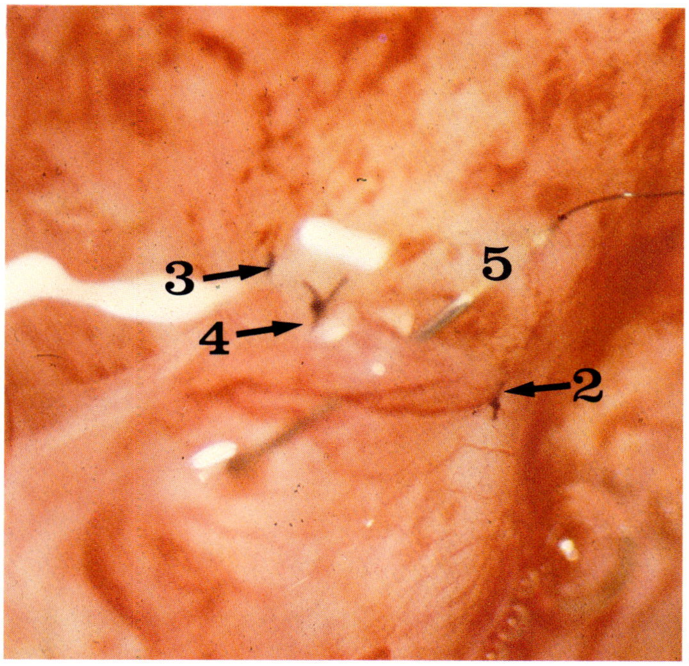

x 20

89

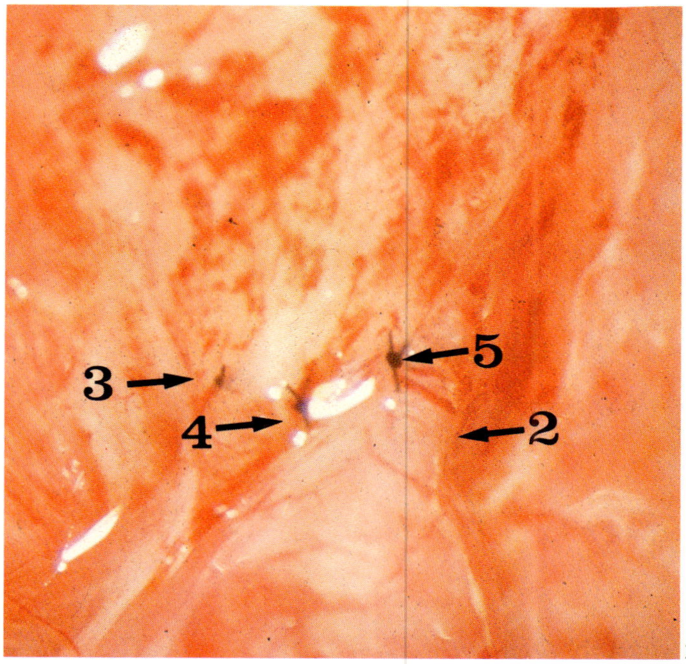

x 16

88 and 89 Completion of the inner layer of the anastomosis
The two tubal edges are now almost completely approximated but in order to get a watertight join on the inner layer a fifth suture is placed between the second and the fourth suture. This is shown in **Figure 88** and the completed inner join in **Figure 89**. The sutures are numbered in their order of placement. Three throws have been put on each knot and the ends cut very short to minimise the amount of foreign material left at the join.

90

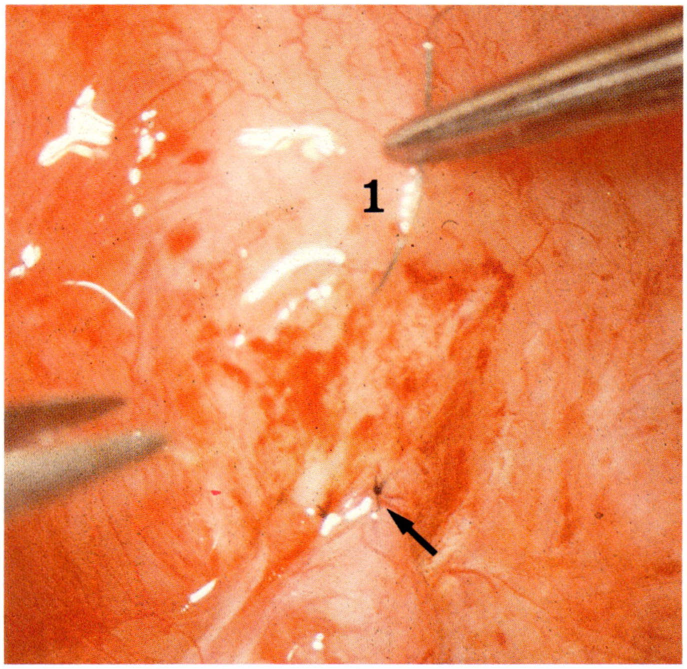

x 12

91

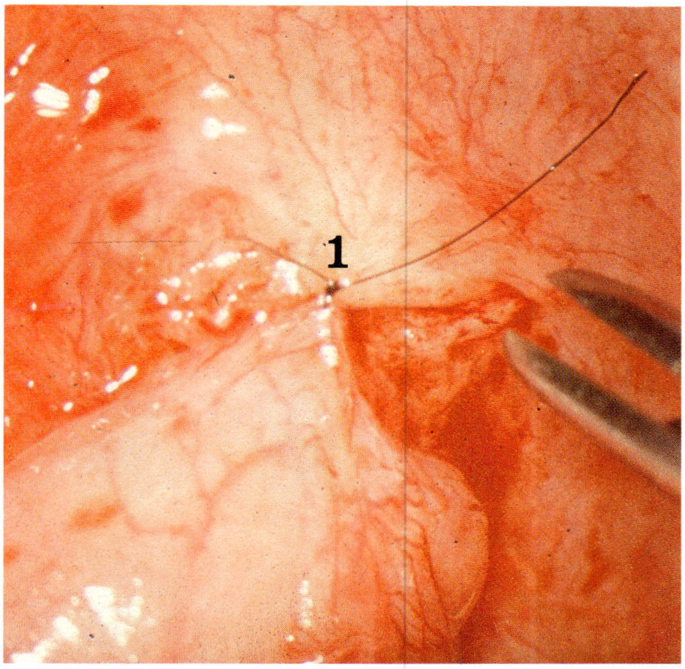

x 16

90 and 91 Beginning closure of tubal peritoneum
The second layer of sutures can now be commenced. 8/0 nylon is still normally used and the suture is placed by taking a bite of peritoneum together with a bite of underlying muscle. In **Figure 90** the first layer of anastomotic sutures is marked with an arrow. Note that the first serosal suture is placed at the 'apex' of the anastomosis, on the antimesenteric border (1). In **Figure 91** the suture is tied and ready to be cut. Note how the tissue gap closes quite easily.

92

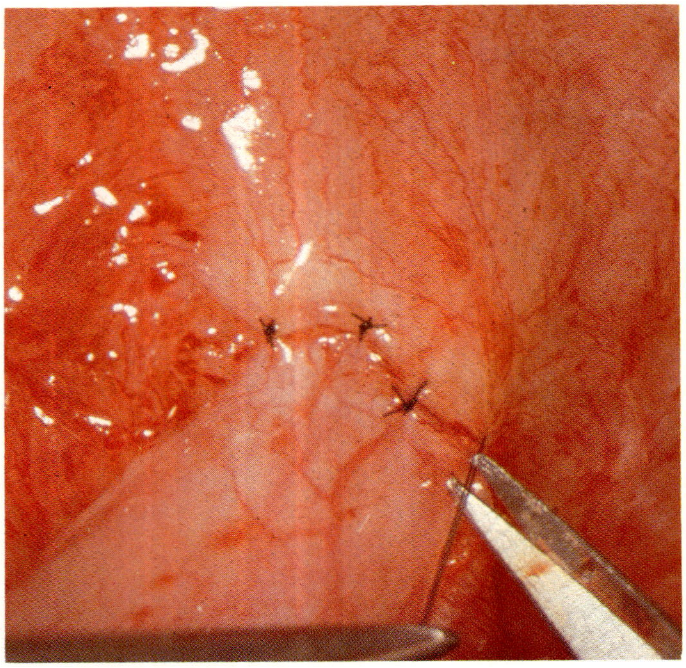

93

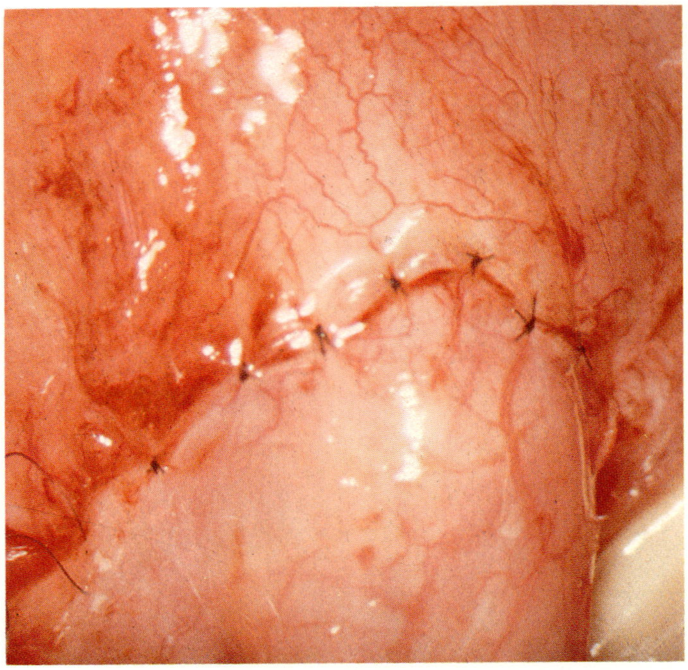

92 and 93 Completion of the peritoneal coat
Interrupted 8/0 nylon sutures are now placed all around the anastomosis. Usually about 12 such sutures are used. The object is to leave no raw area at the anastomosis for adhesion formation. This layer of sutures will also give good support for the join and make abruption very unlikely. It is very important that these sutures are placed in such a way that the join is not kinked. A continuous suture can be used for this outer layer, but if it is, kinking of the join is much more likely to occur.

94

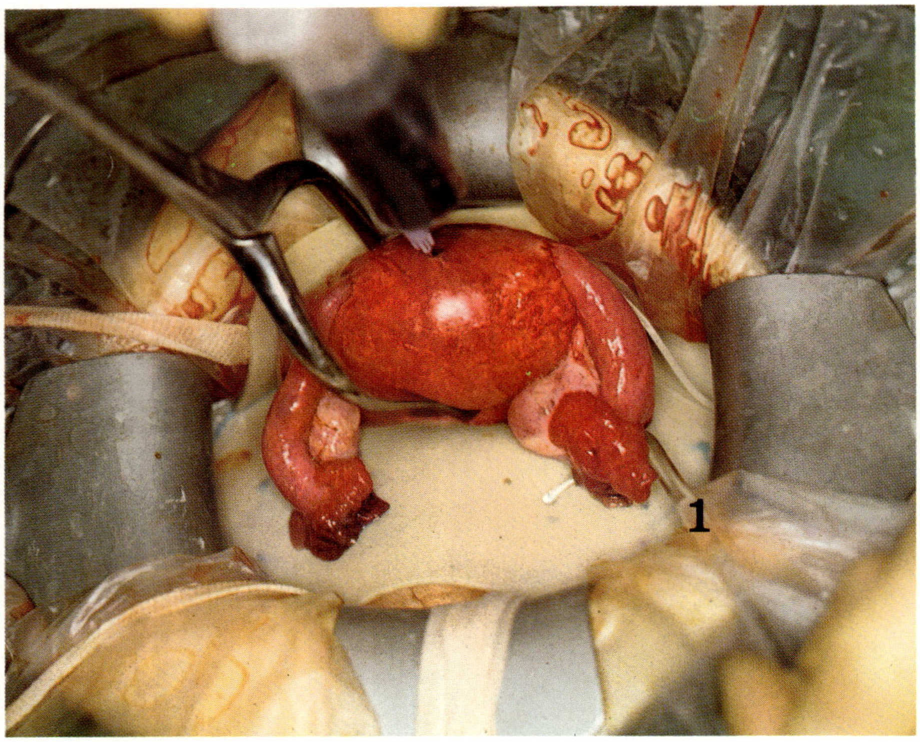

In **Figure 92** the serosal sutures are being placed and cut in turn. In **Figure 93** a suture on the medial side of the join is about to be tied. These sutures will be continued down the side of the tube on either side and any defect in the mesosalpinx will be similarly repaired. Usually at least two or three sutures are required on either side of the mesosalpinx.

94 Bilateral cornual anastomoses completed
The splints can now be removed and dye injected, after clamping the cervix. Dye is injected through the uterine fundus and spill immediately occurs from the fimbrial end of each tube. Note that there is no leakage at the cornual join. The tubes are rather oedematous. This is common after this procedure; the oedema is sometimes related to the tightness of the pack in the pouch of Douglas and there may be a mild degree of temporary venous obstruction. This seems to be quite harmless in our experience. A glass rod (1) elevates the fimbria.

These joins are adequate and the vaginal pack can now be removed and the abdomen closed. Steroids are not necessary in such cases as there is no significant peritoneal damage.

Mid-tubal anastomosis

In the vast majority of cases mid-tubal anastomosis is performed to attempt reversal of previous sterilisation. Although mid-tubal block can occur from other conditions it is rare. Inflammatory causes of mid-tubal blockage are tuberculosis, bilharzia or very extensive salpingitis isthmica nodosa; with these conditions affecting the mid-tube the situation is not usually operable. Very occasionally the mid-tube can be affected by endometriosis and surgery could be considered for this.

The results of mid-tubal anastomosis seem to depend primarily on the excellence of the join; the better the join the more chance of a pregnancy. Patients who have short tubes, and especially a very short ampulla, seem to do less well. Recent evidence (Vasquez, Winston, Boeckx and Brosens 1980) suggests that patients who have been sterilised for more than five years are less likely to conceive after tubal anastomosis than patients who have been sterilised for shorter periods. This may be related to progressive mucosal atrophic changes. In spite of these considerations the most crucial aspect remains the method of sterilisation. The more destructive methods of sterilisation are generally more efficacious but they are more difficult to reverse. This is partly because a greater length of tube is destroyed but also because they are generally associated with more fibrosis and adhesions. Operations which damage the fimbria are particularly difficult to reverse and we are reluctant to attempt sterilisation reversal in any patient following fimbriectomy, even though there are very occasional reports of success in the medical literature. The most reversible method seems to be clip sterilisation and our first 13 patients who have had tubal anastomosis following clip sterilisation have all conceived. Clip sterilisation, by the method of Hulka, Filshie and Bleier, has the advantage of damaging only 3–4 mm of tube. We feel that these clips are most 'reversible' when applied across the isthmus.

95 to 96 Preparation and splinting of cut ends

The steps in mid-tubal anastomosis are basically the same as those already described for cornual anastomosis. We usually transect the isthmic side first and remove any fibrous tissue. Next (**Figure 95**) the polyethylene splint is fed into the isthmus (1) and from thence to the uterus. In this patient about 2 cm of isthmus has been left undamaged. It has already been pointed out that the direction in which the splint is pushed is important – note that it is at first pushed in the same direction as the isthmus travels, i.e. upwards and only downwards when the internal part of the intramural portion is being traversed. In **Figure 95** the surgeon is gently squeezing the cornu between two fingers to flatten out any kinks in the intramural portion – this makes splint introduction much easier.

The muscle of the isthmus has been exposed (arrow) by cutting the serosal coat a little further away from the lumen. This gives plenty of tissue to take good size bites when suturing.

In **Figure 96**, the grooved probe mentioned on page 157 has been inserted through the fimbria, ready to fashion a hole in the ampulla minimising luminal disparity. The ampulla is about 4 cm in length. The peritoneum has been partially stripped from the tip of the blind end of the ampulla (arrow). The very tip of the blind end is now ready for transection, the grooved probe can be advanced to receive the splint and then the probe can be withdrawn through the fimbria, cannulating the whole tube.

95

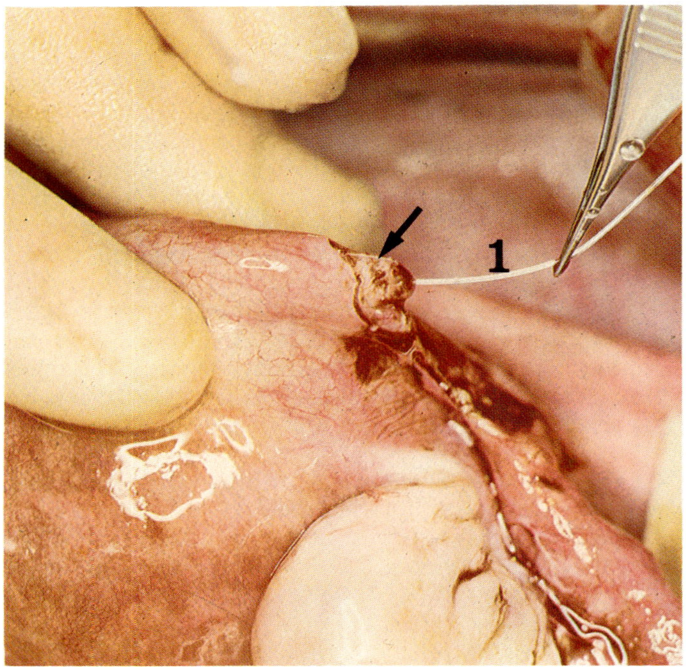

96

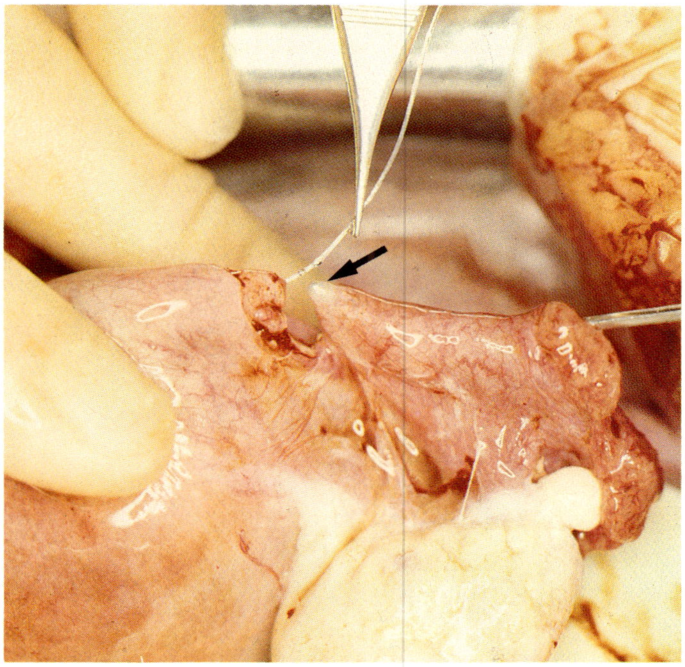

97

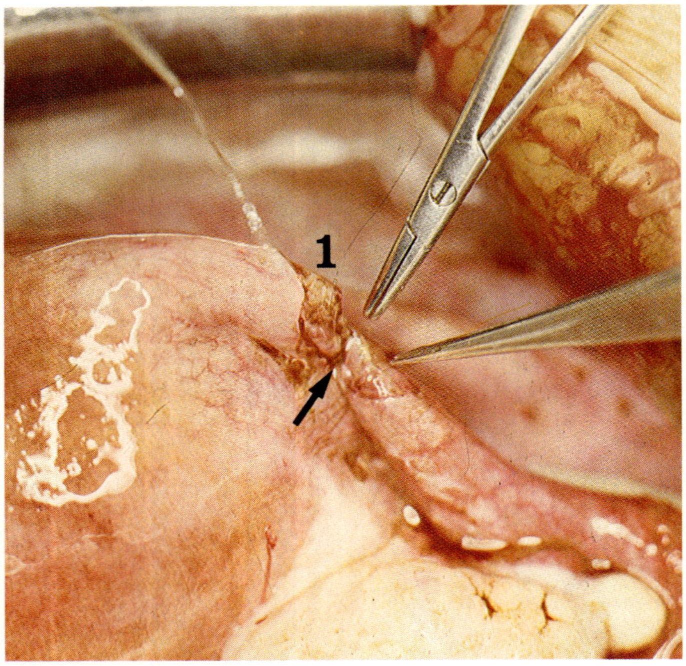

98

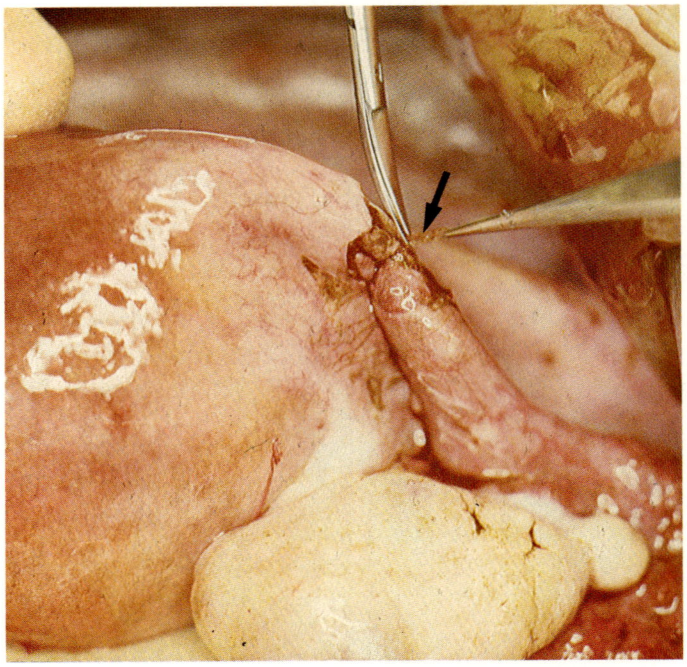

99

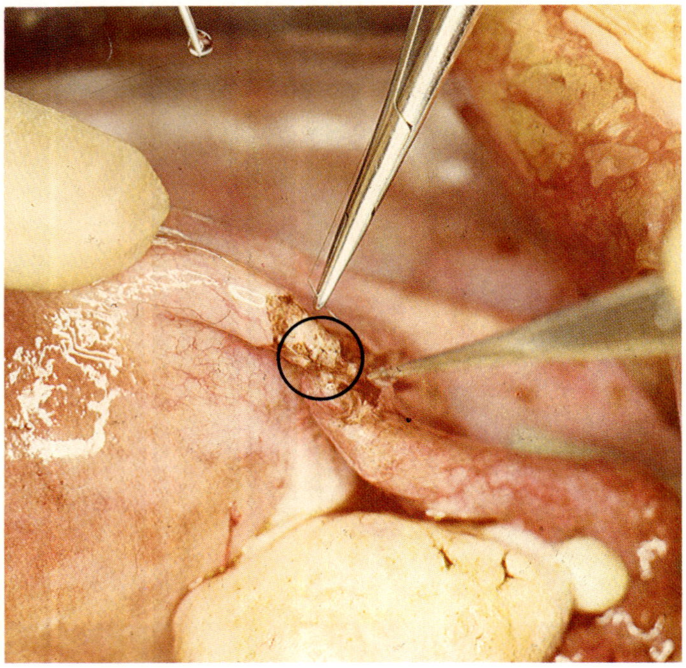

97. Because the cut ends of the two tubal segments lie so well together over the splint, a stay suture of 6/0 prolene is not required in the mesosalpinx of this patient. 9/0 nylon is used for this anastomosis which will be performed in two layers using the same basic technique as that described for cornual anastomosis. The first stitch (arrow) has already been placed at the base of the join, care being taken to avoid the mucosa. The stitch needle has just been passed through the isthmic musculature at the 12 o'clock position (1). Note that whilst this operation is being performed under the microscope at ×4 to ×16 magnification, these photographs are reproduced almost exactly life-size. It becomes quite clear how inaccurate the use of the naked eye is for this procedure.

98. The first layer of sutures is virtually complete. Occasionally one encounters a small area of scar tissue when the anastomosis is only half finished. Using the microscope this can easily be identified and resected (arrow).

99. The muscular (inner) layer of sutures is completed. There are six such sutures in this patient as can be seen in this photograph; they are barely visible to the naked eye. This area is encircled by a thin ring.

100

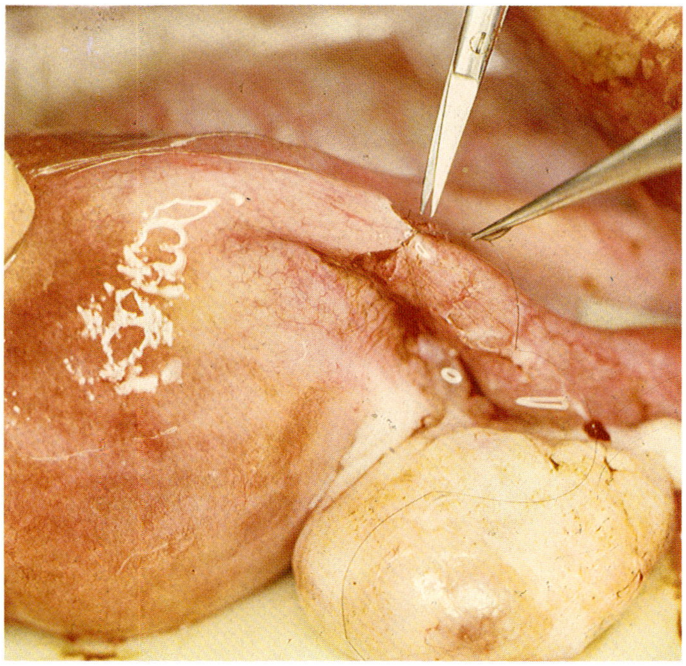

101

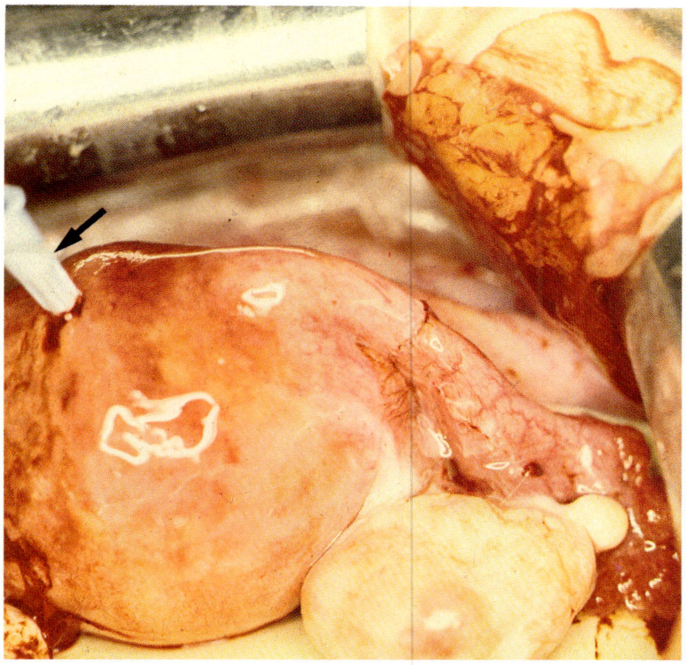

102

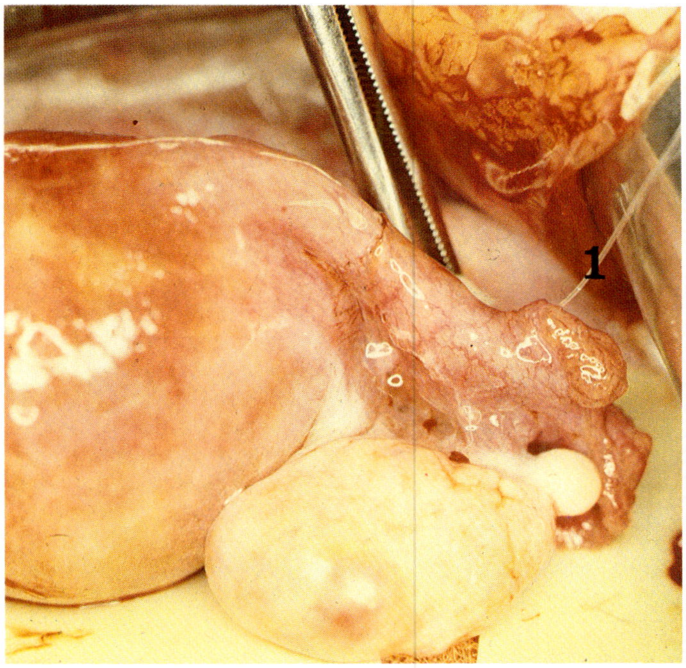

100. The serosal coat of the tube is now repaired with interrupted nylon sutures. We generally suture the medial aspect of the tube first and work around the antimesenteric border. These stitches can be cut quite short with micro-scissors. Continuous suture can be employed but if this method of serosal closure is used very great care must be taken to ensure that the tube is not kinked. As previously mentioned, care must also be taken to avoid raw areas and to ensure that the leaves of the mesosalpinx are adequately reconstructed.

101. Shows the complete right tubal anastomosis (posterior aspect). Note that the peritoneum looks undamaged, there is little blood clot forming on the tissues and most important of all the tube lies nicely in 'a good line'. The blue-topped 22 gauge needle has been left in the uterine fundus (arrow) since the beginning of the entire procedure so that tubal patency can be tested at the end.

102. The splint (1) is withdrawn from the fimbrial end. There seems no point in leaving an indwelling splint in this tube – its presence would in all probability lead to infection. Nowadays we have adopted a policy of leaving a splint in situ postoperatively only if the anastomosis has been especially difficult to establish. In these circumstances we leave a splint in for a maximum of 72 hours only.

103

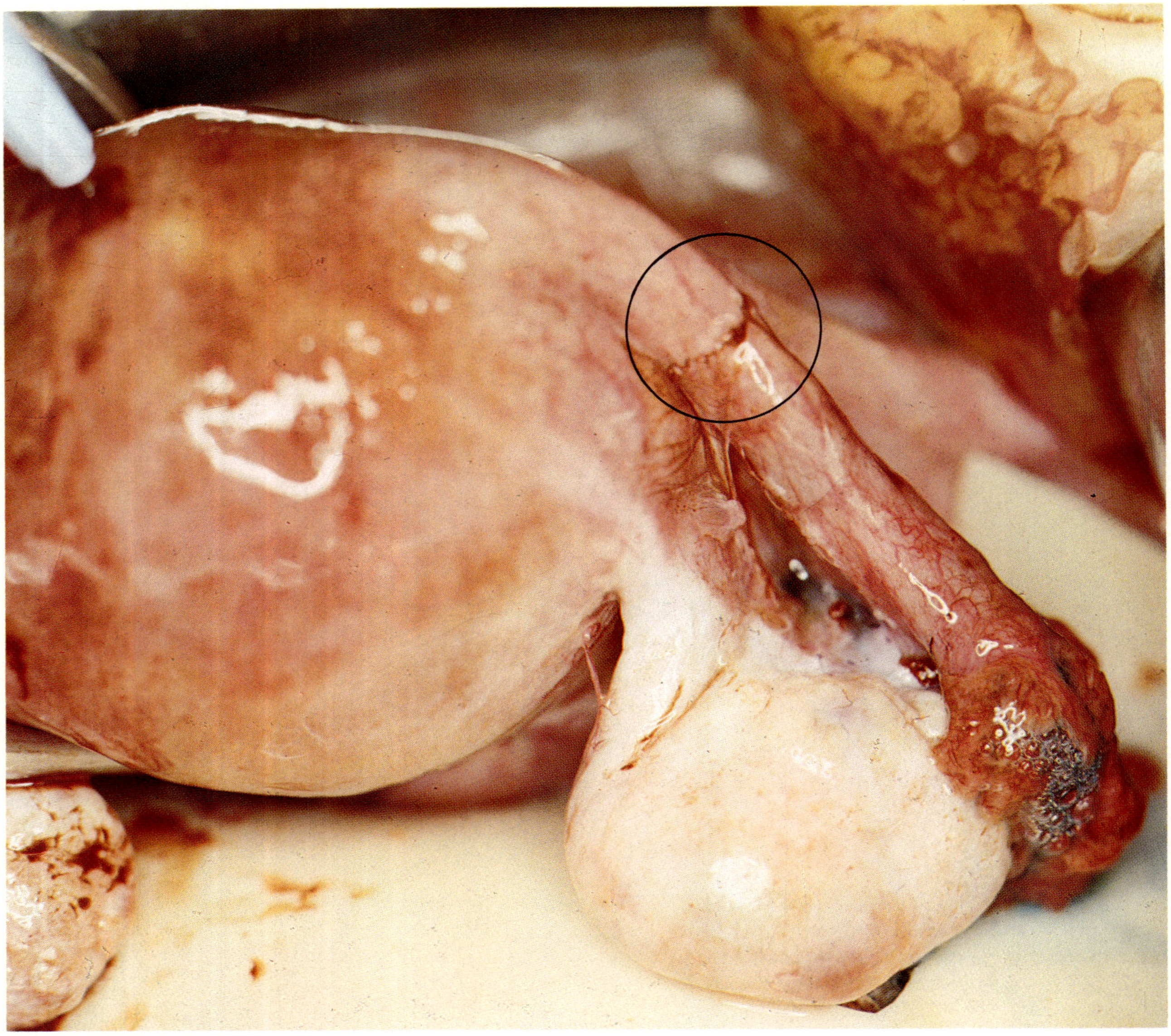

103. The anastomosis is finally completed on the right. Dye is injected and there is prompt spill from the fimbria. The ampulla distends with the pressure of dye but there is no leakage from the join. In the rare event that no dye flows through the anastomosis at this stage, or if there is a major degree of dye leakage around the join, the surgeon has to consider whether he should unpick the stitches and redo the anastomosis. It must be remembered however that if the surgery has taken a long time, severe tubal oedema can affect tubal permeability and a patent anastomosis can appear to be blocked. Unless the surgeon is quite satisfied that oedema is occluding the tube he must do a reanastomosis. Once patency has been tested, the needle in the fundus can be withdrawn. It is an advantage to slide the shaft of this needle alongside the tip of the diathermy electrode as the needle is extracted. This will diathermise the needle track and diminish bleeding. The anastomosis is encircled by a thin ring.

Special problems with tubal anastomosis

(1) Isthmic-ampullary anastomosis with major luminal disparity

Sometimes there may be such scar tissue around the ligated ampullary end that this cannot be removed without transecting the tube. This is particularly likely when large catgut sutures persist in the tubal tissues after some Pomeroy sterilisations. In this situation, the grooved probe technique cannot be used. The ampulla must be transected and fibrous tissue removed. The ampullary side of the anastomosis can be plicated with a few radial sutures before placing the anastomotic sutures. Additionally the inner layer of anastomotic sutures is positioned much further apart on the ampullary side than on the isthmic side. It is sometimes helpful to delay tying some of these sutures until they are all in place. In addition, before commencing the join, we frequently slit the antimesenteric border of the isthmus to create a slightly larger isthmic lumen. This slit need only be between 1–3 mm in length.

104

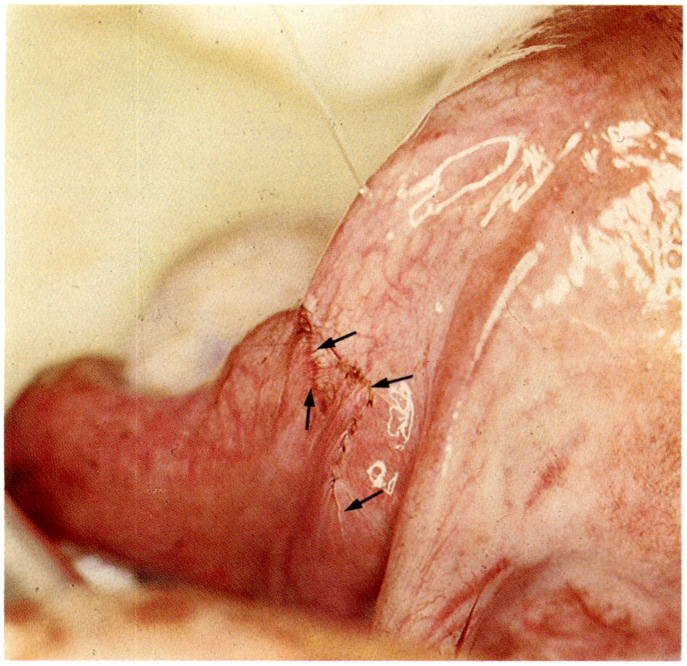

105

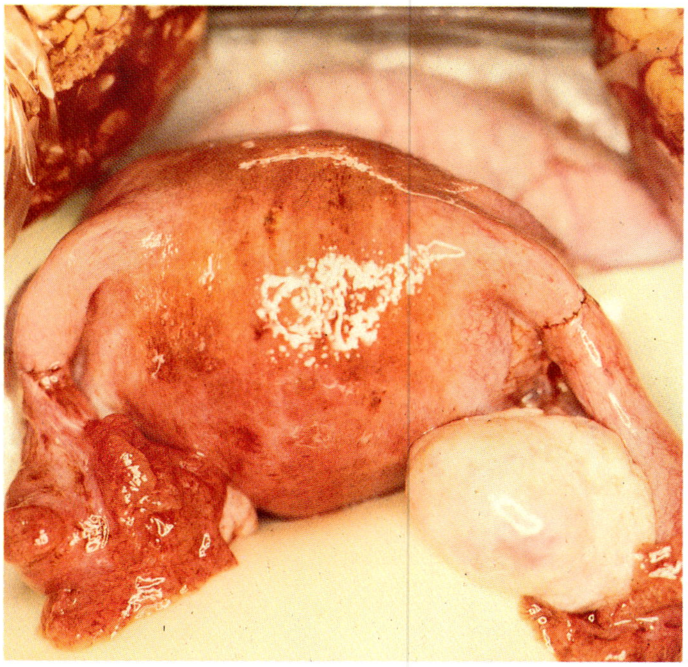

(2) Prolapse of mucosal folds from the ampullary lumen into the wall of the anastomosis

This frequently happens in cases of marked luminal disparity. We try as far as possible to push many of these folds back but frequently this is very tedious and occasionally impossible. It is probably important that this mucosa should not remain in the tube wall – otherwise healing may be impaired and theoretically implantation could occur at this point with a resulting tubal pregnancy. For this reason we tend to trim off persistent prolapsing folds with scissors when necessary. This does not seem to influence the clinical result.

(3) Very short tube

When the damage at sterilisation has been extensive, the tube may be very short after the completion of anastomosis. In tubes with a grossly shortened ampulla, there may be anatomic problems with ovum capture because the fimbriated end is unable to cover the whole of the ovarian capsule at the time of ovulation. Under these circumstances, one may deliberately shorten the ovarian ligament bringing the ovary upwards, closer to the cornu. Plicating stitches of 6/0 prolene are sufficient, and these can be placed in a similar manner to the classical operation of shortening of the round ligaments. Usually, only two or three sutures will be needed. It must be mentioned that the efficacy of this procedure is unproven and that ovum pickup may occur from the pouch of Douglas as well as from the ovarian surface in humans.

(4) Major peritoneal defects

Peritoneal defects are encountered particularly following tubal ligation where ampullary adhesions to the ovary or the fimbria have resulted. It is important to cover these areas; otherwise, the anastomosis may fail due to recurrent adhesions. It is usually possible to mobilise sufficient tubal peritoneum and to stitch this together to avoid raw areas. Tension must be avoided. Usually, interrupted 8/0 nylon sutures are best, and the suture lines should, as far as possible, be linear and longitudinal along the length of the tube to avoid kinking or subsequent stricture. If there are larger raw areas, free peritoneal grafts can be taken and wrapped around the tube. In **Figure 104** there was a major defect in the mesosalpinx due to extensive scar formation. A Z-plasty has been performed using many interrupted 8/0 nylon sutures and complete closure of the peritoneum has resulted (arrows).

(5) Tubes ligated at two or three sites

About 10 per cent of our patients have had their tubes ligated twice or more on the same side. This leaves a 'redundant loop' in the middle of the oviduct. Although we have had considerable success with double (and, on occasion, triple) anastomoses in the same tube, it should be pointed out that the redundant loop is frequently badly damaged. This is probably due to pressure effects in the closed segment. Scanning electron microscopy has shown gross flattening of the mucosa with marked loss of ciliated cells in some cases. A careful examination of the cut ends under high-power magnification of such a segment should be made before deciding whether to resect it completely or to perform an anastomosis at either end of the segment.

Figure 105 shows completed bilateral tubal anastomoses. The peritoneum is clean and glistening and there are no raw areas. The needle track in the uterine fundus has been diathermied and is almost invisible. As might be expected we virtually never see postoperative adhesions when the final result looks like this.

Postoperative management after tuboplasty

Antibiotics

We generally give broad-spectrum antibiotic cover to all patients undergoing surgery for pelvic inflammatory disease. This cover is started the day before surgery and continued for ten days afterwards. We also give similar cover to many patients before hysterosalpingography and laparoscopy particularly if laparoscopy is combined with endoscopic division of adhesions. Antibiotics are not given to patients for reversal of sterilisation except in those exceptional instances where the operation has taken longer than two hours. We generally give tetracycline, 500 mg 6-hourly orally and metranidazole 200 mg 6-hourly. During the operation the tetracycline is given by intramuscular injection and the metranidazole by intravenous infusion. We have had no problem of toxicity in several hundred cases. Before metranidazole became available we gave ampicillin 500 mg 6-hourly. Very exceptionally patients have had diarrhoea or drug rashes following this treatment.

Steroids

Steroid therapy is reserved for those patients who had extensive adhesiolysis or 'difficult' salpingostomies. They are never given following anastomosis or implantation, or if there is the slightest suspicion of latent infection or previous tuberculosis. Our usual régime is: Dexamethazone 6 mg (orally) the night before surgery. Hydrocortisone succinate 200 mg intramuscularly with premedication and once during the operation, giving a total of 400 mg; hydrocortisone succinate 200 mg, two hours after return to the ward. Additionally, hydrocortisone acetate 1.5 G in 50–100 ml of Ringer's solution is left in the pelvis before closure. At night – usually about 10 hours or so after surgery – dexamethazone is commenced by mouth, 4 mg. The first day after surgery the patient takes dexamethazone 2 mg 6-hourly, the second 1.5 mg 6-hourly, the third day 1.0 mg 6-hourly, the fourth day 0.5 mg 6-hourly and the fifth day 0.5 mg twice. This régime seems to slow wound healing a little but we have had minor wound problems with it on rare occasions only. It does not seem to have any long-term effect on adrenal function. We have the strong impression (no hard data) that this régime is valuable *except* when the surgery has been conducted without careful regard to tissue handling – it cannot make up for poor surgical technique.

106

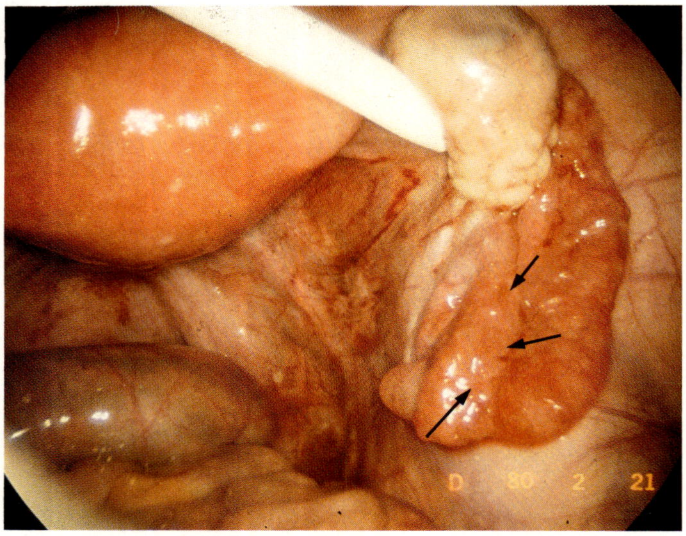

107

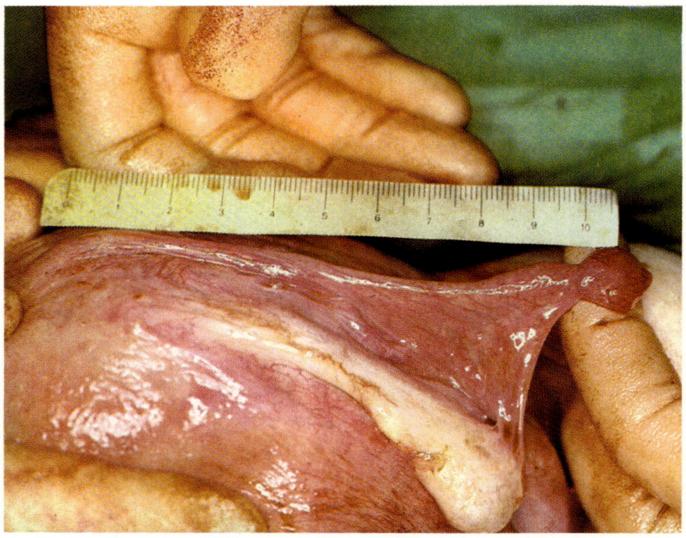

106 and 107 Postoperative appearance

Figure 106 shows a typical result a year later in a patient who required extensive ovariolysis as well as salpingostomy. The fimbria (arrows) are very well healed and the tube is open. Note, however, that the peritoneal vessels are still congested and there may be some low-grade inflammation. Cultures were sterile.

Figure 107 shows a photograph of the uterus at Caesarean section following cornual anastomosis. There is clearly no weakness of the uterine wall and there are no adhesions. The join is invisible. Caesarean section was performed solely because of fetal distress and mild hypertension.

Promethazine
We can find no evidence that this drug has any really valuable *clinical* effect other than being mildly sedative and therefore do not use it to suppress adhesions. Nor do we use dextrans.

Hydrotubation
The value of hydrotubation seems extremely doubtful and we discontinued its use some seven years ago. Our postoperative patency rates have actually improved considerably since then – probably because of better technique. Hydrotubation can be painful and may risk ascending infection, two excellent reasons for not employing it.

Intercourse
We advise patients to resume intercourse about two weeks after surgery or as soon as they feel comfortable. We have many instances where patients have become pregnant immediately and have not had a menstrual period after surgery.

Hysterosalpingography and laparoscopy
We do not do hysterosalpingography after tubal surgery unless we are definitely planning repeated surgery. We prefer to laparoscope patients but only after one year at least has elapsed following surgery and then only if the patient is concerned about persistent infertility or perhaps pain. The author remains unconvinced that laparoscopic adhesiolysis 6–12 weeks after surgery is of any real value. More than 90 per cent of our patients following salpingostomy have at least one patent tube at check laparoscopy one year after surgery (**Figure 106**).

Pregnancy
Patients must be warned about the possibilities of an ectopic gestation. There seems no way at present of preventing this. Our ectopic pregnancy rate is about 9 per cent following salpingostomy and 3 per cent following anastomosis. Abortion, too, is more common and if patients do miscarry we feel that it is important to give broad-spectrum antibiotic cover to prevent tubal infection. In the event of term pregnancy we avoid Caesarean section unless there is an obstetric indication. An exception is tubal implantation where it may be safer than allowing the patient to go in to labour (**Figure 107**).

11: In vitro fertilisation and embryo transfer

This dramatic and new technique (in which preovulatory oocytes are recovered laparoscopically, fertilised in vitro using husband's sperm, the embryo then grown in culture through three or four cleavage divisions and placed in the mother's uterus) has resulted in the birth of a handful of infants to mothers with intractable tubal disease who would otherwise have been considered as hopeless cases of infertility. Steptoe and Edwards (1980) and Lopata et al (1980) have recently described their techniques and successes. The former group pioneered this technique and in 1979 reported that their success rate for in vitro fertilisation of preovulatory eggs was 70 to 80 per cent and that approximately 90 per cent of the fertilised eggs yielded embryos which cleaved normally in tissue culture. These embryos could be maintained in an apparently healthy state for up to 5 days in vitro. In 1977–78 Edwards and Steptoe were able to transplant into the uterus during the early luteal phase of a natural menstrual cycle four such embryos which resulted in pregnancy. Only two however culminated in live births.

It is the authors' intention to discuss the technical aspects of this technique. The medical management of these patients, which has been recently described in detail by Edwards and Steptoe (1980), will be briefly considered.

Indication for embryo transfer

The technique opens up the possibility of regaining fertility in women with severe and permanent tubal or peritubal disease and in those with absence of the fallopian tubes as a result of surgery. It is also possible as Lopata et al (1980) suggest, that the procedure may be of value to couples who cannot conceive due to unexplained infertility, sperm antibodies in the female circulation and/or genital tract, cervical 'hostility', and oligospermia.

Initial investigation and selection of patient

Laparoscopy

Laparoscopy is the major diagnostic method in assessing the condition of the pelvis. The procedure seeks the answer to two questions in patients who may be *potential* candidates for embryo transfer. The first is whether tubal surgery is still possible and if it is not the second is whether laparoscopic ovum recovery is technically possible. If it is possible the amount of residual tube must be assessed. If a significant amount remains, even as a cul de sac, the possibility of ectopic implantation exists. Steptoe and Edwards (1976) suggest that the cornual portion of the tube should be obstructed at this initial laparoscopy or that the remaining damaged portion be excised at laparotomy. If the latter is performed then adhesiolysis and elevation of the ovaries is performed so as to allow easier ovum recovery.

Assessment of ovulation

The menstrual cycle is assessed hormonally as described earlier (page 13) to determine whether ovulation is occurring and if so its 'quality' and the stage at which it occurs in the cycle. In Edwards and Steptoe's recent work reliance was placed on rapid methods of determining LH as a guide to ovulation. Three hourly specimens of urine were analysed for LH by the Hi-Gonavis (Mochida Pharmaceutical) method; tests were started in the follicular phase and continued until the LH surge was obvious.

Other investigations

The uterus of the potential recipient is measured by a sound and a calibrated catheter during preliminary investigation which also must include blood tests for various transmittable diseases such as toxoplasma, rubella, cytomegalovirus, hepatitis-B virus, herpes and syphilis. A Papanicolaou smear is also taken.

The husband's semen is examined at an early stage with particular emphasis placed on sperm motility.

Counselling

The psychological stability of the couple should be assessed since the success rate for this complicated and invasive procedure is still small. They should be aware of all the stages of the technique and be able to cooperate effectively, and have a realistic understanding of the prognosis.

Ovum recovery

Preovulatory stimulation

In the initial stages of the Steptoe and Edwards' study, follicular growth was induced by gonadotrophic hormone injection; this being considered important in regulating follicle growth and subsequent ovulation. It also allowed multiple oocytes to be aspirated from their follicles prior to actual ovulation. In 1977 they abandoned this method of superovulation because it resulted in abnormal hormone secretion. They subsequently relied on recovery of mature oocytes developing during the natural cycle.

Timing of ovum collection during the natural cycle

The patient is admitted to hospital in the middle of the follicular phase when urine collections are tested. A daily rising urinary oestrogen level of about 40 μg/24 hours suggests impending ovulation. At this stage three-hourly urinary LH estimations are commenced. The time for ovum 'pick-up' by laparoscopy is set from the start of the LH surge and is usually some 15–27 hours after the LH rise is detected. All of Steptoe and Edwards' pregnancies occurred where 24 hours had elapsed between the LH surge and aspiration. A technique using ultrasonography to determine follicle growth and maturation is discussed on page 172; this method may act as a confirmatory indicator of ovulation and thereby reduce the number of wrongly timed laparoscopies (**Figures 5** to **7**).

Steptoe and Edwards (1980) noted that follicle aspiration is more successful when undertaken at night than during the day. The technique is shown in **Figures 1** to **4**, and **8** to **9**.

Laparoscopy

Premedication and general anaesthesia are used as in routine laparoscopy. The gas mixture used was 5 per cent carbon dioxide + 5 per cent oxygen + 90 per cent nitrogen, the same composition as that used for embryo culture.

1 and 2 Preparation for follicle aspiration

In **Figure 1** the apparatus is displayed. The laparoscope is introduced just below the umbilicus and is seen (1) with a Palmer holding forceps (2) inserted in the right iliac fossa. This forceps grasps the ovarian ligament and rotates the ovary to reveal the follicle, ripe for aspiration. The needle (3) used for aspirating the preovulatory follicle is a 12.5 cm long 20 gauge spinal needle with a 45° bevel which will be passed through a 16 gauge intravenous cannula with its original needle. As seen in **Figure 1**, it is connected via manometer tubing (5) to a 10 ml 'Pyrex' beaker (6) acting as a collecting chamber. Suction is provided by a further piece of manometer tubing (7) and a third entry hole in the rubber bung acts as a bypass valve (8) allowing the operator to control the suction with his fingertip. In **Figure 2** the aspiration needle (3) is now passed down the cannula which has been inserted in the midline half way between the umbilicus and the symphysis pubis. The operator is monitoring its intra-abdominal progress via the laparoscope (1). The Palmer forceps (2) has already been applied to the ovarian ligament and is held by an assistant.

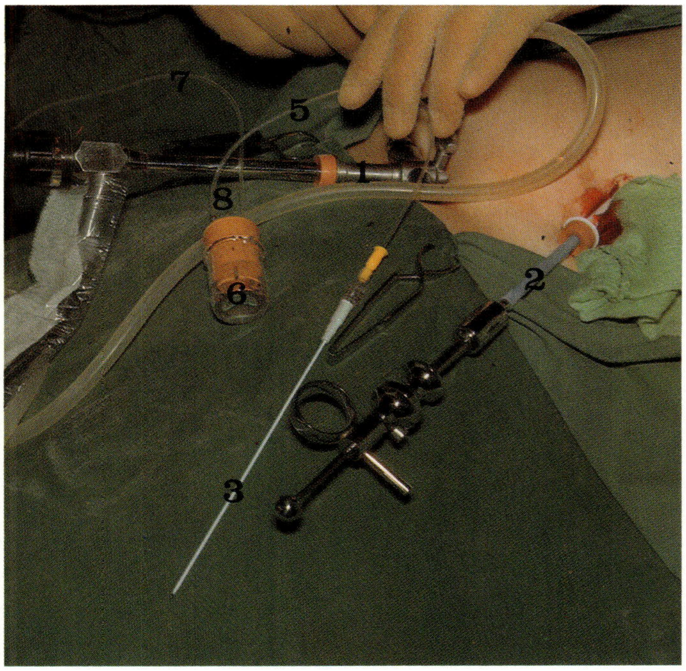

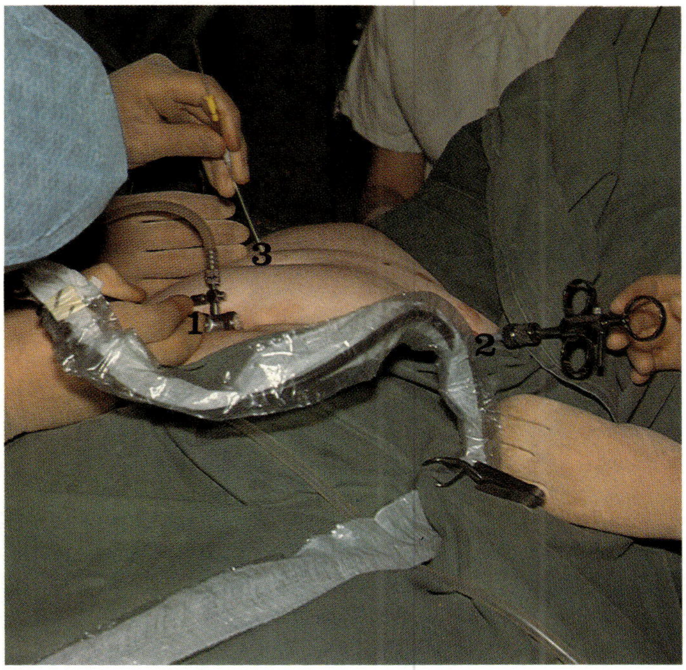

3

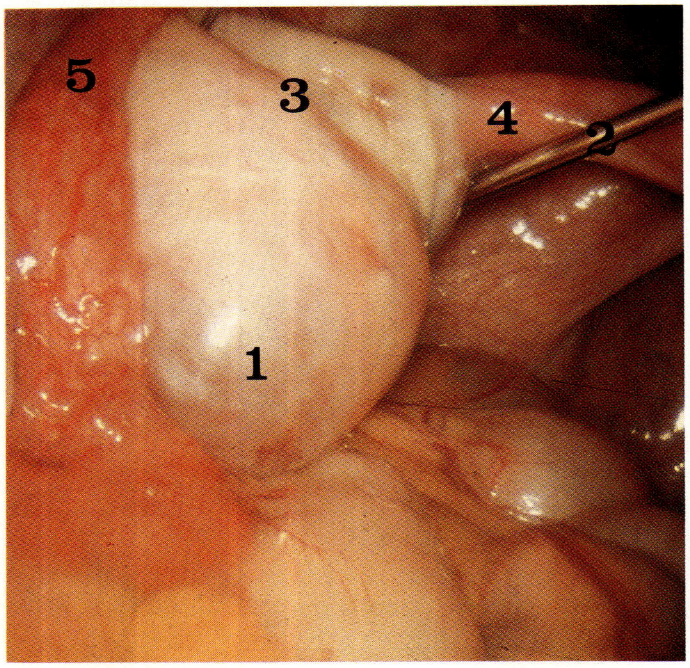

4

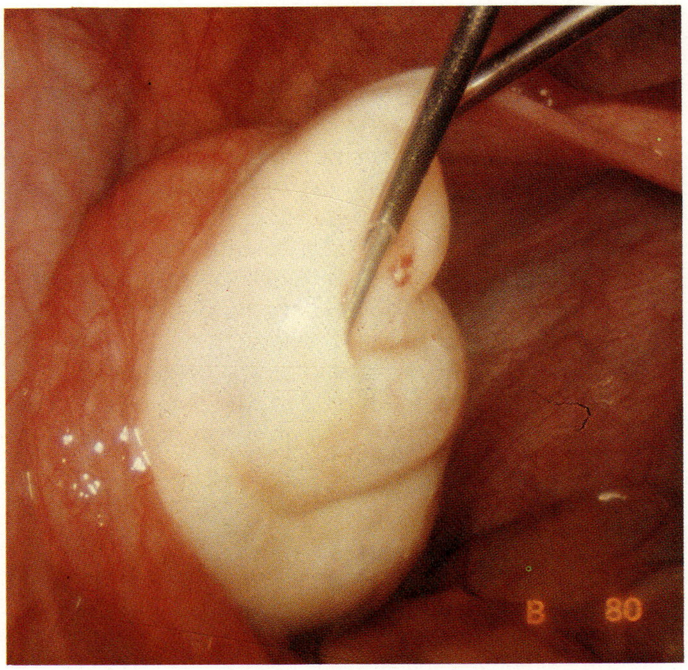

3 and 4 Follicle aspiration
In **Figure 3** the follicle (1) is seen ready to be aspirated. The grasping forceps (2) in this particular case is situated behind the ovary (3) and below the ovarian ligament (4), and has succeeded in rotating the ovary so as to make follicle puncture easier. The fallopian tube is at (5) and the follicle appears as a thin-walled pink swelling, varying in size from 0.5 cm to 3 cm. In **Figure 4** the follicle has been punctured. Usually this is done directly through an avascular area or through the adjacent ovarian stroma so as to prevent leakage of fluid from the distended follicle. Prior to follicle puncture the aspirating needle is cleared of blood and tissue cells by the passage of a medium containing heparin.

Ultrasonic determination of follicle growth

It is now possible to measure follicular growth by ultrasonography (US). Recent evidence from Kerin et al (1981) has shown that in the 5 days prior to ovulation the follicle increases in size from 12 to 23 mm as measured by US. The mean peak diameter of the ovulating follicle was 23.2 ± (SEM) mm (range 18–29 mm) as taken within 24 hours of the LH peak.

5 to 7 Ultrasonographs of follicular growth
Using a B-mode scanner and the full bladder technique of Hackeloer (1979), serial transverse sections of the pelvis show the progressive increase in follicle size as seen on day 8 (**Figure 5**), day 11 (**Figure 6**) and day 15 (**Figure 7**) of the menstrual cycle. The bladder and uterus are marked and the follicle is labelled (1).

5

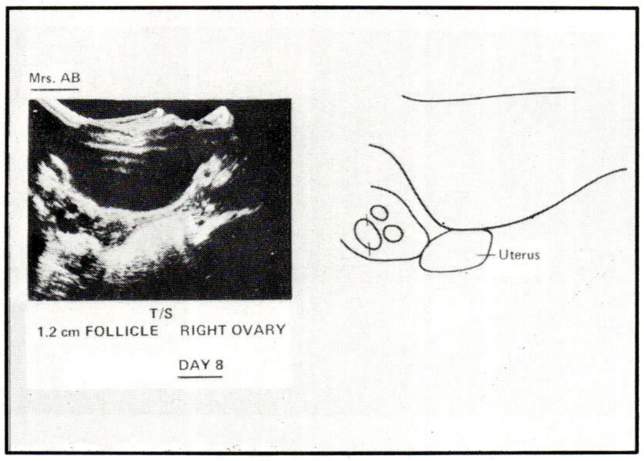

6

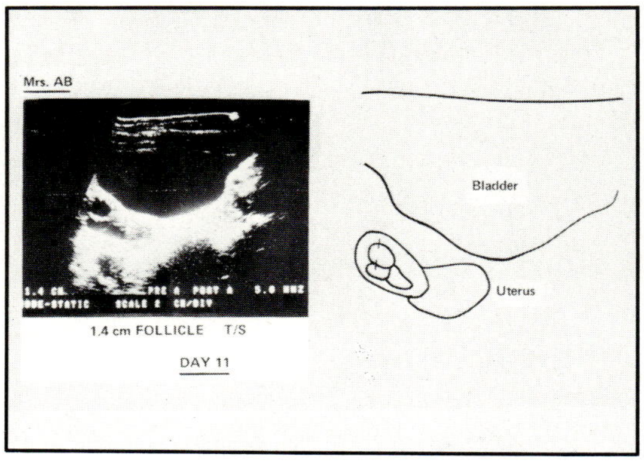

7

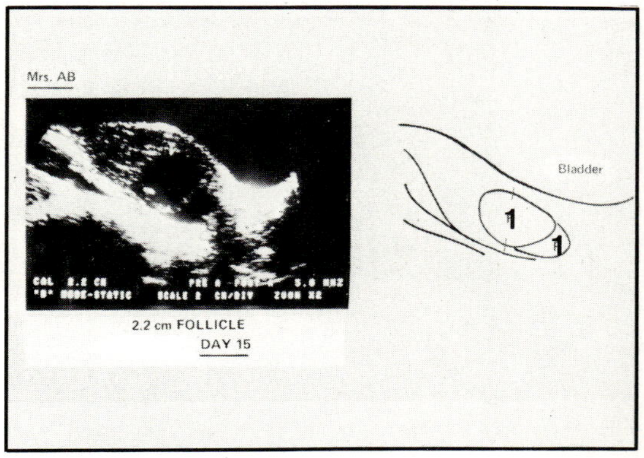

8
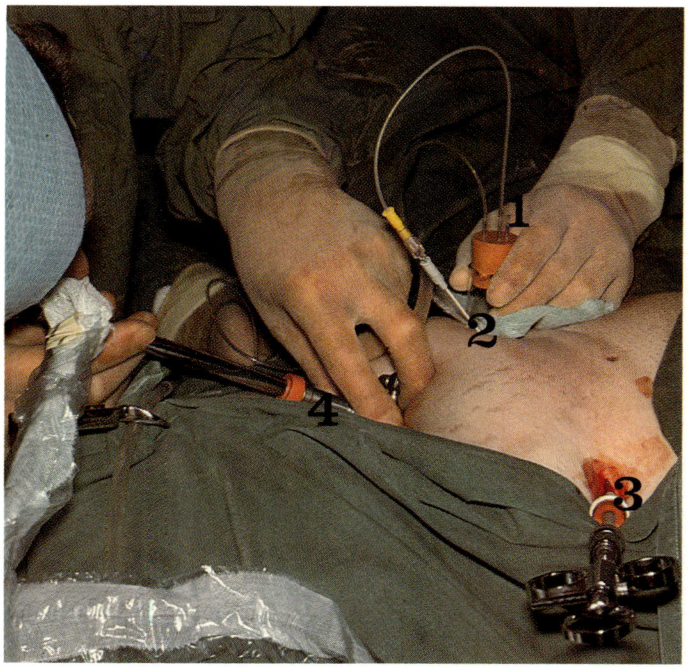

9
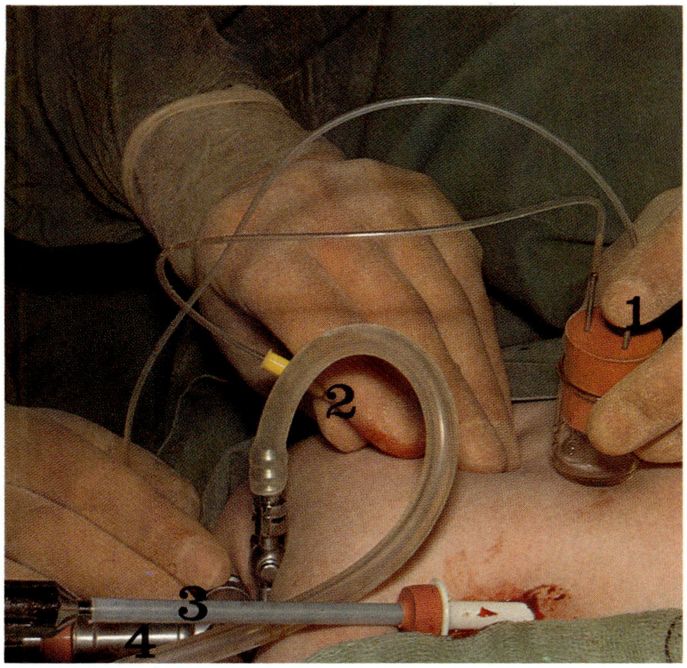

8 and 9 Follicle aspiration
In **Figure 8** the aspiration needle is in situ with its position confirmed by the operator. In **Figure 9** aspiration is occurring and controlled by an assistant's finger on the bypass valve (1). The aspiration needle is at (2), the holding forceps at (3) and the laparoscope at (4). Aspiration is stopped if blood is present around the needle point or in the tubing leading from the aspiration needle to the collecting chamber. The vacuum used should not be above 12 cm Hg in order to avoid damage to the oocyte. A steady flow of gas mixture is required to provide a clear space for the operator.

Handling of ovum
The collecting vessel containing the follicular fluid is taken from the operating theatre to a culture room in which full sterile precautions are observed and there is laminated AVR flow, ultraviolet light and full protective clothing. In Steptoe and Edwards' study the interval between the time of removal of the collecting chamber from the aspiration device and its examination under an examining microscope, was 60 seconds.

Oocytes are detected in the collecting chamber under a low-power stereo microscope. If the follicle is aspirated cleanly then the oocyte is identified quickly, but if contaminated with blood the search for the oocyte is lengthy. Second aspiration of the follicle is sometimes necessary. Preovulatory oocytes with their distinct corona radiata and viscous follicular fluid surrounds are easily seen.

The oocyte is transferred through several culture solutions to remove the erythrocytes and blood plasma if contamination has occurred. Otherwise as in **Figure 10** the aspirated oocytes with two or three drops of medium (1) will be placed in the insemination droplet (2).

Fertilisation

The semen sample is obtained from the husband by masturbation just before commencing laparoscopy and the specimen is examined microscopically to confirm sperm activity. A small sample of semen is suspended in the same media as used for the oocyte afterwards and the seminal plasma is removed by gentle centrifugation.

Oocytes are transferred (as seen in **Figure 10**) into suspensions of sperm held in microdrops, the drops usually containing 1.0 to 1.5×10^6 sperm per ml. The mixture is incubated at 37°C in an atmosphere of 5 per cent CO_2 + 5 per cent O_2 + 90 per cent NO_2 (pH 7.2) for 6 to 18 hours. The culture is examined every 3 hours to assess any change in the corona and cumulus cells and in the viscous fluid surrounding the oocyte.

Certain morphological features indicate fertilisation. These are, an extruded second polar body, cytoplasm of the egg contracting from the zona pellucida, and a male and female pronucleus in the cytoplasm during the late stage of fertilisation approximately 12 to 18 hours after insemination.

Embryo cleavage

After the insemination period the pronucleate egg is transferred into an equilibrated droplet of culture medium under paraffin, for cleavage. Cell division continues and occurs at defined intervals of time so that at 35–46 hours the embryo should contain 2 cells,

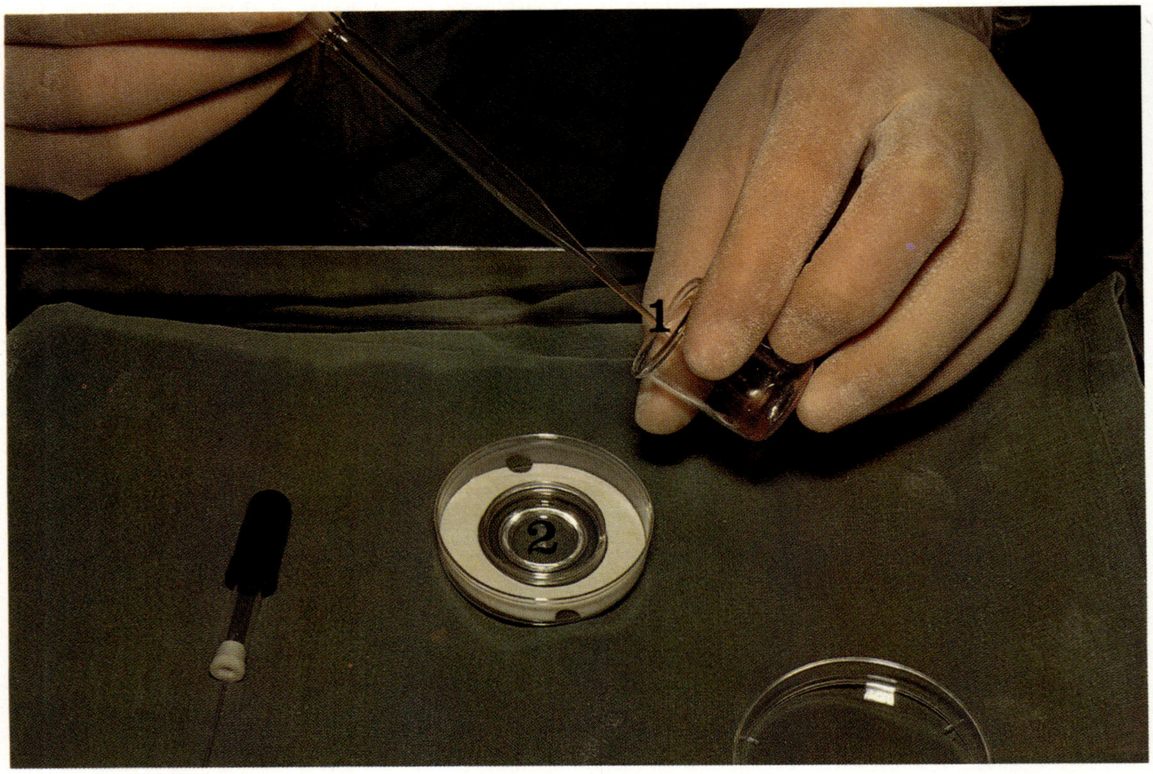

10 Transfer of oocyte to insemination suspension
The aspirated oocytes with two or three drops of medium (1) are about to be placed in the insemination droplet (2).

4 cells being present at 51–63 hours with 8 cells by 68–86 hours. Sixteen cell stage should be obtained by 84–112 hours after insemination. This means that human embryos must be maintained in vitro for 3–4 days before implantation is attempted at the 8–16 cell stage.

Embryo placement

The placement of the embryo into the uterus via the cervix is undertaken without anaesthesia and using a similar technique to that used for AID (page 176). The embryo is loaded into a smooth polythene cannula of 1.3 mm diameter in culture medium under microscopic control. Steptoe and Edwards (1980) recommend holding it 2 cm from the end of the cannula so that expulsion of between 0.05–0.09 ml of the fluid would carry it from the cannula into the uterine cavity.

The loaded cannula is passed into the endometrial cavity so that it lies 1 cm from the fundus. The contents are gently expelled and left to disperse for a few seconds after which the cannula is gently removed and examined to check that the embryo has been successfully expelled. The patient is kept in bed for 10 hours thereafter. Embryo transfer seems to be more successful at night; 4 out of 21 women treated at night conceived whereas none of 11 embryos transplanted during the day survived.

Results

To date only Edwards, Steptoe and Purdy (1980) have released details of their study, in which 4 pregnancies occurred. Fertilisation and cleavage occurred in 34 instances and 32 embryos were implanted. Sixty-eight laparoscopies were performed in order to obtain 44 mature eggs for in vitro insemination. Of these only 34 (77.3 per cent) were fertilised and developed to the 8–16 cell stage. Four pregnancies resulted, with 2 live children; the remaining 2 pregnancies ended in miscarriage, one after an amniocentesis and the other was of a triploid fetus.

It has recently been announced that 4 further pregnancies have been obtained by the team led by Wood and Lopata in Melbourne, Australia.

Conclusions

On the present rate of 6 per cent success (2 live births in 32 embryo transfer) it is doubtful if this technique has yet reached a stage for universal employment. It is, however, the authors' belief that in vitro fertilisation and embryo transfer will in the years to come develop into a technique which will bring relief to many women at present suffering permanent infertility. For this reason they have included these techniques in this volume.

12: Artificial insemination

The artificial introduction of foreign genetic material in the form of sperm into the female genital tract is a simple task but it is associated with complex ethical and moral problems that are well outside the scope of this text. It is the object of the authors to present, for completeness of this volume, a brief resumé of the practice and principles involved in artificial insemination whether of the common donor (AID), or the uncommon husband (AIH) type. An excellent review of the non-clinical aspects of the problem has been published by the Royal College of Obstetricians and Gynaecologists working party on AID (RCOG 1976).

1

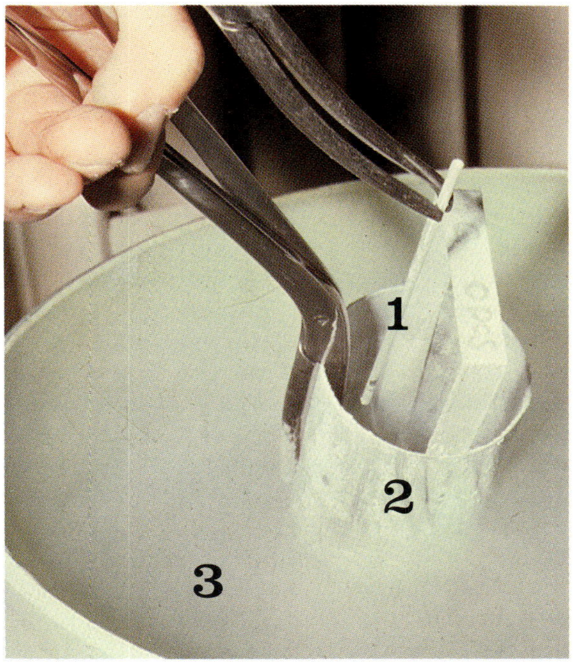

Selection of recipients

It is estimated that the partners in two of every 1000 contracted marriages request AID; representing approximately 4 per cent of those marriages where infertility is due to a male factor.

Couples requesting AID will have undergone a certain degree of self selection before reaching the referral centre. However even though they have arrived at this stage, a certain amount of selection is still needed. Two questions must be considered: the general suitability of both partners for AID and their own reproductive status.

An assessment of the general suitability of the couple for AID is difficult, and it is advisable that they be given general information concerning AID; a suitable introductory leaflet is reproduced in full as Appendix D. Some expert counselling is necessary if a correct assessment is to be made. Special emphasis should be placed on a critical survey of the parental environment and the possible effect that this will have on future children. During such counselling sessions it is important to emphasise the 40–50 per cent failure rate of AID, as undue optimism by the doctor can lead to severe emotional problems when failure occurs following unrealistic expectations.

1 Storage system
A standard storage system. The frozen semen in the form of a pellet is contained in a plastic straw (pailette) (1). The straw is a very economic form of storage and is simple to thaw and prepare. The straws, suitably labelled, are placed in a small metal cannister (2) which is immersed and stored in a liquid nitrogen tank at −196°C (3).

2

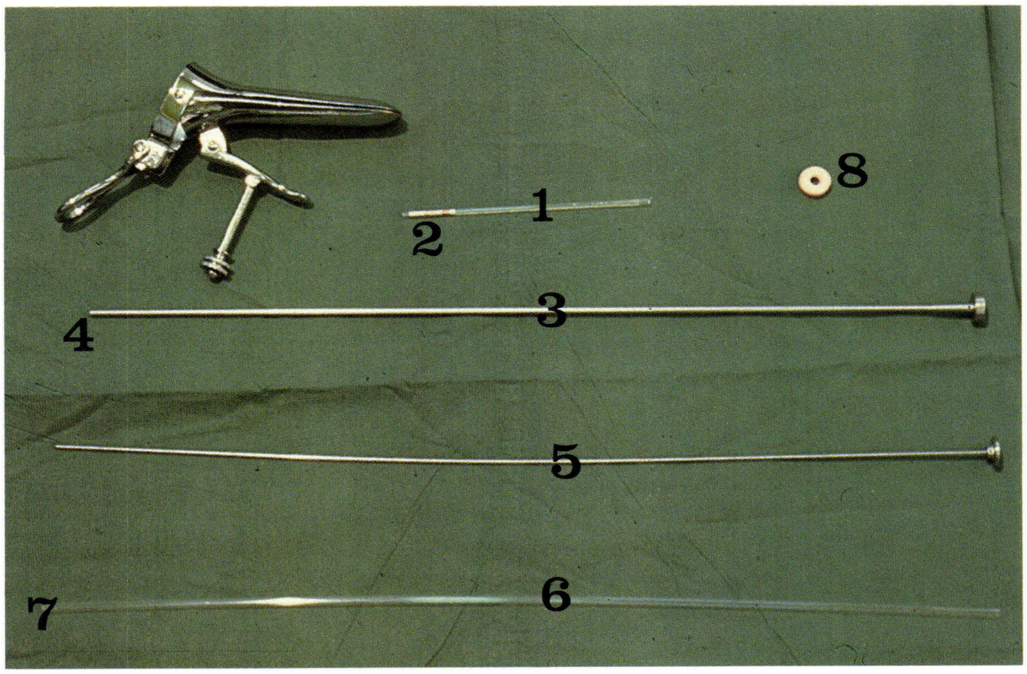

2 Insemination equipment
The straw (1) containing the frozen pellet (2) is placed into a metal delivery tube (3) at its proximal end (4). An introducer (5) is then inserted into the delivery tube and a plastic cover tube (6) with a bevelled non-traumatic end (7) is placed over the metal tube. A small rubber valve (8) is passed down over the metal and plastic cover tube to act as a lever allowing the controlled extrusion of the semen content.

Investigations of recipients

The male partner will probably have untreatable azoospermia or defective spermatogenesis leading to oligozoospermia with a substantial period of infertility. These conditions have been considered earlier (page 17) and a detailed discussion of the analysis of the semen sample is also presented elsewhere (Appendix A). Some gynaecologists insist that two years of regular intercourse must elapse before the wife of an oligospermic male (especially with decreased sperm motility) is considered for AID. Before using AID they estimate the ability of the husband's sperm to penetrate his wife's preovulatory mucus and rarely it will be normal. This probably accounts for the occasional cases (approximately 8 per cent, Matthews 1980) where conception occurs in couples awaiting adoption or AID.

The woman must be fully examined as explained earlier (page 19); this examination always including a laparoscopy. Templeton and Kerr (1977) found significant pelvic abnormalities which would have affected ovum 'pick-up' in 5 of 27 healthy women requesting AID.

3

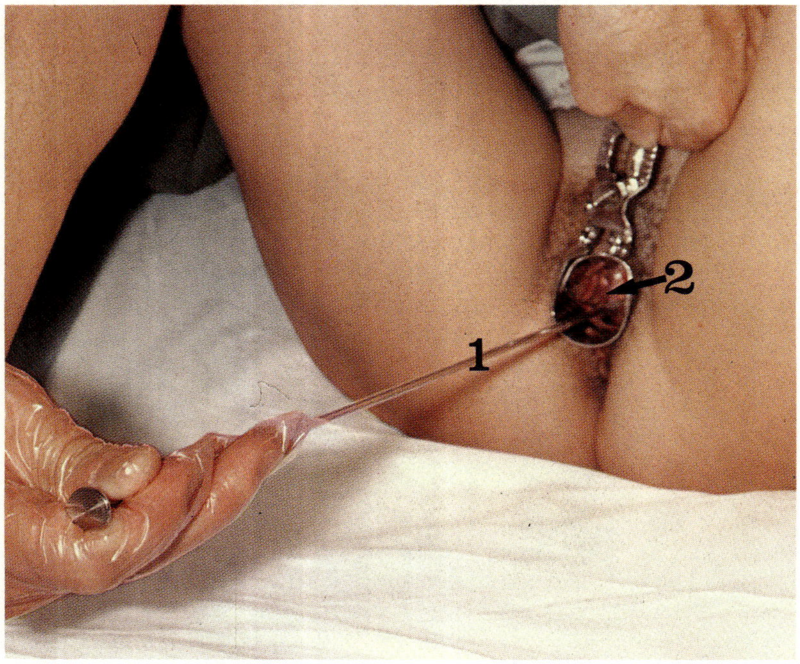

4

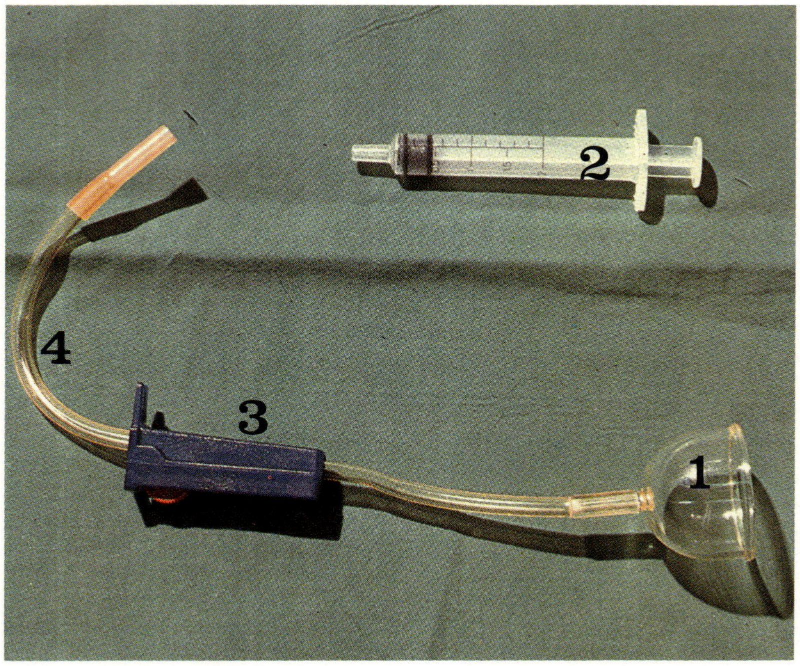

Insemination techniques

Timing of insemination

Detection of the time of ovulation is of the upmost importance in AID and the various methods for the determination of ovulation have been discussed earlier (page 14). The physical and observable changes in cervical mucus are commonly used and also the basal body temperature chart. The hormonal changes of ovulation with the preovulatory rise in plasma oestrogens followed by the dramatic rise in plasma LH, are more accurate and are widely employed. Rapid methods for detecting the LH rise in plasma, by radioimmuno and radioreceptor techniques have also been used while more recently the ultrasonographic estimation of follicular growth (as described in the preceding chapter) provides probably the most accurate estimation of the time of ovulation. Any disturbance in ovulation should be corrected by appropriate therapy as described earlier (page 16); some gynaecologists even induce a 'timed' ovulation with clomiphene in those women with an irregular cycle length.

Introduction of semen into genital tract (Figures 2–4)

3 and 4 Insemination techniques

In **Figure 3** the inseminating device (1) is seen placed just inside the ectocervix (2) allowing the contents of the now thawed pellet of semen (approximately 0.25 ml to 0.5 ml) to be placed in the most suitable position for rapid sperm transport. Some authors believe that the pericervical area is a more suitable position than the ectocervix; others introduce the specimen into the uterine cavity although this latter technique may be associated with frequent painful uterine cramps. Whatever method is used the woman should remain recumbent and preferably with her buttocks supported for at least 15 minutes to avoid seepage of sperm into the lower vagina.

In **Figure 4** a small plastic cap in which the semen is deposited (1) is attached by suction to the cervix. Suction is produced by a syringe (2) and maintained by a simple adjustable tap (3). The specimen is introduced along a 2 ml volume filling tube (4); samples of less than 2 ml need to be inserted directly into the cap.

How often to inseminate?

It is difficult to perform multiple inseminations with fresh semen unless one has an organised service; it is easier with preserved semen when the usual practice is to inseminate frequently during the periovulation period. This entails between 2 and 5 inseminations immediately before, after and coinciding with ovulation. The optimum number of inseminations in a cycle is still the subject of controversy.

Each unsuccessful attempt at AID should be reviewed critically since the continued failure of the technique quickly induces a state of stress in the recipient and her partner and in the former may be detrimental to her ovulatory process. Matthews (1980) showed that between 15 and 25 per cent of women in his AID programme developed either anovulation or defective ovulation during therapy. After 8 unsuccessful cycles, the prospects of conception are very poor and further treatment is usually of little avail.

Selection of donor

It is essential in the practice of AID that both the recipient and the doctor have total confidence that the semen to be used has had the highest possible standards of medical care applied to its source and its substance. Anything less would compromise ethical standards and could lead to legal challenge.

An endeavour is usually made to match donor and recipient in respect of obvious physical, intellectual and racial attributes. Medical screening includes blood grouping, venereal disease investigations, haemoglobin patterns, presence of Australia antigen and karyotyping. The latter is an expensive test and chances of finding a serious abnormal autosomal defect in a phenotypically normal donor are small (i.e. 3–4/1000) but it is considered by some to be important when measured against the number of recipients associated with multiple semen samples from the donor. This subject is discussed in detail by the RCOG working party report (1976).

Collection and storage of specimen

The specimen to be used can either be freshly collected or reconstituted from a preserved sample. Preservation is by freezing and is based on the fact that glycerol is a potent and effective protector of semen from cryo-injury.

The methods used in the cryo-preservation are applied in this order:

- addition of the cryo-protective medium (CPM)
- a short period of equilibration
- cooling (20°C to 5°C) and freezing (5°C–20°C) processes
- storage (−196°C) in liquid nitrogen (**Figure 1**).

Specimens when required for insemination are usually thawed rapidly and following a 15 minute period of equilibrium at 35°C are ready for use. An efficient coding system must be in force for each specimen. Limited information is available concerning retention of fertility after long-term storage but some authors have recorded conceptions after storage of between 3 and 10 years (Sherman 1973).

Results

For the average couple having AID, the chances of producing a live child are between 50 and 60 per cent. A further 10 per cent will conceive, thus leaving 30 to 40 per cent still infertile. It is estimated that 15 to 20 per cent of all AID recipients will conceive in the first cycle of treatment while three-quarters of all conceptions occur within the first six cycles.

There is no obvious difference in conception rates when using fresh or frozen semen (Steinberger and Smith 1973), although one of the highest success rates (72 per cent) reported by Chong and Taymor (1975) was achieved when using a fresh specimen technique.

Artificial insemination by husband (AIH)

This entails the collection, possible storage and delivery of the husband's sperm by direct artificial insemination as already described, or through the use of a cervical cap (**Figure 4**).

The subject of AIH is controversial and many question whether it has a place in clinical practice. There are a number of possible indications:

- where the semen cannot be deposited in the vagina because of organic causes such as epispadias.
- retrograde ejaculation as a result of bilateral sympathectomy, diabetes mellitus, lumbar disc disease, paraplegia or drug therapy.
- paraplegia.
- 'cervical hostility' and the condition in which sperm agglutinating or immobilising antibodies are found in the serum of partners of a prolonged infertility. Intrauterine insemination in these controversial cases would seem logical but reports of significant success are not available.
- questionable semen 'quality'.
- as a prophylactic measure before vasectomy, chemotherapy or irradiation.

Successful results from AIH are few. Dixon et al (1976) obtained only a 9.5 per cent success rate after treating 158 patients; one-half with direct insemination and the other with a cervical cap. There was no difference in success rate for each group. There is as yet no evidence as to whether the first (sperm rich) portion or the total ejaculate is the more successful inseminant. Recent reviews of the subject are by Finegold (1980), Glass (1980), Beck and Wallach (1981) and Philipp and Carruthers (1981).

Appendix A: The infertile male

1. Causes of oligo/azoospermia

Disorders of testicular control
Defects of LH/FSH secretion
Hyperprolactinaemia

Primary testicular disorders
Idiopathic
Varicocele
Chromosomal disorders, i.e. Klinefelter's syndrome
Cryptorchidism
Physical and chemical agents, i.e. drugs
Orchitis (traumatic or infective)
Chronic illness
Immunological disorders
Immotility due to absence of dynein arms

Duct obstruction
Congenital
Inflammatory
Associated with bronchiectases

Accessory duct disorders
Prostatitis
Vesiculitis
Congenital absence of vas/vesicles

Coital defects
Low frequency
Use of lubricants
Impotence
Hypospadias
Retrograde ejaculation

Psychological factors

2. The semen specimen – its collection and assessment

(a) Collection
Written instructions given to the patient should emphasise the following:

- sample collected after 2–7 days of abstinence.
- if the specimen is abnormal then 2 or 3 more should be collected at weekly or biweekly intervals due to the wide variation in sperm production in the one individual.
- delivery should be made to the laboratory within 2 hours.
- the specimen is collected by masturbation into a clear glass or plastic container which must be prewarmed to room temperature. Glass bottles should be washed with detergent, then rinsed in distilled water and dried. No rubber stoppers or condoms must come near the semen sample.
- coitus interruptus is not to be used to collect the sample as it is likely that the first part of the specimen with the highest concentration of sperm will be lost.

(b) Assessment
It is essential that an experienced laboratory undertake the examination of the specimen. The error of measurement of many of the parameters, especially sperm motility and morphology, is high due to the subjective nature of the observation. This means that abnormal results must be interpreted with caution and repeat samples obtained.

Each sample must be assessed on the basis of its collective characteristics as for instance oligospermia is frequently associated with an increase in abnormal sperm forms and a reduction in sperm motility.

The following characteristics of the sample are examined:

(i) General appearance
Ejaculated semen is liquid but coagulates immediately to a gel. It will then liquify within a further 20 minutes and thereafter remain in a viscous state. If liquification does not occur and the sample remains in a partially viscous state then sperm are unable to achieve normal motility and due to the thick semi-solid mass of the specimen a sperm count is difficult. The cause of this abnormal viscosity is not known and may indicate a disorder of accessory gland function.

(ii) Volume
One to four ml is found in about 80 per cent of men; a larger volume than this may also indicate a disorder of the accessory gland.

(iii) Sperm concentration (millions/ml)
Estimates between 15–40 million/ml are considered to represent the lower limit compatible with normal fertility. Counts below this level are in no way incompatible with potential fertility and the evaluation of future fertility must not depend solely on sperm concentration; due attention must be given to the following parameters.

(iv) Total sperm concentration
The usually accepted lower limit of normal is 50 million.

(v) Sperm motility
This is an important characteristic and is determined subjectively by grading the forward progression made by the largest number of sperm. The gradations are 'none, poor, good and excellent'. In the normal semen specimen more than 50 per cent of sperm should show good or excellent motility. Some authors insist that it is the quality of forward motion that is important. It is suggested by other authors that men with abnormal motility specimens should have them repeated after 48–72 hours of sexual abstinence with analysis within 30 minutes to determine whether their initial quantitative and/or qualitative motility is good but rapidly declines, or is poor from the start.

(vi) Sperm morphology
In a stained smear the normal sperm has an oval head and a single tail piece. Abnormalities in morphology are classified according to various sperm head configurations, i.e. large or small size, amorphous or double, or of an abnormal shape. The majority of fertile men have more than 60 per cent and four-fifths have more than 70 per cent of normal oval forms. Variations occur in relation to intercurrent illness or stress when a preponderance of tapered shapes and amorphous forms persist.

(vii) Evidence of infection
An excessive number of leukocytes, particularly polymorphs and other cellular debris (i.e. bacteria, epithelial cells or immature germ cells in the stained smear) indicate genital tract infection.

(viii) Fructose concentration
Seminal vesicle function can be measured by this test but has marked individual variations, i.e. 4–28 mmol. If it is low or absent it may indicate obstruction to the vesicle ducts, i.e. after infection, or congenital absence of the vesicles and/or vasal agenesis.

The reader is advised of a recent publication by the World Health Organisation's special programme for research, development and research training in human reproduction – a monograph entitled Laboratory manual for the examination of human semen and semen-mucus interactions *(eds. Belsey, M.A. et al, Press Concern, Singapore, 1980).*

3. Management of treatable and untreatable causes

Management of treatable causes
The number of patients who can be treated for conditions in which there is a chance of improving fertility is small. It is therefore essential that these conditions be diagnosed and treated when present. They are:

- Varicocele
- Obstruction of the epididymus
- Infection of genital tract
- Gonadotrophin deficiency
- Hyperprolactinaemia

Treatment for *varicocele* should be reserved for those with subfertility who possess a clinically palpable varicocele or a subclinical one detected by Doppler flow measurement or retrograde venography. *Obstruction* of the epididymus results in azoospermia, normal sized testes and normal FSH levels. Clinical examination may reveal either congenital absence of the vas and no fructose in the semen or an enlarged head of epididymus which may be tender. Further diagnostic aids such as vasography and biopsy may be done but the results for reparative surgery (i.e. vaso-epididymostomy) are not encouraging, i.e. 5–30 per cent. *Infection* may be diagnosed from a history of acute/sub-acute genital tract inflammation resulting in a high number of leukocytes in the semen (>5 million per ml) with occasional reduction in motility, increase in agglutination and variations in semen volume. Pretreatment is given in the form of antibiotics which are concentrated in seminal secretions (i.e. dimethylchlortetracycline, erythromycin and trimethoprim-sulphamethoxazole combination). *Gonadotrophin deficiency* is very uncommon; men with hypogonadotrophic hypogonadism can possibly be rendered fertile by gonadotrophin replacement therapy. *Hyperprolactinaemia* is also uncommon and sometimes associated with a pituitary adenoma (prolactinoma).

Management of untreatable and 'idiopathic' causes
Several disorders of spermatogenesis result in irreversible infertility. In these the germ cells are absent or fail to differentiate beyond a certain stage. Although the cause in many cases is unknown, there are certain well known associations such as orchitis, mumps, cryptorchidism, chromosomal abnormalities, cytotoxic drugs and irradiation. These conditions must be recognised and a realistic appraisal given to the couple.

Half of the men with no obvious cause for their semen abnormality, are designated as an *'idiopathic group'*. Various forms of empirical treatment have been given to this group with occasional success. Such agents as testosterone (rebound therapy), clomiphene, gonadotrophins, mesterolone, steroids and thyroxine have been tried.

The major need for understanding male infertility is additional research with precise definition of obvious causative conditions and the establishment of randomised controlled clinical trials to evaluate the various therapeutic regimes.

Further details of treatment for individual causes (as listed in the flow charts on pages 20 and 180) are given on page 180.

4a. Schema for investigation and treatment of the infertile couple

(cont. from page 20)

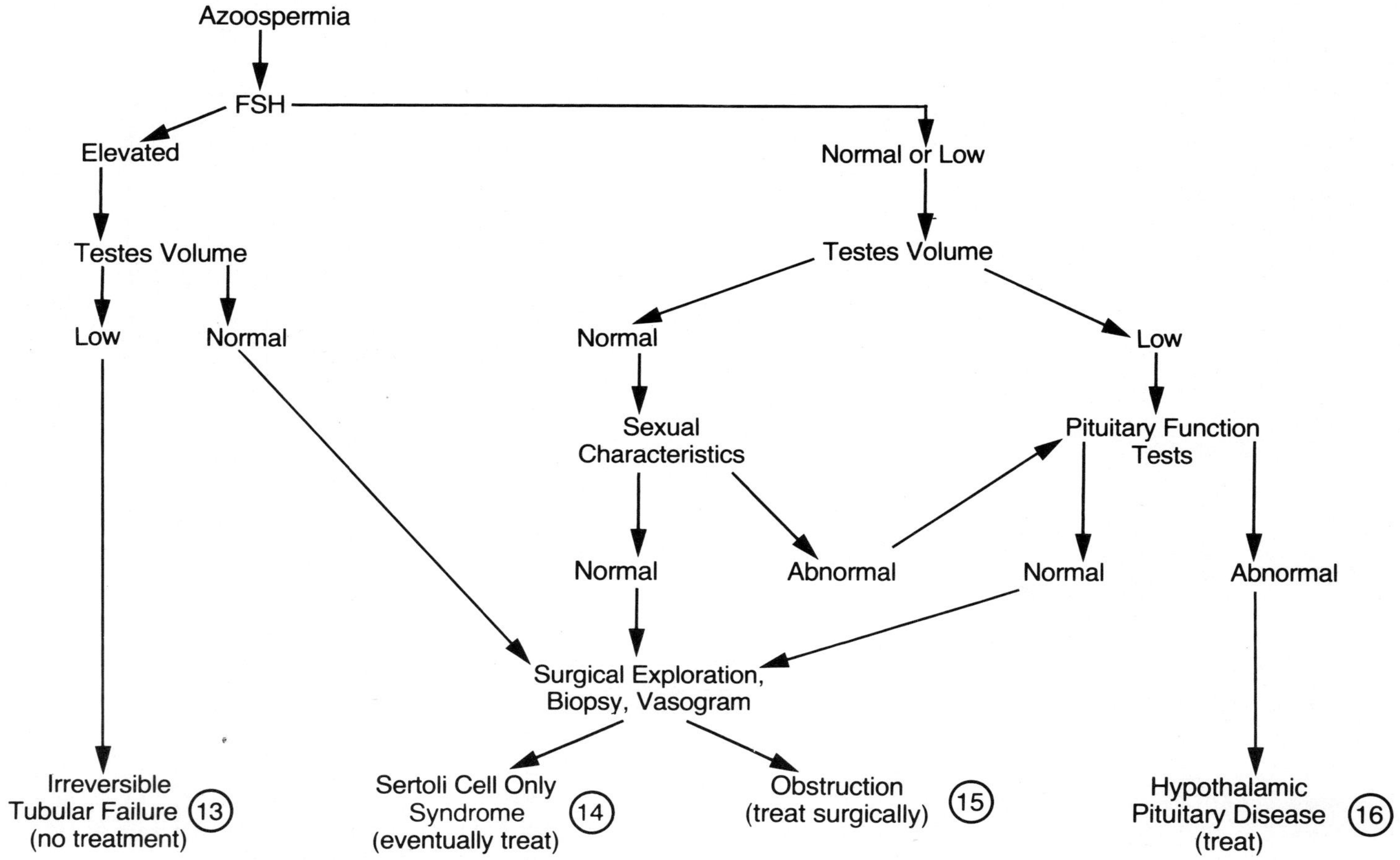

4b. Details of treatment of individual causes (as featured in the flow charts above and on page 20)

(1) Sexual dysfunction, including sexual impotence or anejaculation (ejaculatory failure) should be treated by means of sex therapy.

(2) Varicocele treatment should only be offered if semen analysis is abnormal. Treatment aims at complete interruption of reflux in the internal spermatic vein(s).

(3) Idiopathic epididymal-testicular failure with teratozoospermia has poor prognosis and generally is resistant to treatment.

(4) Male adnexitis (prostatovesiculitis) should be treated with antibiotics against aerobic strains (dimethylchlortetracycline, erythromycin and trimethoprim-sulpha methoxazole combination, semisynthetic penicillins), and/or against anaerobic strains (metronidazole), together with an anti-inflammatory drug (Indomethacine, Naproxen). Recovery to normal sperm quality however is rather uncommon.

(5) Immunological infertility is mostly due to sperm agglutination but may occur without this phenomenon. Treatments proposed are intrauterine insemination of isolated, non-agglutinated spermatozoa, or immunosuppressive doses of corticosteroids.

(6) Idiopathic testicular failure will be treated preferentially with an anti-oestrogen (Tamoxifen 20 mg/day or Clomiphene citrate 25 mg/day); other treatments proposed have not yet been proved to be effective in (placebo) controlled trials.

(7) Hypothalamo-pituitary hypofunction may be treated with HMG (3×150 U/week) + HCG (500 U/week). Pituitary tumours need adequate medical or surgical management followed by gonadotropin treatment.

(8) Partial epididymal obstruction may be due to fibrocystic degeneration or chronic (silent) infection. Surgery should be considered, together with antibiotic and anti-inflammatory treatment.

(9) Irreversible lesions are either intratesticular fibrosis (sequellae of orchitis or testicular haemorrhage), or meiotic abnormalities, or idiopathic maturation reduction (Sertoli cell dysfunction?).

(10) If anejaculation is exclusively coital, and no psychological contraindication is present, artificial insemination with husband's semen may be offered.

(11) In retrograde ejaculation due to sphincter dysfunction a three week treatment trial with imipramide may be considered. If not successful in normalising ejaculation, artificial insemination with alcalinised post-orgasm urine can be attempted.

(12) In the presence of normal findings at routine semen analysis, an *in vitro* penetration test (either Kurzrock Miller or Kremer capillary test) should be performed. If this is normal and infertility remains unexplained, an *in vitro* penetration test of zona free hamster eggs may further prove valuable. Impaired *in vitro* penetration in cervical mucus may point to an immunological factor in male or female, or to other causes of cervical hostility.

(13) Irreversible tubular lesion may be due to Klinefelter's syndrome, Sertoli cell only syndrome, acquired testicular atrophy after testicular torsion, orchitis, cryptorchidism or arterial occlusion (hernia operation). AID or adoption may be offered.

(14) After exclusion of meiotic disturbances, and in the presence of idiopathic maturation arrest at the spermatid level, treatment with either HMG + HCG, or HCG alone, or the androgen rebound method, may be attempted. Chances of success are however poor.

(15) If testicular biopsy reveals full spermatogenesis, epididymo-vasostomy or vaso-vasostomy may be attempted. Alloplastic spermatocele is experimentally implanted in congenital agenesis or acquired complete obstruction of the vasa deferentia, provided the epididymus is healthy.

(16) After full investigation of hypothalamus and pituitary, hypogonadotrophic hypogonadism will be treated with HMG (3×150 U/week) + HCG (1×500 U/week) generally yielding satisfactory results.

Appendix B: Diagnosis of utero-tubal disease

SIGNIFICANT FINDINGS IN PATIENTS WITH INFERTILITY (PRIMARY AND SECONDARY) WITH NO CLINICALLY DETECTABLE ABNORMALITY

Condition	Primary Infertility		Secondary Infertility	
	study (1)*	(2)†	(1)	(2)
	number 209	520	70	155
	%		%	
Normal	68	62	40	49
Abnormal				
Peritubo-ovarian adhesions with patent tubes	9	5	30	5
Pelvic adhesions *plus*				
– bilateral tubal block	4	8	16	16
– unilateral tubal block	2	9	4	12
Distal tubal block	4	3	4	2
Apparent isthmic tubal block	3	—	1	—
Ovarian endometriosis	5	9	1	4
Miscellaneous (i.e. fibroids, congenital abnormalities)	5	4	4	12

*Templeton & Kerr (1977).
†Duignan et al (1972).

Appendix C: Surgery of the fallopian tube

1. Basic pre and postoperative considerations in tubal surgery

1 Investigation and treatment of both partners should always be complete before surgery is undertaken. Hysterosalpingography and laparoscopy should have been done in all cases.

2 The patient and her husband must be realistic about the results of tubal surgery and be prepared to accept the risk of ectopic pregnancy following such surgery.

3 Recent infection contraindicates operation. There should be no signs of active inflammation in the three months preceding operations and ESR and blood levels should be normal.

4 Surgery should be done in the mid-proliferative phase of the menstrual cycle as this is the anabolic and regenerative stage. The outside possibility of disturbing an early pregnancy is also avoided.

5 Antibiotic cover is essential except possibly in tubal reanastomosis where there should be no question of infection. It should be given for at least 14 days postoperatively.

6 It has not been the authors' custom to use steroids since it is considered that they interfere with healing; a case could however be made for their use to prevent adhesions following salpingolysis and salpingostomy. A suitable regime is given in Chapter 10, page 168.

7 Ventrosuspension following tubal operations is not recommended. Any advantages are likely to be outweighed by the risks of peritoneal trauma and adhesion.

8 Postoperative hydrotubation has not been used by the authors and the literature indicates a trend towards its omission.

9 Laparoscopic examination six weeks following operation is considered unjustifiable although the case for later laparoscopy to view results is discussed on page 169.

10 Personal postoperative follow-up is essential.

2. Suggested FIGO classification of tubal surgery (Miami classification)

I. Tubal implantation
A. Isthmus
B. Ampulla (i.e. when isthmus removed)

II. Tubal anastomosis
A. Cornual – to isthmus
– to ampulla (isthmus absent)
B. Isthmic – to isthmus
– to ampulla
C. Ampulla – to ampulla

III. Salpingoneostomy
A. Terminal (opening outer point of tube)
B. Medial (mid-ampulla)
C. Isthmic (includes linear salpingostomy)

IV. Fimbrioplasty
A. Deagglutination
B. Incision of fibrous ring
C. Incision of tube wall

V. Adhesiolysis
1. Mild: 1 cm of tube/ovary involved
2. Moderate: partially encapsulated tube/ovary
3. Severe: complete encapsulation of tube/ovary

VI. Combinations
A. Different operation right and left tube
B. Different operations on same tube

VII. Other
A. Transplantation
B. Estes procedure (Estes 1924)
C. Insertion of prosthetic tube (Taylor 1971)

Appendix D: Artificial insemination – a guide to the infertile couple

(This is the text of a booklet issued by the Royal College of Obstetricians and Gynaecologists, London, 1979, and reproduced with their kind permission)

Artificial insemination has been practised in the United Kingdom for many years. Each year several hundred children are born following this procedure, bringing a great deal of happiness to the parents.

Artificial insemination can be carried out using the husband's own sperm, in which case it is known as AIH (Artificial Insemination by Husband), or another man's sperm, in which case it is known as AID (Artificial Insemination by Donor). The semen used in both cases may be either stored frozen, or freshly produced.

AID (Artificial Insemination by Donor)
This booklet is concerned with AID. This is available to happily married couples who both agree that they want children but where for a variety of reasons it is inadvisable or impossible to use the husband's sperm. In other words AID is an alternative to adoption when the main factor leading to infertility or avoidance of pregnancy is on the male side. This may be because the husband is unlikely ever to father a child due to low sperm fertility, or if there is a very high risk of the couple producing an abnormal baby, or because the husband's and wife's blood groups are incompatible and sensitisation has occurred. It is important to exclude any treatable cause of infertility before AID is considered and certain simple tests will have to be carried out initially by the doctor on both you and your husband. Further tests may be needed during the course of treatment.

Selecting AID donors
The donors are carefully selected. They are required to be intelligent, fit and healthy and on questioning to have given no family history of hereditary disease. They must all be of very high fertility and every specimen of semen is checked before it is used to make sure that it reaches an acceptable standard.

Matching donors
Most centres will try, as far as possible, to use a donor who has the same physical characteristics as your husband.

Confidentiality
The clinic is organised and your notes are kept in such a way that confidentiality is preserved. For example, the name of the donor is kept strictly confidential, so that there is no way in which you can learn his identity, and similarly, your name will not be known to the donor.

Treatment
The treatment itself is straightforward and painless. It will be carried out by a doctor or nurse who will insert a simple instrument into your vagina to place the sperm in the mucus at the neck of the womb. You will probably be asked to rest for a short time after this has been done. It is important not to douche or bath immediately before or after treatment. However, it is all right to carry on with sexual intercourse as usual, unless the doctor advises against this.

Timing
Once the couple have decided that they would like AID treatment, it is done during the fertile period each month. The most fertile time is likely to be about fourteen days before your next period is due, and before the small rise in body temperature which follows ovulation. You may notice an increase in vaginal discharge at this time.

Pregnancy following AID
Once you have conceived through AID your pregnancy should follow a normal course. Having AID will not effect your chances of having a normal pregnancy, normal delivery and normal baby. This is so whether your doctor uses fresh or frozen semen. However, every pregnancy carries some risks, and AID does not protect you from these. You can still have a miscarriage or a baby with some defect but the chances of this happening are certainly no greater than usual.

Legal aspects
There are no laws against AID in the United Kingdom, and provided it is carried out with the husband's consent it cannot constitute grounds for divorce on the basis of unreasonable conduct.

Legitimacy of the baby
There is at present no legal guide for the registration of the AID baby. Strictly speaking, a baby conceived by AID should be registered as 'father unknown' and since it would then be illegitimate, the parents should adopt it. However, babies born within a marriage are presumed to be legitimate and provided you do not abstain from intercourse during the period in which AID was carried out there can be no certainty that any child conceived is not your husband's. We hope that some definite guidance, by the courts or by Parliament, will eventually be given to couples having AID. You should consider seeking the advice of a solicitor; he could also advise you about any possible problems concerning inheritance of property.

Telling your child
Unless you decide to tell your child, there is no reason for him (or her) ever to know that he (or she) was conceived by AID. Whether or not you do so is entirely up to you.

Success rate
Most women who become pregnant do so within six months. A small proportion of women will never become pregnant with this treatment, and some clinics put a limit on the length of time they will treat you.

Risks of infection
Many couples ask if there is any chance of suffering from a sexually transmitted infection following donor insemination. There is virtually no chance of this happening, because all donors are carefully screened and each semen sample is checked before use. In the highly unlikely event of such an infection occurring, treatment with antibiotics is possible.

Consent Form

for Completion by the Husband and Wife

To: Dr ....

We, ... (*husband*)

and .... (*wife*)

of .... (*full address*)
hereby request and authorise you or a suitably trained member of your staff to inseminate artificially

.... (*wife*)
by means of semen supplied by a donor selected by you. The possible medical consequences of the procedure have been explained to us by

Dr ....
and we have, in addition, read the booklet entitled 'Artificial Insemination', a copy of which we have initialled and which is attached to this consent form.

Signature of Husband ....

Signature of Wife ....

Dated this .... *day of* .... 19..........

Signature of Witness ....

Address ....

Occupation ....

Please Note

The form should be completed by the husband or wife in their own handwriting. The Witness may be any person other than the doctor named above.

Appendix E: Documentation of investigations and management of the infertile couple

A comprehensive protocol is presented which is suitable for the clinical documentation of the investigation and management of an infertile couple. The recorded data are appropriate for computer recording and similar protocols have been successfully employed in a number of European clinics. It is very detailed and serves as a guide to what questions should be asked at the interview and what the physical examination of each partner entails. It also provides information on the nature of the investigations which may be required.

The interview should be conducted in as informal and relaxed an atmosphere as possible. Completion of some of the data, especially that related to the sexual history, may with advantage be left to the end of the interview or even later. An attempt to complete the collection of all the information during the actual interview can lessen rapport with the patient and her husband and may lead to their becoming apprehensive or embarrassed. One has to be careful to avoid such a development and delicate questions can profitably be postponed to subsequent interviews.

1. General information

Includes presenting problem, coital and contraception details, menstrual and reproductive history.

Hospital clinic number ....

Names of couple

male (family).......................... *(given)* ....

female (family).......................... *(given)* ....

Age (completed years)

male ....

female ....

Ethnic group/race

male ....

female ....

Present occupation and duration

male ....(years)

female ....(years)

Duration of marriage/union ....(years)

Presenting problem

Primary infertility ....

Secondary infertility (same partner) ....

Secondary infertility (different partner) ....

Number of months trying to conceive ....

Previous infertility investigations

male ....

female ....
(give exact details)

Sexual history

Number of previous marriages ....

Frequency of vaginal intercourse
(per week) over last six months ....

Knowledge of fertile time (yes/no) ....

Ejaculation (yes/no) ....

Penetration (yes/no) ....

Dyspareunia (yes/no) ....

Enjoyable for male (yes/no) ....

female (yes/no) ....

Douches (yes/no) ....

Contraceptive history
Times used (never, premarital, only in previous marriage, only in present marriage, during previous and present)

....

Type used (pill, IUD, condom, withdrawal, rhythm – natural, other)

method ....

length ....(months)

Menstrual cycle disturbance while taking and/or after stopping oral contraception ....

....

Menstrual history

Age at menarche ....(years)

Amenorrhoea (primary/secondary) ....(months)

Cycle length (average) ....(days)

shortest in previous two years ....(days)

longest in previous two years ....(days)

Duration of menstrual flow (average for previous six months) .... (days)

Dysmenorrhoea (yes/no) ....

Reproductive history

Pregnancy during present marriage/union (yes/no) ....

Time since last pregnancy ....(months)

Results of pregnancies (in present marriage/union, and previous to present marriage/union)

(number)

livebirths	present..........	previous..........
stillbirths	present..........	previous..........
spontaneous abortions (weeks)	present..........	previous..........
induced abortions	present..........	previous..........
ectopic pregnancies	present..........	previous..........
molar pregnancies	present..........	previous..........

Outcome of last pregnancy

livebirth ....

stillbirth ....

spontaneous abortion ....(weeks)

induced abortion ....

ectopic pregnancy ....

molar pregnancy ....

2. Specific information – female

Includes family, gynaecological, medical, surgical and social history.

Family history

History of any of the following (yes/no); if yes, give details (tuberculosis, thyroid disease, diabetes mellitus)

....

Gynaecological history

History of sexually transmitted disease (yes/no); if yes, give details

(e.g. syphilis, gonorrhoea, lymphogranulomata, herpes genitalis, chlamydia, mycoplasma, non-specific, other)

....

time since last episode ....(months)

number of episodes ....

History of pelvic infection ....

time since last episode ....(months)

number of episodes ....

Medical history

History of weight loss/gain (yes/no); if yes, give details

....

History of any of the following (yes/no); if yes, give details

(tuberculosis, thyroid disease, radiotherapy/cytoxic therapy, diabetes mellitus, other)

....

....

Surgical history

Tubo-ovarian surgery (yes/no); if yes, list type and outcome

....

Uterine surgery (yes/no); if yes, list type and outcome

....

Abdominal surgery (yes/no); if yes, list type and outcome

....

if appendicectomy, was it complicated/uncomplicated

....

Social history

Alcohol consumption ....(gm/day)

Tobacco consumption ....(cigarettes/day)

History of addictive drug consumption (yes/no); if yes, give details

....

3. Specific information – male

Includes family, genito-urinary, medical, surgical, sexual and social history.

Family history

History of any of the following (yes/no); if yes, give details

(tuberculosis, thyroid disease, diabetes mellitus)

....

Genito-urinary history

History of sexually transmitted disease (yes/no); if yes, give details

(e.g. syphilis, gonorrhoea, lymphogranulomata, chlamydia, mycoplasma, herpes genitalis, non-specific urethritis, other)

....

time since last episode ....(months)

number of episodes ....

History of pelvic organ infection (yes/no); if yes, give details

(epididymo-orchitis, prostatitis, other) ....

....

time since last infection ....(months)

History of mumps orchitis (yes/no); if yes, was it pre- or post-puberty

....

Medical history

History of any of the following (yes/no); if yes, give details

(tuberculosis, diabetes mellitus, thyroid disease, parasitic infestation, bronchiectasis, neurological disease, radiotherapy or cytoxic therapy)

....

Surgical history

History of any of the following (yes/no); if yes, give details

(orchidopexy, herniorrhaphy/otomy, varicocele, ligation, vasectomy, bladder neck surgery, tubular surgery, testicular trauma)

....

Sexual history

Number of pregnancies from previous marriages/unions

....

Time since last fertilisation ....(years)

Problems with erection (yes/no) ....

Problems with ejaculation (yes/no) ....

Social history

Alcohol consumption ....(gm/day)

Tobacco consumption ....(cigarettes/day)

History of addictive drug consumption (yes/no); if yes, give details

....

4. Examination – female

General

Height ....(cm)

Weight ....(Kg)

Blood pressure ....

Secondary sexual characteristics (normal/abnormal)

....

Hair distribution (normal/abnormal) ....

Breasts – discharge or galactorrhoea ....

Any evidence of dysfunction of the following organ systems (yes/no); if yes, give details

(thyroid, adrenal, cardiovascular, respiratory, gastro-intestinal, neurological)

....

Pelvic examination

Vulva (normal/abnormal – if abnormal, describe)

....

Clitoris (normal/abnormal) ....

Hymen (normal/abnormal) ....

Vagina (normal/abnormal) ....

discharge (yes/no); if yes, list type

(e.g. trichomonal, monilial, other) ....

Uterine prolapse (yes/no) ....

Cervix (normal/abnormal) ....

Uterus (normal/abnormal) ....

Adnexae (normal/abnormal) ....

5. Investigations – female

General

Full blood count (inc. ESR) ....

Full urinalysis ....

Tests of tubal patency

Hysterosalpingography ....

Laparoscopy (diagram/photograph)

(indicate the presence of any adhesions, endometriosis, and describe the status of both tubes and their patency)

....

....

Assessment of endometrial cavity (optional – see page 36) (either as determined by D & C or hysteroscopy with emphasis placed on the presence of intrauterine adhesions, submucous fibroids, congenital malformations, polypi etc)

Hormonal investigations (see pages 13–14)

test *date, results and comments*

Plasma FSH ....(IU/L)

Plasma LH ....(IU/L)

Plasma oestradiol ....(pg/ml)

or

24 hour urine excretion of total oestrogens

....(n mol/24 hr)

Plasma progesterone ....(ng/ml or n mols/L)

day of cycle obtained ....

Plasma prolactin ....(mIU/L)

repeat (if elevated) ....

Thyroxine ....(n mols/L)

Basal body temperature chart (see comments, page 14)

(generally indicative of ovulation/anovulation/other?)

Other investigations (dependent on diagnosis, see page 20)

which may include

Endometrial biopsy ....

Leucocyte karyotype ....

Ovarian biopsy ....

Visual fields ....

Skull x-ray, CAT scan ....

Other tests of pituitary function, i.e. LHRH test

....

Dexamethasone test (Cortisol) ....

5B. Diagnosis prior to treatment commencement (see page 20)

....

....

....

6. Examination – male

General

Height ....(cm)

Weight ....(Kg)

Blood pressure ....

Secondary sexual characteristics (normal/abnormal)

....

Hair distribution (normal/abnormal) ....

Gynaecomastia (yes/no) ....

Urogenital system

Inguinal examination (normal/abnormal – if abnormal, describe)

(e.g. scars, lymphadenopathy) ....

Penis (normal/abnormal – if abnormal, describe)

(e.g. hypospadias, phimosis etc) ....

Testes (normal/abnormal – if abnormal, describe)

(e.g. tenderness, consistency, position – scrotal, inguinal, elsewhere)

....

volume (as measured by Prader orchidometer)

right ....(ml)

left ....(ml)

Vasa deferentia (normal/abnormal – if abnormal, describe)

(e.g. non-palpable, thickened, tender etc) ....

....

Epididymitis (normal/abnormal – if abnormal, describe)

(e.g. non-palpable, thickened, tender, cystic, nodular etc)

....

Scrotal swellings (yes/no – if yes, type) ....

Varicocele – if present, is it

grade I (valsalva positive) ....

grade II (palpable) ....

grade III (visible) ....

is it detectable by the Doppler blood flow technique (yes/no) (see page 19) ....

Rectal examination – prostate (normal/abnormal – if abnormal, describe)

(e.g. enlargement, consistency, tenderness)

....

7. Investigations – male

General

Full blood count (including ESR) ....

Full urinalysis ....

Seminal fluid analysis

	Volume (ml)	Density ($\times 10^6$/ml)	Motility (%)	Abnormal forms (%)	WBC (yes/no)
1st					
2nd*					
3rd*					

**Note the number of days between specimens*

Immunological tests of mucus/sperm interaction (if indicated)

....

Seminal fluid biochemistry (if indicated)

(including pH, fructose, acid phosphatase)

....

Seminal fluid culture (if indicated) ....

Prostatic secretion culture (if indicated) ....

Post coital urine – sperm present (if indicated)

Hormonal investigations (if indicated)

test — *date, results and comments*

Plasma FSH ....(IU/L)

Plasma LH ....(IU/L)

Plasma testosterone ....(n mols/L)

Prolactin ....(mIU/L)

repeat (if elevated) ....

Other investigations (dependent on diagnosis, see page 20)

which may include

Leucocyte karyotype ....

Testicular biopsy ....

Vasogram ....

Retrograde venography (internal spermatic vein) see page 19

....

Thermography (scrotal) see page 19 ....

Visual fields ....

Skull x-ray ....

Other tests of pituitary function, i.e. LHRH test

7B. Diagnosis prior to treatment commencement (see page 20)

....

....

....

8. Treatment, response and management

The documentation of the progress of treatment and the response to different therapeutic regimes is difficult. The authors have therefore reproduced a schema for such follow-up recordings of the couple which has been successfully used in the infertility clinic at King's College Hospital, London.

Female Treatment Codes

00 = under investigation	10 = myomectomy
01 = none	11 = uterine reconstruction
02 = clomiphene	12 = cervical cautery
03 = bromocriptine	13 = wedge resection
04 = ethinyl oestradiol	14 =
05 = HCG	**Tubal Surgery**
06 = Pergonal/HCG	15 = macrosurgery
07 = A.I.H.	16 = microsurgery
08 = AID waiting list	17 = salpingolysis (only)
09 = A.I.D.	18 = salpingostomy
	19 = reanastamosis
	20 =

Ovulation	Response Codes	Management Codes
1 = no	**Pregnancy**	0 = start treatment
2 = yes	0 = none	1 = continue treatment
3 = uncertain	1 = pregnant	2 = increase dose
	2 = abortion	3 = stop all treatment
	3 = ectopic	4 = add 2nd treatment
	Cervical mucus	5 = add 3rd treatment
	4 = no change	6 = change treatment
	5 = improved	7 = rest
	6 = decreased hostility	8 = ignore cycle since no intercourse at fertile time
	Others	9 =
	7 = patent tubes post surgery	
	8 = drop out	
	9 =	

Cycle	Treatments						Ovulation	Response	Management
1									
2									
3									

Male Treatment Codes

0 = under investigation
1 = none
2 = androgens
3 = antibiotics
4 = clomiphene
5 = bromocriptine
6 =
7 = ligation of varicocoele
8 = "tubular" surgery
9 =

Management

1 = continue treatment
2 = increase dose
3 = stop all treatment
4 = add 2nd treatment
5 = change treatment
6 = rest
7 =
8 =
9 =

DATE STARTED TREATMENT	40					

MONTH	Treatments		Seminal Fluid Analysis: S.F.A. done 1=no 2=yes 3=dropout	Volume ml	Density $\times 10^6$ ml			Motility %		Abnormal Forms%		WBC 1=no 2=yes	Management
1													
2													
3													

Appendix F: References and suggested further reading

1: The problem of the infertile couple – a guide to diagnosis and management

References

Belsey, M. (1980). Infertility; Etiology and Natural History. In, P. Rowe and R. Ramarozaka (eds.): *Diagnosis and Treatment of Infertility, W.H.O. Workshop, Nairobi, 1980*. pp.11–42. Pitman Press, Bath.

Brown, J. B., Pepperell, R. J. and Evans, J. H. (1980). Disorders of ovulation. In, R. J. Pepperell, B. Hudson and C. Wood (eds.): *The Infertile Couple*. pp.7–42. Churchill-Livingstone, London.

Chatfield, W. (1970). The investigation and management of infertility in East Africa. *East African Medical Journal* **47**, 212.

Comhaire, F. (1980). The surgical treatment of male infertility. In, P. Rowe and R. Ramarozaka (eds.): *Diagnosis and Treatment of Infertility, W.H.O. Workshop, Nairobi, 1980*. p.85. Pitman Press, Bath.

Garrow, L. (1979). Weight penalties. *British Medical Journal* **2**, 1171.

Hudson, B., Baker, D., and de Kretser, D. (1980). The abnormal semen sample. In, R. J. Pepperell, B. Hudson and C. Wood (eds.): *The Infertile Couple*. pp.70–111. Churchill-Livingstone, London.

Jacobson, L. and Westrom, L. (1969). Objectivized diagnosis of acute pelvic inflammatory disease. *American Journal of Obstetrics and Gynecology* **105**, 1088.

Jacobson, L. (1980). Differential diagnosis of acute pelvic inflammatory disease. *American Journal of Obstetrics and Gynecology* **138**,7, 1006.

Lenton, E., Weston, G. A. and Cooke, I. D. (1977). Problems in using basal body temperature recordings in an infertility clinic. *British Medical Journal* **1**, 803.

Kormano, M., Kahanpa, A. and Svinfufvud, U. et al. (1970). Thermography of varicocele. *Fertility and Sterility* **21**, 558.

Kovacs, G. T., Newman, G. B. and Henson, G. C. (1978). Post coital tests – what is normal? *British Medical Journal* 1, 818.

Westrom, L. (1975). The effect of acute pelvic inflammatory disease on fertility. *American Journal of Obstetrics and Gynecology* **121**, 5, 709.

Westrom, L. (1980). Incidence, prevalence and trends of pelvic inflammatory disease and its consequence. *American Journal of Obstetrics and Gynecology* **138**, 7, 880.

Vasquez, G., Winston, R. M. and Boeckx, W. (1980). Tubal lesions subsequent to sterilization and their relation to fertility after attempts at reversal. *American Journal of Obstetrics and Gynecology* **138**, 1, 86.

Suggested further reading

Edwards, R. G. (1980). *Conception in the Human Female*. Academic Press, London.

Givens, J. R. (1979). *The Infertile Female*. Year Book Medical Publishers, Chicago.

Gold, J. J. and Josimovich, J. B. (1980). *Gynaecologic Endocrinology*. 3rd ed. Harper and Row, Hagerstown.

Hall, R. G., Anderson, J., Smart, G. and Besser, M. (1980). *Fundamentals of Clinical Endocrinology*. Pitman Medical, Tunbridge Wells.

International symposium on pelvic inflammatory disease, Atlanta, Georgia (1980). *American Journal of Obstetrics and Gynecology* **138**, 7, 2, 845 (Special Issue).

Laboratory Manual for the Examination of Human Semen and Semen-Cervical Mucus Interaction (1980). M. A. Belsey, R. Eliasson and A. J. Gallegos et al. (eds.). (W.H.O. Study Group). Press Concern, Singapore.

Lunenfeld, B. and Insler, V. (1978). *Diagnosis and Treatment of Functional Infertility*. Grosse, Berlin.

Pepperell, R. J., Hudson, B. and Wood, C. (1980). *The Infertile Couple*. Churchill-Livingstone, Edinburgh.

Reproduction (1979). R. V. Short (ed.). *British Medical Bulletin* **35**, 2, 97.

Speroff, L., Glass, R. H. and Kase, N. G. (1981). *Clinical Gynaecologic Endocrinology and Infertility*. 3rd ed. Williams & Wilkins, Baltimore.

Yen, S. S. and Jaffe, R. B. (1978). *Reproductive Endocrinology; Physiology, Pathophysiology and Clinical Management*. Saunders, Philadelphia.

2: Techniques for the investigation and diagnosis of utero-tubal disease

References

Alexander, G. D. and Coe, F. E. (1969). Anaesthesia for pelvic laparoscopy. *Anaesth. Analg.* (Cleve) **48**, 14.

Barbot, J. (1980). Contact hysteroscopy: another method of endoscopic examination of the uterine cavity. *American Journal of Obstetrics and Gynecology* **136**, 721.

Brown, D. R. and Fishburne, J. (1976). Ventilatory and blood gas changes during laparoscopy with local anaesthesia. *American Journal of Obstetrics and Gynecology* **124**, 741.

Cumming, D. and Taylor, P. (1980). Combined laparoscopy and hysteroscopy in the investigation of the ovulatory infertile female. *Fertility and Sterility* **33**, 5, 475.

Duignan, N. M., Jordan, J. A. and Coughlan, B. M. (1972). One thousand consecutive cases of diagnostic laparoscopy. *Journal of Obstetrics and Gynaecology of the British Commonwealth* **79**, 1016.

Edstrom, K. and Ternstrom, I. (1970). The diagnostic feasibility of a modified hysteroscopic technique. *Acta. Obstet. Gynecol. Scand.* **49**, 327.

Frangenheim, H. (1972). *Laparoscopy and culdoscopy in gynaecology.* Butterworth & Co., London.

Keirse, M. and Vandervellen, R. (1973). A comparison of hysterosalpingography and laparoscopy in infertility. *Obstetrics and Gynaecology* **41**, 685.

Kistner, R. W. and Patton, G. W. (1975). *Atlas of Infertility Surgery.* p.37. Little, Brown & Co., Boston.

Israel, R. and March, C. M. (1976). Diagnostic laparoscopy: a prognostic aid in the surgical management of infertility. *American Journal of Obstetrics and Gynecology* **125**, 7, 969.

Leeton, J. and Talbot, J. (1973). Study of laparoscopy and hysterosalpingography in 100 infertility patients. *Australia and New Zealand Journal of Obstetrics and Gynaecology* **13**, 169.

Maathuis, J. B., Horbach, J. G. and Van Hall, E. (1972). A comparison of the results of hysterosalpingography and laparoscopy in the diagnosis of fallopian tube dysfunction. *Fertility and Sterility* **23**, 428.

Mattingly, R. F. (ed.) (1977). *Te Linde's Operative Gynaecology.* 5th ed. p.232. J. B. Lippincott & Co., Philadelphia.

Oelsner, G., Amnon, D. and Insler, V. (1974). Outcome of pregnancy after treatment of intra-uterine adhesions. *Obstetrics and Gynaecology* **44**, 361.

Penfield, A. J. (1977). Laparoscopic sterilization under local anaesthesia. *Obstetrics and Gynaecology* **49**, 725.

Peterson, E. P. (1971). Anaesthesia for laparoscopy. *Fertility and Sterility* **22**, 695.

Philipp, E. E. and Carruthers, G. B. (1981). *Infertility.* p.93. Heinemann Press, London.

Rosenfeld, D. (1979). A study of hysteroscopy as an adjunct to laparoscopy in the evaluation of the infertile woman. In, J. M. Phillips (ed.): *Endoscopy in Gynecology.* p. 337. American Association of Gynecologic Laparoscopists, Downey, California.

Swolin, K. and Rosencrantz, M. (1972). Laparoscopy vs hysterosalpingography in sterility investigation. *Fertility and Sterility* **23**, 270.

Taylor, P. J. (1977). Correlations in infertility symptomatology, hysterosalpingography, laparoscopy and hysteroscopy. *Journal of Reproductive Medicine* **18**, 339.

Templeton, A. A. and Kerr, M. G. (1977). Laparoscopy as the primary investigation in the subfertile female. *British Journal of Obstetrics and Gynaecology* **84**, 760.

Wadhwa, R. K. and Katz, D. (1979). General anaesthesia for laparoscopy and physiology of pneumoperitoneum. In, J. M. Phillips (ed.): *Endoscopy in Gynecology.* p.113. American Association of Gynecologic Laparoscopists, Downey, California.

3: Anatomy and instruments

Reference

Dewhurst, C. J. (1970). Fetal sex and development of genitalia. In, E. E. Philipp, J. Barnes and M. Newton (eds.): *Scientific Foundations of Obstetrics and Gynaecology.* pp.173–181. William Heinemann Ltd., London.

Suggested further reading

Aydelotte, M. B. (1978). Developmental anatomy. In, H. J. Buchsbaum and J. D. Schmidt (eds.): *Gynecologic and Obstetric Urology.* pp.1–21. W. B. Saunders Co., Philadelphia.

Beazley, J. M. (1974). Congenital malformations of the genital tract (excluding intersex). In, *Clinics in Obstetrics and Gynaecology* **1**, No. 3. pp.571–592. W. B. Saunders Co., London.

Forsberg, J. G. (1978). Development of the human vaginal epithelium. In, E. S. E. Hafez and T. N. Evans (eds.): *The Human Vagina.* pp.3–19. North Holland Biomedical Press, Elsevier.

4: Psychological factors in infertility surgery

Suggested further reading

Berger, B. M. (1977). The role of the psychiatrist in a reproductive biology clinic. *Fertility and Sterility* **28**, 141.

Christie, G. L. (1980). The psychological and social management of the infertile couple. In, R. J. Pepperell, B. Hudson and C. Wood (eds.): *The Infertile Couple.* pp.229–247. Churchill-Livingstone, London.

Kaltreider, N. B. and Margolis, A. G. (1977). Childless by choice: a clinical study. *American Journal of Psychiatry* **134**, 179.

Mai, F. M. M., Munday, R. M. and Rump, E. E. (1972). Psychiatric interview comparisons between infertile and fertile couples. *Psychosomatic Medicine* **34**, 431.

Platt, J., Ficher, I. and Silver, M. (1973). Infertile couples: personality traits and self-ideal concept discrepancies. *Fertility and Sterility* **24**, 972.

Wiehe, V. R. (1976). Psychological reactions of infertility. *Psychological Reports* **38**, 863.

6: Operations on the cervix

References

Jones, J. M., Hibbard, B. and Sweetnam, P. (1979). The outcome of pregnancy after cone biopsy of the cervix – a case control study. *British Journal of Obstetrics and Gynaecology* **86**, 913.

McDonald, I. (1980). Cervical cerclage. *Clinics in Obstetrics and Gynaecology* **7**, 3, 461. I. MacGillivray (ed.). W. B. Saunders Co., London.

Shirodkar, V. N. (1968). Long term results with the operative treatment of habitual abortion. *Obstetric and Gynaecological Survey* **23**, 553.

Shirodkar, V. N. (1960). Habitual abortion in the second trimester. In: *Contributions to Obstetrics and Gynaecology*. p.1. Livingstone, London.

7: Operations on the uterus

References

Babaknia, A., Rock, J. A. and Jones, H. W. (1978). Pregnancy success following abdominal myomectomy for infertility. *Fertility and Sterility* **30**, 644.

Barter, R. H. and Parks, J. (1958). Myoma uteri associated with pregnancy. *Clinical Obstetrics and Gynecology* **1**, 519.

Jones, H. W. Jnr. (1977). In, R. F. Mattingly (ed.): *Te Linde's Operative Gynecology*. 5th ed. pp.309–318. J. B. Lippincott Co., Philadelphia.

Jones, H. W. and Wheeless, C. R. (1969). Salvage of the reproductive potential of women with anomalous development of the mullerian ducts: 1868–1968–2068. *American Journal of Obstetrics and Gynecology* **104**, 348.

Jones, H. W. and Rock, J. A. (1980). Other factors associated with infertility: Endometriosis externa, fibromyomata uteri. In, R. J. Pepperell, B. Hudson and C. Woods (eds.): *The Infertile Couple*. pp.147–161. Churchill-Livingstone, Edinburgh, London and New York.

Kaufman, R. H., Adam, E. and Binder, G. (1980). Upper genital tract changes and pregnancy outcome in offspring exposed in utero to DES. *American Journal of Obstetrics and Gynecology* **137**, 299.

Suggested further reading

Kistner, R. W. and Patton, G. W. Jnr. (1975). In: *Atlas of Infertility Surgery*. pp.65–92. Little, Brown & Co., Boston, Massachusetts.

Malone, L. J. and Ingersoll, F. M. (1968). Myomectomy in infertility. In, S. J. Behrman and R. W. Kistner (eds.): *Progress in Infertility*. 1st ed. p.115. Little, Brown & Co., Boston.

Williams, E. A. (1978). Uterus septus and uterus bicornis unicollis. In, D. H. Lees and A. Singer (eds.): *Clinics in Obstetrics and Gynaecology* – Gynaecological Surgery. pp.509–512. W. B. Saunders Co., London.

8: Operations on the ovary

References

Cohen, M. R. (1976). Endoscopy. In, R. B. Greenblatt (ed.): *Recent Advances in Endometriosis*. Proceedings of a Symposium. Augusta, Georgia, 1975. *Excerpta Medica*. Amsterdam.

Cooke, I. D. (1978). The current status of infertility surgery. In, D. H. Lees and A. Singer (eds.): *Clinics in Obstetrics and Gynaecology* – Gynaecological Surgery. pp.591–620. W. B. Saunders Co., London.

Garcia, C. R. and David, S. S. (1977). Pelvic endometriosis: infertility and pelvic pain. *American Journal of Obstetrics and Gynecology* **129**, 740.

Greenblatt, R. B., Borenstein, R. and Hernandez-Ayup, S. (1974). Experiences with Danazol (an antigonadotrophin) in the treatment of infertility. *American Journal of Obstetrics and Gynecology* **118**, 783.

Jones, H. W. and Rock, J. A. (1980). Other factors associated with infertility: endometriosis externa, fibromyomata uteri. In, R. J. Pepperell, B. Hudson and C. Wood (eds.): *The Infertile Couple*. pp.147–161. Churchill-Livingstone, Edinburgh, London and New York.

Kistner, R. W. and Patton, G. W. (1975). *Atlas of Infertility Surgery*. p.186. Little, Brown & Co., Boston.

Meldrum, S. I., Clark, K. E., Rubenstein, L. M. and Lebherz, T. B. (1977). The relationship of prostaglandins to infertility associated with endometriosis. Abstract, *Pacific Coast Fertility Society*.

Williams, T. and Pratt, J. H. (1977). Endometriosis in 1000 consecutive celiotomies: Medicine and Management. *American Journal of Obstetrics and Gynecology* **129**, 245.

9: Operations on the fallopian tube

References

Brosens, I. and Vasquez, G. (1976). Fimbrial microbiopsy. *Journal of Reproductive Medicine* **16**, 171.

Cooke, I. D. (1978). Current status of infertility surgery. In, D. H. Lees and A. Singer (eds.): *Clinics in Obstetrics and Gynaecology*. Vol. 5, No. 3. pp.591–603. W. B. Saunders Co. Ltd., London and Philadelphia.

Douglas, C. (1978). Tubal uterine implantation. In, I. Brosens and R. Winston (eds.): *Reversibility of Female Sterilization*. pp.85–88. Academic Press, London and Grune & Stratton, New York.

Gomel, V. (1977). Tubal reanastomosis by microsurgery. *Fertility and Sterility* **28**, 59.

Grant, A. (1971). Infertility surgery of the oviduct. *Fertility and Sterility* **22**, 496.

Hanton, E. M., Pratt, J. H. and Banner, E. A. (1964). Tubal plastic surgery at the Mayo Clinic. *American Journal of Obstetrics and Gynecology* **89**, 934.

Horne, H. W., Clyman, M. and Debrovner, C. et al. (1973). The prevention of post operative pelvic adhesions after infertility surgery. *International Journal of Fertility* **18**, 109.

Kistner, R. W. and Patton, G. W. (1975). Utero-tubal implantation. In, R. W. Kistner and G. W. Patton Jnr. (eds.): *Atlas of Infertility Surgery*. pp.122–145. Little, Brown & Co., Boston.

Marik, J. (1977). Microsurgical repair of hydrosalpinx. In, J. Phillips (ed.): *Microsurgery in Gynecology*. p.126. St. Louis, A.A.G.L.

Mattingly, R. F. (1977). Cornual implantation. In, R. F. Mattingly (ed.): *Te Linde's Operative Gynecology*. 5th ed. pp.326–327. J. B. Lippincott Co., Philadelphia.

Shirodkar, V. N. (1960). Habitual abortion in the second trimester. In: *Contributions to Obstetrics and Gynaecology*. p.1. Livingstone, London.

Shirodkar, V. N. (1966). Factors influencing the results of salpingostomy. *International Journal of Fertility* **2**, 361.

Siegler, A. M. (1969). Salpingoplasty: classification and report of 115 operations. *Obstetrics and Gynecology* **34**, 339.

Siegler, A. M. (1978). Reversibility of tubal sterilization. In, I. Brosens and R. Winston (eds.): *Reversibility of Female Sterilization*. pp.73–77. Academic Press, London.

Swolin, K. (1975). Electromicrosurgery and salpingostomy: long term results. *American Journal of Obstetrics and Gynecology* **121**, 418.

Umezaki, C., Katayama, K. P. and Jones, H. W. (1974). Pregnancy rates after reconstructive surgery of the fallopian tubes. *Obstetrics and Gynecology* **43**, 418.

Westrom, L. (1980). Incidence, prevalence, and trends of acute pelvic inflammatory disease and its consequences in industrialized countries. *American Journal of Obstetrics and Gynecology* **138**, 7, 880.

Williams, E. A. (1978). Results of reversal of female sterilization. In, I. Brosens and R. Winston (eds.): *Reversibility of Female Sterilization*. pp.85–95. Academic Press, London and Grune and Stratton, New York.

Winston, R. M. L. (1977). Micro-surgical tubo-cornual anastomosis for reversal of sterilization. *Lancet* **1**, 280.

Winston, R. M. L. (1978). The future of microsurgery in infertility. In, D. H. Lees and A. Singer (eds.): *Clinics in Obstetrics and Gynaecology, Gynaecological Surgery*. pp. 607–620. W. B. Saunders Co. Ltd., London.

Winston, R. M. L. and Margara, R. A. (1980a). Techniques for the improvement of microsurgical tubal anastomosis. In, P. G. Crosignani and B. L. Rubin (eds.): *Microsurgery in Female Infertility*. pp.25–34. Academic Press, London.

Winston, R. M. L. (1980b). Microsurgery of the fallopian tube; from fantasy to reality. *Sterility and Fertility* **34**, 6, 521.

10: Microsurgery for infertility

References

Caspi, E., Halperin, Y. and Bukovsky, I. (1979). The importance of periadnexal adhesions in tubal reconstructive surgery for infertility. *Fertility and Sterility* **31**, 296.

Diamond, E. (1979). Lysis of postoperative adhesions in infertility. *Fertility and Sterility* **31**, 287.

Eddy, C. A., Asch, R. H. and Balmaceda, M. P. (1980). Pelvic adhesions following microsurgical and macrosurgical wedge resection of the ovaries. *Fertility and Sterility* **33**, 557.

Garcia, C-R. and Mastroianni, L. (1980). Microsurgery for treatment of adnexal disease. *Fertility and Sterility* **34**, 5, 413.

Hedon, B., Wineman, M. and Winston, R. M. L. (1980). Loupes or microscopes for tubal anastomosis? An experimental study. *Fertility and Sterility* **34**, 264.

Israel, S. L. (1951). Total linear salpingostomy. *Fertility and Sterility* **2**, 505.

Margara, R. A. (1980). Hammersmith Hospital, London W.12. Unpublished experimental data.

Siegler, A. M. and Kontopoulos, V. (1979). An analysis of macrosurgical and microsurgical techniques in the management of the tuboperitoneal factor in infertility. *Fertility and Sterility* **32**, 377.

Swolin, K. (1967). Beitrage zu operativen Behandlung der weiblichen Sterilitat. Experimentelle und klinische studien. *Acta Obstet. Gynecol. Scand.* (Suppl. 14) **46**, 1.

Winston, R. M. L. (1980). Microsurgery of the fallopian tube. From fantasy to reality. *Fertility and Sterility* **34**, 521.

Winston, R. M. L. (1980). Evaluating instruments for gynecologic microsurgery. *Contemporary Ob-Gyn* **15**, 153.

Vasquez, G., Boeckx, W., Winston, R. and Brosens, I. (1980). Human tubal mucosa and reconstructive microsurgery. In, P. G. Crosignani and B. L. Rubin (eds.): *Microsurgery in Female Infertility*. p.41. Academic Press, London.

Vasquez, G., Winston, R. M. L., Boeckx, W. and Brosens, I. (1980). Tubal lesions subsequent to sterilization and their relation to fertility after attempts at reversal. *American Journal of Obstetrics and Gynecology* **138**, 86.

11: In vitro fertilisation and embryo transfer

References

Edwards, R. G., Steptoe, P. C. and Purdy, J. M. (1980). Establishing full term human pregnancy using cleaving embryos grown in utero. *British Journal of Obstetrics and Gynaecology* **87**, 737.

Lopata, A., Johnston, J., Leeton, J. and McBain, J. (1980). Use of in vitro fertilisation in the infertile couple. In, R. J. Pepperell, B. Hudson and C. Wood (eds.): *The Infertile Couple*. p.209. Churchill-Livingstone, Edinburgh.

Steptoe, P. C. and Edwards, R. G. (1976). Reimplantation of a human embryo with subsequent tubal pregnancy. *Lancet* **1**, 880.

Steptoe, P. C., Edwards, R. G. and Purdy, J. M. (1980). Clinical aspects of pregnancy established with cleaving embryos grown in vitro. *British Journal of Obstetrics and Gynaecology* **87**, 757.

Hackeloer, B. J., Fleming, R., Robinson, H. P. *et al* (1979). Correlation of ultrasonic and endocrinologic assessment of human follicular development. *American Journal of Obstetrics and Gynecology* **135**, 122.

12: Artificial insemination

References

Beck, W. W. and Wallach, E. E. (1981). When therapy fails – artificial insemination. *Contemporary Ob-Gyn* **17**, 113.

Chong, D. and Taymor, M. (1975). Sixteen years experience with therapeutic donor insemination. *Fertility and Sterility* **26**, 791.

Dixon, A. and Avidan, D. (1976). Experience with A.I.H. – report of 158 patients. *Fertility and Sterility* **27**, 528.

Finegold, W. J. (1980). *Artificial insemination with Husband's Sperm*. Charles Thomas, Springfield.

Glass, R. H. (1980). Complications and pitfalls of AID. *Clinical Obstetrics and Gynaecology* **23**, 667.

Mathews, C. D. (1980). Artificial insemination – donor and husband. In, R. J. Pepperell, B. Hudson and C. Wood (eds.): *The Infertile Couple*. p.182. Churchill-Livingstone, Edinburgh.

Nachtigall, R. D., Faure, N. and Glass, R. H. (1979). Artificial insemination of husband's sperm. *Fertility and Sterility* **32**, 141.

Philipp, E. and Carruthers, B. (1981). *Infertility*. p.225. Heinemann Medical, London.

Royal College of Obstetricians and Gynaecologists (1976). Artificial Insemination, *Proceedings of the 4th Study Group*. RCOG, London.

Sherman, J. K. (1973). Synopsis of the use of frozen human semen since 1964. *Fertility and Sterility* **24**, 772.

Steinberger, E. and Smith, K. D. (1973). AID with fresh and frozen semen – a comparative study. *Journal American Medical Association* **223**, 778.

Templeton, A. A. and Kerr, M. G. (1977). Laparoscopy as the primary investigation in the subfertile female. *British Journal of Obstetrics and Gynaecology* **84**, 760.

Contents of other volumes in the Gynaecological Surgery series

Volume 1: Vaginal Operations

Volume 2: Abdominal Operations For Benign Conditions

1 **Surgical Anatomy and Instruments**

2 **Opening and Closing of Abdomen**
Lower abdominal transverse incision
Midline (subumbilical) incision

3 **Abdominal Hysterectomy**
Basic technique
Conditions demanding modification of basic hysterectomy technique:
Broad ligament fibroid
Cervical fibroid
Pelvic endometriosis
Chronic pelvic inflammatory disease (including hysterectomy for frozen pelvis)
Accompanying vaginal vault prolapse
Supravaginal (subtotal) hysterectomy
Removal of residual cervix

4 **Myomectomy**

5 **Tubo-Ovarian Surgery**
Ovarian cystectomy
Salpingo-oophorectomy
Tubal ligation

6 **Endometriosis**
Conservative pelvic surgery, including ventrosuspension

7 **Operation for Acute Pelvic Inflammatory Disease**

8 **Appendicectomy**

9 **Laparoscopy**
Basic technique
Sterilisation procedures

10 **Cysto-urethropexy**
(Marshall–Marchetti–Krantz procedure)

11 **Ligation of Internal Iliac Artery**

12 **Drainage of Abdominal Wound Haematoma**

13 **Abdominal Closure of Pelvic Fistulae**
Vesico-vaginal fistula
Recto-vaginal fistula

Volume 3: Operations For Malignant Disease

1 **Instruments and Surgical Anatomy**

2 **Carcinoma of Vulva**
Biopsy of the vulva
Local vulvectomy
Radical vulvectomy
Radical vulvectomy with pelvic lymphadenectomy
Local excision of recurrent vulval carcinoma

3 **Cervical Carcinoma**
Preclinical Carcinoma
Colposcopy and cervical biopsy
Local destructive techniques:
Electrodiathermy
Cryosurgery
CO_2 laser
Cone biopsy
Abdominal hysterectomy with removal of vaginal cuff
Clinical Carcinoma
Examination, staging and biopsy
Radical hysterectomy with pelvic lymphadenectomy (Wertheim's Hysterectomy)

4 **Uterine Carcinoma**
Diagnostic dilatation and curettage
Extended hysterectomy
Radical hysterectomy and partial vaginectomy with pelvic node biopsy

5 **Ovarian Carcinoma**
Surgical clearance of pelvic growth (total hysterectomy and salpingo-oophorectomy)
Extensive surgical removal of abdomino-pelvic growth

6 **Surgical Management of Recurrent Pelvic Malignancy**
(following failed radio-therapy)

7 **Radiation Therapy for Gynaecological Cancer**
(by Dr F.E. Neal)
Insertion of intrauterine and intravaginal radiation sources
External irradiation sources
Lymphography

Volume 4: Surgery Of Vulva And Lower Genital Tract

1 **Surgical Anatomy**

2 **Surgery of Congenital Abnormalities**
Imperforate hymen causing cryptomenorrhoea
Longitudinal vaginal septum
Para-vaginal cyst
Construction of an artificial vagina
Williams' vulva-vaginoplasty operation

3 **Operations on the Urethra**
Urethral caruncle
Prolapsed urethra
Para-urethral cyst
Urethral diverticulum
Reconstruction of terminal urethra

4 **Surgery of Bartholin Duct/Gland**
Marsupialisation
Excision

5 **Operations for Contraction of Vaginal Introitus**
Fenton's operation
Vaginoplasty

6 **Repair of Complete Perineal Tear**

7 **Closure of Recto-vaginal Fistula**

8 **Surgery of the Chronic Vulvar Dystrophies**
Local vulvectomy
Laser excision

9 **Vaginal Abnormalities as Sequelae of Maternal Diethylstilboestrol Treatment**

10 **Surgical Treatment of Vulvar Condylomata**
Diathermy excision
Cryosurgery
Laser excision

11 **Injuries to the Vulva**
Forensic aspects of vulvar injuries
(by Professor Alan Usher)

12 **Haemorrhoidectomy**

Volume 6: Surgery Of Conditions Complicating Pregnancy

1 **Anatomy, Physiology and Surgical Instruments**

2 **Termination of Pregnancy**

3 **Management of Abortion**
Inevitable and incomplete abortion
Missed abortion
Septic abortion and septic shock

4 **Management of Recurrent Abortion**
Cerclage
Myomectomy
Uteroplasty

5 **Ectopic Pregnancy**
Ruptured tubal pregnancy – salpingectomy
Intra-tubal pregnancy – conservation of tube
Surgery of abdominal pregnancy

6 **The Acute Abdomen in Pregnancy**
Acute appendicitis
Acute intestinal obstruction
Other acute abdominal crises

7 **Ovarian Cysts and Fibroids Complicating Pregnancy**
Very large ovarian cyst
Twisted ovarian cyst
Ovarian cyst obstructing labour
Uterine fibroids

8 **The Control of Haemorrhage in Operative Obstetrics**

9 **Caesarean Section**
Lower segment operation

10 **Hysterectomy for Uterine Rupture and/or Persistent Haemorrhage during Pregnancy and Labour**
Caesarean hysterectomy
Subtotal and total hysterectomy

11 **Automobile Accidents, Assault and Other External Uterine Traumata**

12 **The Positive Cervical Smear in Pregnancy**

13 **Gestational Trophoblastic Disease**

14 **Amniocentesis**

15 **The Contribution of the Specialist Anaesthetist**

Index

I

L

M

O